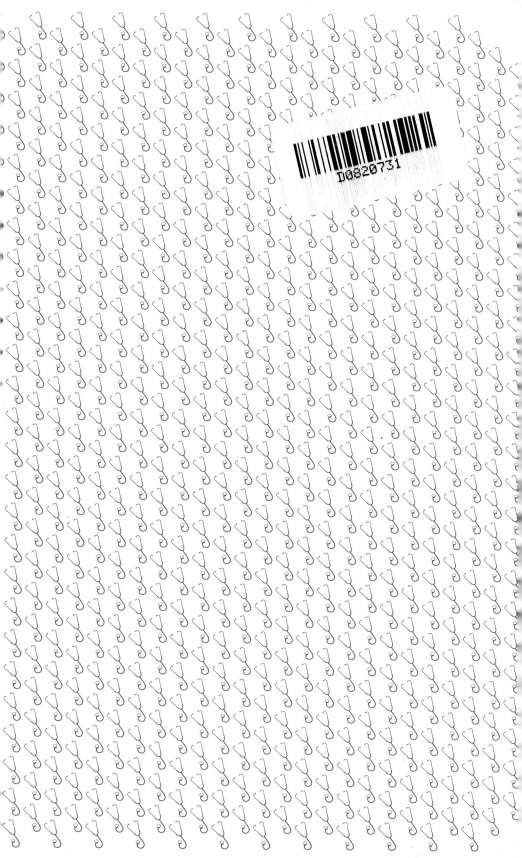

ACKNOWLEDGEMENTS

Thank you to all of the physicians who shared their lives and time to make *White Coat Wisdom* a reality.

Special thanks go to Doctors Richard Roberts, Dennis Costakos, Darold Treffert, John Frantz, Mary Frantz, Michael Miller, John Frey and Sandra Osborn, who were constantly assisting me in the process of writing this book, whether it was regarding medical ethics issues, marketing ideas, proofing or recommendations for reviewers, etc.

Thanks also to my wife, Maureen, who cared for our young girls much more than her share, as I worked on this manuscript over several years. For help in understanding the publishing business, as well as marketing principles, thanks to Neil deGrasse Tyson, PhD, Brian Jud, Chris DeSmet, Marshall Cook, Robert Ian, Randall Davidson, Richard Rehberg, Norman Gilliland, Roger Rathke, Marian Edsall, Jeff Mayers, Joan Strasbaugh and Scott Edelstein.

To my primary editor, Walter Kleine, thank you for your expertise and encouragement. The efforts of my professional reviewers, C. Everett Koop, MD, Nancy Dickey, MD, Kurt Stange, MD, and journalism Professor Richard Roth are greatly appreciated. You made this a better book, as did lay reviewers Bessie Busalacchi, Eric Korbitz, Rita Flock, Sandra Allen, William Rock and Tammy Ripp.

Thanks also to Susan Manning, JD, whose enthusiasm and legal advice were especially valuable. I am grateful to Jeff Nelson for encouraging me to find a way to honor Kenneth Viste, Jr., MD in this book, despite the fact that I wasn't able to interview Dr. Viste before his death.

Finally, I extend my appreciation to graphic designers Steve Agard and Melissa Sargent of Opacolor, for their technical advice and expertise, as well as Natalie Boon of Boon Information Services, Canada, for her indexing skills.

White Coat Wisdom

*Extraordinary doctors talk about
what they do, how they got there and
why medicine is so much more than a job*

Stephen J. Busalacchi

Apollo's Voice

Apollo's Voice

Apollo's Voice, LLC
P.O. Box 628044
Middleton, WI 53562-8044

5 4 3 2 1

FIRST EDITION

Printed in the United States of America

Busalacchi, Stephen J.
White coat wisdom : extraordinary doctors talk about what they do, how they got there and why medicine is so much more than a job / Stephen J. Busalacchi. -- 1st ed.
p. cm.
Includes index.
LCCN 2007905422
ISBN-13: 978-0-9794222-01
ISBN-10: 0-9794222-05

1. Physicians--Anecdotes. 2. Medicine--Anecdotes. 3. Physician and patient--Anecdotes.   I. Title.

R705.B87 2008   610'.92'2
                       QBI07-600287

To order, visit www.whitecoatwisdom.com
Page design by Steve Agard and Melissa Sargent of Opacolor
Illustrations by Samantha L. Flock
Cover design by Shinanthi Kelly of Vedic Design
Indexing by Natalie Boon, Boon Information Services, Canada

The author is donating a portion of all royalties from sales of this book to the Wisconsin Medical Society Foundation, in memory of Kenneth Viste Jr., MD.

WEBSITE LINKS

After reading White Coat Wisdom, you may wish to learn more about the individual physicians presented, or their causes. See the links section of www.whitecoatwisdom.com.

"Life becomes harder when we live for others,
but it also becomes richer and happier."

—Albert Schweitzer, MD

For my three favorite girls in all the world,

Olivia, Serena and Maureen,

and for my parents

Sam T. Busalacchi

and

Bess M. Busalacchi

TABLE OF CONTENTS

IV. Performing Artists

V. Life On Call

VI. Frayed Net

VII. Physicians who Listen

VIII. Medicine on Trial

IX. World Class

X. Grave Matters

XI. Tribute

Postscript

INTRODUCTION

Many years ago when I was a radio reporter, I attended a news conference at Madison's University of Wisconsin Hospital, where two doctors, a PhD scientist and a physician, were announcing results from their research. It involved genetic links to alcoholism, and whether some of us were more susceptible to the disease than others. In terms of their communication styles, the contrast between the two would have been no less distinct had one of them spoke Mandarin Chinese. The scientist, who was clearly the lead researcher, dominated the presentation's opening, occasionally referring to the Periodic Table of Elements posted behind him as well as formulas written on the blackboard. Reporters, who are generalists, and sparsely trained in the sciences, looked completely baffled. I certainly was.

Then, Michael Fleming, MD spoke, and as he did, heads began to slowly nod. One could almost see light bulbs go on across the room. Meanwhile, the PhD scientist, sensing that he had lost the room, interjected with more highly technical explanations that caused those bulbs to abruptly dim yet again. An impatient television reporter with a booming voice finally ended all doubt about who we wanted to hear from when he interrupted the scientist in mid-sentence and shouted, "Doctor *Fleming*, I'd like to hear what you...."

On my way out of the room, I told one of the hospital PR people what a great job Dr. Fleming had done, and that she should make it her life's work to "make sure the other guy doesn't get anywhere near a microphone again."

That may have been an overly harsh assessment, but the truth is not everybody, no matter how brilliant, can effectively communicate complex information. That's not to say they can't learn to do it. But physicians are often among those best equipped to translate such information because they're used to explaining technical concepts to laypeople. After all, they speak to patients every day as part of their job.

In addition to tapping doctors as translators of science information in my news reporting, I had come to love hearing them express themselves verbally, with all the nuance of tone, volume, pacing and passion.

"It doesn't come easily and it doesn't grow in the Christmas tree," said Munci Kalayoglu, MD {chapter 30}, a transplant surgeon from Turkey, regarding the skills necessary to perform such operations. I loved his version of that expression! Kalayoglu uses English phrases in the most charming ways, while always getting his point across clearly.

With all of this in mind, I only *thought* about writing this book—for about 15 years. Then, in mid 2004, I actually got going. What finally nudged me into motion was a brief, yet energizing conversation with a Rotary Club friend at a Super Bowl party. Our conversation turned to books and I mentioned my oral history idea. The concept of hearing physician stories directly from doctors themselves really seemed to captivate this guy. His face lit up as he enthusiastically proclaimed, "I'd read that! You have to do it," said Ed Fink, an attorney.

Oddly enough, that serendipitous vote of confidence turned out to be the excuse I needed to finally begin exploring what it would take to actually pull this off. The first major step I took was in hiring a literary attorney because I didn't want any question regarding publication rights if I were to begin this time consuming odyssey. Having made that financial investment, I was then compelled to keep advancing to the next stage. I compiled a list of eloquent doctors I had come to know over the years and started sending e-mails to see how many would be interested in sharing their experiences. Almost everybody immediately agreed to participate, and many said they'd be "honored" to do so.

This book was possible because of the type of work I have done for the past 25 years, which has put me in close touch with a great number of physicians who have come to trust me. Initially, I came to know them through news reporting, when I covered medicine for Wisconsin Public Radio. Soon after I took over WPR's medical beat in the mid 1980s, it quickly occurred to me just how articulate, compassionate and thoughtful physicians tend to be—interview after interview. *There had to be a great story behind each of them*, I thought.

Secretly, I often wondered what being a doctor was really like. I was impressed by their intellectual gifts, as well as their passion for medicine. What's it like to actually save somebody's life? For a living? How do you develop the confidence to cut somebody open and repair a problem? This book was the excuse to hear all about it first hand without applying to medical school! The fact is science is not my forte, and to paraphrase Woody Allen, I wouldn't want treatment from anybody who graduated from a medical school that would accept me as a student.

Being a fan of Studs Terkel's oral histories, and like Terkel, a radio interviewer, I knew doctors would be perfect subjects for this kind of book. They're not only knowledgeable, but they're used to conveying that knowledge to laypeople.

I also admired the reasoning by which physicians made their points. Listen carefully to politicians and others quoted publicly regarding any manner of issues, and oftentimes they fail to make a strong case for their point of view. The comment may sound good, but frequently there's little substance backing it up. Doctors, on the other hand, tend to express their opinions about issues based on evidence, because that's how they're trained. The same tends to be true with university professors, whom I also interviewed regularly. Even when I didn't agree with their conclusions, I still respected their opinion because it was thought out so carefully.

I'm not sure if my journalism background has anything to do with it, but I've never had any trouble communicating with doctors, either. Some, if not many, patients are intimidated by physicians. When I was in my early 20s, I needed surgery to help me breathe better. I reported early in the morning to the hospital, and was prepped, lying in bed ready for the operation. Seven hours later, I was still waiting.

It turns out my surgeon had a difficult case he was trying to stabilize and he kept coming into my room periodically throughout the day to give me updates on when my surgery would begin. Finally, at the end of the day, the surgeon, Dr. Charles Ford, had successfully dealt with the other patient and was ready for me. He apologized for the delay and offered to let me go home and do the operation on another day.

But I wasn't the least bit chagrined, given the urgency with the other patient. I said, "Look doc, all I've been doing is lying around all day. I'm just fine. But you're the one putting in a 12-hour day. If doing my surgery now is the last thing you want to do, no problem. I'm out of here. Go home and relax. I'll come back another time when you're fresh. On the other hand, if you feel good and still want to do it, let's go."

Doctor Ford smiled, and assured me that he felt good and would be happy to do the operation. When he left the room, his nurse whispered to me, "Good for you! Nobody talks to doctors like that." I was a little puzzled by her reaction and I thought, *Why not?* I meant no disrespect. I was just being honest with him.

In later life as a medical reporter, I had no difficulty asking challenging questions of doctors, and they always seemed to enjoy fielding them. What I learned was that once you engage anyone in conversation about something they know well, you'll be amazed at the stories they'll tell you, as well as *how* they will tell you.

I saw *White Coat Wisdom* as something everybody could relate to, in that we all have self-interest in maintaining our good health and most everybody has a personal doctor. In fact, almost everybody has, or should have a close relationship with his or her doctor by nature of the intimacy and trust inherent in the process of getting one's health needs assessed and addressed.

But how many people really know their doctors? How did these physicians get to where they are? What motivated them? What obstacles did they need to overcome? My goal was to personalize the profession by focusing on a few dozen physicians I had come to know through the years who have medical interests that are particularly salient, thereby combining biography with intriguing medical topics. This would be their chance to tell their story. My intent was to stay out of the way and let them speak.

This book became a more realistic endeavor after I left radio in 1997 for public relations. I began working for the Wisconsin Medical Society as its PR Director, which put me in closer contact still with even more physicians. But now, I was really getting to know them, and many had become personal friends.

One of the challenges was in selecting whom to feature in the book. To further complicate matters, every time I mentioned this project, somebody enamored with his own physician would inevitably tempt me with, "You have to interview Doctor…" I readily concede that there are a plethora of other fine, well-spoken doctors who could have just as easily filled these pages. Nevertheless, my intent was to feature a good mix of physicians of varying generations, with diverse backgrounds and specialties, although *White Coat Wisdom* in no way purports to cover the full gamut of medicine, specialties or demographics. But it is a start.

Only four doctors declined to participate, and another passed away before we could schedule time together. I'll always regret my procrastination in scheduling that interview with Kenneth Viste, Jr., MD. He not only was a good friend of many years, but multi-talented, glib, and knowledgeable. And he never hesitated to help me with whatever issue I was working on, either as a reporter or a PR professional. {See the Tribute chapter} That's why a portion of the profits from *White Coat Wisdom* will always go to the Wisconsin Medical Society Foundation, in honor of Dr. Viste's memory and to encourage the development of more doctors like him.

Despite my misstep in not recording that Viste interview, what you are about to read are first person accounts from noteworthy physicians that may well change your life and perspectives. You will have greater appreciation for what it takes to succeed in this profession {or any profession} and what your doctor did to learn his or her craft. But more importantly, you will learn and be entertained by their unique experiences, where human lives are always hanging in the balance.

In addition to a relentless drive to succeed, learning, spirituality and serendipity seem to be the threads that are woven through each of the medical lives described here. Medical school is only a step in the process. They become real healers later, through experience, compassion and continual learning.

For many of those interviewed, spirituality seems to ground them because they're often thrust into circumstances well beyond the control of a mere mortal. The serendipity comes in to play in how most of them chose their specialties. Buying a microscope led to a surgery career, an old jalopy drove another into family practice, while just hanging out with a fun group of doctors turned into a life in gastroenterology!

I am a wiser person for having listened to these doctors and for hearing about what they've learned on their journey. These conversations may even inspire some readers to pursue medical school or choose a particular specialty, if they're already training to be doctors. And physicians themselves may well be enlightened by the experiences and backgrounds of these *White Coat Wisdom* colleagues who may have a much different professional or personal background than they do.

We all might live a few years longer, too. Thank you, Ed!

I

No Strain, No Gain

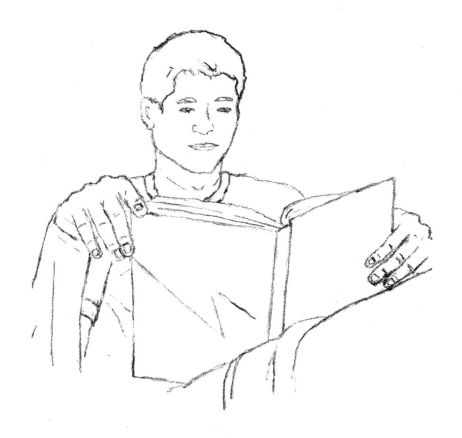

"In order to succeed, your desire for success should be greater than your fear of failure."

—Bill Cosby

CHAPTER ONE

TOP "GUNNER"

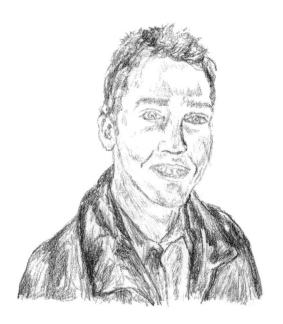

"My brain just wasn't used to memorizing such a large amount of material, and that changes as time goes on. I felt like my brain's capacity had increased somehow."

Anderson Bauer, MD
Medical College of Wisconsin, Milwaukee

I used to think journalism students cornered the market on curiosity, until I learned more about medical students. Imagine picking up a saw and cutting through a human head to learn about what's inside. Now that's curiosity.

Such imagery is appropriate for a discussion of how very intelligent young people become doctors after four years of medical school and two or more years of on the job training. The sheer amount of information they must absorb makes for a brain dump of facts that challenges the brightest scholars. But somehow, they manage to keep studying an ungodly amount of hours to learn what's necessary. They're determined to put it all together so they can some day heal your grandson, sister, friend, or you.

Anderson Bauer is the perfect candidate for this job description. Affable, articulate and sharp, you just know he's got what it takes to succeed in such a demanding profession. Besides his raw intelligence, Anderson's been blessed with many family role models who've also embarked on a journey that began in medical school.

But no matter what their background, how stellar their grades or how determined they are to succeed, it takes the assistance of a lot of others to help medical students achieve their goal of becoming doctors. Their most important supporters are the patients who allow these students the chance to explore medicine through their bodies. Unfortunately, not every patient is so tolerant.

I met Anderson when he was a medical student serving on the Wisconsin Medical Society's Board of Directors. He describes what life is like in the throes of med school.

This guy came in. He had some symptoms that were GI-related and when that happens, they want you to do a rectal exam.

"Alright sir, we need to do a rectal exam."

"What?"

"A rectal exam—We need to stick our fingers in your bottom."

"What? Are you crazy? I'm not going to let you do that. You people here, you're all butt crazy."

Needless to say, I didn't perform a rectal exam.

They like to tell us you need to perform a rectal exam unless you have no fingers and the patient has no rectum. We don't do it for fun or anything like that, or just for practice.

Do you ever get, "I don't want to be a guinea pig," when they see you're a young looking guy?

All the time. But people are usually very nice and say, "Sure. You can do it." It's unfortunate that we have to practice on somebody, but we're not given any sort of a role where we can cause serious damage or cause major problems. If we can get that experience, that helps us, which is going to help their children, their grandchildren, everybody who's coming down the line.

It's really easy to be timid and worrisome about that, but you just got to go in there and get the experience. The really awkward parts are when you're doing more sensitive examinations, like any exams in the genital or urinary areas. Nobody wants it done to them, period, much less by this young med student coming in who doesn't have a grey hair on his head.

Doing the history and the physical is really the key basis for everything. You need to understand the story of a patient. Okay, so how did this present? How long has this been going on? How is this different from normal? Did anything happen at that time which may have caused this? Then, you find out whether they had any other illnesses at this time. Are there any major family illnesses that might be causing this? Cancer, strokes, diabetes? What medications are you on? What allergies do you have?

In the beginning, they make you go through an entire review of systems. Have you lost any weight? Do you have any fevers, unusual malaise lately? Runny nose or coughing up blood or any masses in your mouth, any enlarged lymph nodes?

As time goes on, you don't have to ask as many questions because you understand what questions are important. But in the beginning, they want you to get experience going through everything.

Then, you see if there are any other problems that they didn't mention. Initially, that may line up with what they're talking about now. Once you have the whole story, you're priming yourself for what you want to look for on the exam.

To do a full history and physical, it could take me an hour, two hours, depending on how in depth you get into it. Are you checking the reflexes on every possible muscle? There are just so many things you can check.

When you do the physical, there are some areas that are a little more sensitive than others. I was told in pediatrics, you do not do a rectal exam on a child, period, unless there's very obvious pathology. It's hard enough to get adults to go through with it. They teach us how to do that in the second year. They start going through the whole procedure. You have a mentor that you practice with. My mentor actually let me do a history and physical on him. It was a rather nerve-wracking experience, but a great learning experience. But he could say when you feel somebody's abdomen, and you're trying to feel the liver, you have to breathe in and out like this, so you can really feel that edge of the liver. That's a real basic skill, your history and physical, and that's your information to work with. Then, you can put together your differential diagnosis and tease out what's most likely. Maybe you'll have to go to the labs and images too, to help out.

What about examining the opposite sex? Is that more complicated?

I would say so. The most awkward person to examine would be an attractive member of similar age of the opposite sex—a really good looking girl comes in and she's also 24. This is just another issue that people have to deal with. We're professionals. We've just got to do the exam.

It's so much easier when it's a real little baby. There are really no issues when you're examining a newborn. They're just kind of laying there and you do your exam. No big deal.

You're in the middle of this now. How long has it been since you've wanted to be a doctor?

Both my parents are physicians. They actually met at the Medical College of Wisconsin, so I grew up a child of two doctors. My mom's an emergency room physician. My dad is an orthopedic surgeon. And it was classic suburb life. I'm the fourth of five children.

I frequently went to the hospital with my dad. He's always rewarded me by giving me chicken nuggets and a happy meal. I'd go on rounds with him and see his patients in the morning. I eventually did see one of his surgeries, but that wasn't until I was in college.

I thought about it a lot, whether it was something I wanted to do because of my parents, or because I wanted to do it. Medicine is a career well suited to me. Just what it is, is the reason I went to medical school. By the time high school was coming towards a close, I was very much set on wanting to become a doctor.

What were your parents' reactions to that?

My mom is the kind of person who stands back. You can tell what she feels, but she won't say anything. "I like medicine, but you have to make your own decision."

My dad is more open about it. He'd always say, "Your great grandmother always said, 'Medicine—that's a noble profession.'" I must have heard that story about one thousand times. He was always saying, "Being a doctor's great. When are you going to start applying?"

I'd say, "Calm down. It's something that I want to do. You don't have to push me into it."

Any other family members go into medicine?

Quite a few. I have a great grandfather who was a doctor. He had seven children. Four of them became doctors. One of my dad's sisters is a doctor. One of my mom's sisters is a doctor. My oldest brother's a dentist and then the second brother's a pediatrician. My roommate said that I'm "old medicine."

Tell me what it was like to get into medical school?

I went to UW Madison for undergrad. It seems that half of everybody you meet is pre-med. Everyone wants to go into medical school and all the advisors will say, "Well, just wait and see."

I had a general chemistry course, which was filled with all those premeds, and I remember studying for that first test and thinking, *Okay, I'll see where I fit it. See how things turn out.* I put in a pretty good effort studying for that test and all the results came back and I ended up getting the highest score in the class. I was excited to pan out pretty well in the group. {Laughs}

There's a lot of anxiety going through it. You want to make sure you get this certain grade point. You want to make sure you get that certain M-CAT *score. It's one of those things where you see things start to fall into place. You get a little more confidence in it. By the time I got my M-

* Medical College Admissions Test

6

CAT scores back and my grade point I was applying with, I felt pretty good about getting into medical school.

What kind of student, what kind of person does it take to qualify for medical school?

People would recommend having a 3.8 grade point or a 30 on the M-CAT or above. Those are shoe-in kind of numbers, but you can have, you know, 3.5 GPA. You could have a 27 M-CAT. I'm aware of several people who have such numbers and get into medical school and I'm confident will be good doctors. They bring to mind the personality that would fit well with a doctor.

It's very interesting watching my classmates go through medical school with me now, and you can hear certain people, "Oh that person's going to be a great doctor, a lot of confidence." Some of the characteristics are someone who is very comfortable with people and being able to communicate all the science that we learn. Keeping in mind what the patient's perspective is, understanding where he's coming from—those tend to be the qualities that will help people become good doctors.

The first two years are primarily and almost completely basic science, which is essentially just classroom work, biochemistry, physiology, pathology and all that. The first year is the most basic science, biochemistry and cell and tissue biology, those kinds of things that really, you're down at the molecular level. You're not as close to making the connection to patient care at that point. That can be very brutal at times, because you think of what you got into medical school for, and you look forward to taking care of patients, and you see yourself walking around and making diagnoses. At that point, you're really just sitting around in a study room or a coffee shop.

In the very first semester you start off with anatomy, so I guess that's supposed to pull you in to everything. That was a great course. I had seen cadaver labs three or four times before. The first time it feels a little eerie, but after a while you just get used to it and you see what its purpose is.

People will tell you to leave a sheet over the face in the beginning, until you get to that part of the exam. The face is a very personalizing, human aspect of a cadaver, but you just start to realize that, okay, this is a cadaver. I'm very thankful that someone would donate their body to let me do this. It's an incredible way to learn anatomy, especially in the first two years when you go through and you know, pick up a heart and look at where all the arteries and veins and nerves attach, the different chambers of the heart.

It was always taught in a way that we got the lecture on it first. You'd see all the pictures and then you go into the body and look at the different structures. I really enjoyed that part.

They always refer to the pickers and the hackers. The pickers are the ones who finely dissect out every little piece. "Oh, I got this artery and conserved all the branches off of the artery and I got every nerve going to that organ."

Then, you have the hackers who are more, "Okay, I got a lot of stuff, gotta get going. If I miss an artery on this side, the body's symmetrical, so it's on the other side." That's just fine. It's fun in anatomy lab to go through all that. A very community based experience where all the students are in the lab and people will go from body to body and ask, "Do you have anything good on your body?" During that time, you'll throw in, "What are you doing this weekend?"

Are you a picker or a hacker?

Ideally, thought I was gonna be a picker, but it was hard to go in there and get everything. It's not worth it. I quickly became accustomed to, if I missed it on one side, it's all on the other. You can get through stuff a lot faster. This is the first time we've been dissecting things. If I was a professional dissector, which I doubt even exists, I'd be more concerned about getting everything, more concerned about getting every little piece.

If I knew somebody had a really good section of the body, I wouldn't worry about dissecting that as finely. I remember our foot. No one else had a really good foot. And my team dissected out every tendon and every nerve and every artery, so other people would come and look at our foot to study from. If somebody had a better thigh, then I would go look at their thigh and study off of that part.

In our case, there were five students to each body and then you start off with the chest and the back and then slowly work your way around the body to different areas. You understand what your body's good for. Like if you have a male who's in good shape, they tend to have really good muscles. If you have a skinnier person, thin, muscles aren't very well developed, they might be a really good body to dissect. Sometimes they'll even tell us what they died from. If it's lung cancer, you know that when you open up that chest, you're likely to see black all over the lungs.

But I think it's something where for everyone, it at least crosses their mind about who this person is. They had a family and they had a life. That fades. I just found myself more focused.

They do take the brains and then we look at those in our neuroanatomy course in the second semester of the first year.

When you go to dissect the head, you need to get through the skull. You need to take a saw and take off the cap of the skull and take out the brain. But then when you want to go further inside the skull, we take a saw and saw right through the middle of the head. When I told my brother this, "You did what?" {laughs} "Sawing through people's heads?"

"Yeah, that's what we do."

It's one of those things. How else would you get to see everything inside? You need to do it. It's unbelievable to think that less than a percent of the population is that intimate with dissecting anatomy and going into pretty much of every corner of somebody's body.

At the end, we had a ceremony in honor of the people who donated their bodies. It's put on every year. Two or three students are selected to organize it, and we have a couple speakers talking about the importance of respecting the bodies and respecting the people who donated their bodies. I helped write a poem for it, and some of the students here played a couple of music pieces. It's just one of those things to kind of take time out and reflect on the experience.

Then, the second year, it gets a little better and you start having some courses that are easier to relate to patient care, like pathology, so you learn what the diagnoses are. You learn what the mechanisms are behind the disease, and you learn pharmacology. You learn all about the drugs that you're going to prescribe. In microbiology, you learn about all the bacteria and the parasites and the fungus-related diseases that you'll be diagnosing in patients, so it kind of bridges you that way. And then, at the end of your second year, you have a step one board exam, which tests you on all your basic science knowledge and they try to relate it more to the clinical aspect of medicine.

It's very exciting as you move forward to see it. It becomes more and more patient-related, and you're just champing at the bit to relate this to what you're actually going to be doing. It eventually does get that way, but you do need that foundation.

The first year prepares you for the second year. The second year prepares you for getting into your clinical years. And the board exam, I would think most medical students would say that's the most miserable time of their medical school career, because pretty much everybody just shuts themselves off from the rest of the world and studies for three weeks straight at the end of the second year.

We were there on Memorial Day and there was nobody else in the entire medical school, anywhere. Businesses were closed, and here it was jam-packed and you couldn't even find space in school to study because we were all there plugging away getting ready for our board exam.

A lot's on the line.

Oh definitely. If you fail, you can take it again. But it's just not anything that you want to go through. Your step one board scores are something that can play a major factor into what type of residency you can get into.

It really can be overwhelming. Life can be pretty simple when you're in medical school because you have very clear things that you need to get done and those things take up a lot of time. But you can get so overwhelmed with school at times that when emotional issues come up in people's lives, it's almost like they just don't have the energy to deal with it.

There are just certain points where you have a lot of exams at a given point or let's say you're studying for boards and something comes up outside of that. We're all in a point of development in our lives where some people come in married, but a lot of people are searching out for that special someone. People are buying homes, making some major life decisions and sometimes it's like you don't have any social energy left in the tank and you just see people can crash.

It's a situation where we're all in it together so you see a lot of people helping each other out and being there for one another. That's one of the reasons people can make a lot of really good friends in medical school—that common bond. You'll even hear people say, "My parents, my friends, my girlfriend doesn't understand." We understand it.

We're still worried about being competitive candidates for residencies, so in addition to knowing the basic concepts, you've got to know more and more detail in order to do better on the exam compared to the other medical students. You're sitting there at the end and you know that time is so precious right before coming up on an exam, and I've got to take this whole weekend or maybe a whole week, depending on how the exams are. I just need to study as much as I can before that.

{People ask} "Haven't you been studying all along?"

"Well, I have been studying all along too, but I really needed to be primed up for these exams that are coming up tomorrow or at the beginning of next week."

"Nobody else studies like this."

Our favorite thing is, "Well, my friend in dental school isn't studying this much." That always gets us going. That's something where other medical school students know how valuable that 24 or 48 hour period can be for somebody for studying.

I'm a type of person who, when the game's on the line, you gotta step it up. At MCW {Medical College of Wisconsin}, we tend to have four sets of exams in a given semester. I'll, on a typical Saturday and Sunday, try to get there about five-thirty, six in the morning and then I'll usually study, depending how desperate, usually until at least 10, 11 or 12, if necessary, in the evening. I usually just bring food with me and go into the study room and just sit there, put my chair in the corner of the room and just study as much as I could and try not to be distracted by other people.

On Sunday, I'll still take my break for church in the morning, but otherwise I keep studying. On the night before an exam, some people pull all-nighters. I did that a few times, but I like to get at least two hours, three hours of sleep the night before an exam.

I study until about midnight, go home. Study a little more. Go to sleep for a little bit. I always thought it was worth going through the rituals, like getting ready for bed because somehow, in my mind, oh, you're getting ready for bed, like you're going to sleep for a whole night. Then, wake up and do my routine for getting up in the morning, which is probably just completely ridiculous. Some sort of mental battle, like you just went to bed for the whole night, even though my getting ready for bed routine is like close to half the amount of sleep I got that night.

People who go to medical school really want to be there. It's no mystery that it's going to take a lot of work and it's going to take a lot out of you. I'll be working with people and using all the knowledge that I obtained about the human body and how people work. I can really make a huge impact on a lot of people's lives.

It's a long road. My favorite joke with little kids is, "What grade are you in?"

{In a kid's voice} "I'm in third grade."

"I'm in 19th grade." {Laughs} You can see the fear in their eyes, going to school for that many years.

It's theoretically going to pay off and the more studying you do, the more you learn. Once you're done with the exam, you catch up on sleep and everything else.

What are you cramming in your brain?

Oh, definitely a lot of memorizing. I remember one of my interviews. They asked some question along the lines of, "So do you think it's more important to memorize concepts or details?" which is just a loaded type interview question.

I said, "Well of course, the concepts are the most important. When you're a doctor, you need to think through things and reason things out."

If you have hundreds of bacteria, but you know what the more likely ones are, you still have all these things in your brain. There's no concept behind the name of a bacteria or a disease or an x-ray finding. You can use those to guide your details and use your details to guide your concepts.

Yeah, there's a lot of memorizing involved and I heard a lot of theories behind it. Some say, well, you only tend to remember 20 to 25% and after a year or two years, so the more you can grasp in there with those details, the more likely you are to really remember the concepts when you come out of it.

I wish it were all conceptual thinking, and ideally that would be so nice, but it's just like anything. You have to memorize details about things, so that if you're going in on a surgery, you can't forget about an artery that's sitting there because you might not want to cut that if you're not supposed to. You do need to have the balance of the concepts and the details.

Do you ever find yourself questioning, why are they making me learn this?

Oh definitely, and it's on two levels. The first level is no matter what detail you're memorizing, it's just fun to complain about it to your fellow classmates.

"This is so stupid. Why would I ever need to memorize this?" We're all happy that we all agree about that.

I do admit that there are certain details that you need to memorize, but there's still a lot that I'm still not buying. I'm getting more and more into the clinics now and I'm thinking to myself, *there is really no point in learning a lot of that detail—no point whatsoever.*

Healthcare is very spread out into general, primary care, then, you have your specialists. You'll see the primary care take their knowledge so far and they'll say, this is just out of my realm. I'm not very familiar with these details and that's where you depend on the specialists. They see a lot of it, and they're very focused on it.

Any idea then, why they walk you through that?

We get taught by the PhDs, mostly in the basic science years. That's not true for all courses. But for courses like biochemistry, it's PhDs that are teaching it. I don't blame 'em. They've put so much time into their careers and they know so much and it would be hard for me to say, "Oh well, that's just not important. You don't need to know that." There are things that they don't make us memorize. But when they're trying to decide what to include in their lecture and what not to include, which could be important, what's not important, but has clinical relevance, but only is one out of a million cases, somebody's got to be the judge. If they have 50 minutes to fill, then they're going to put that detail in there and we'll have to memorize it.

But it's a tough balance where I don't think anybody knows what's exactly right or wrong, and I'd be willing to bet that there are variations between the curriculum of the different medical schools and what details that they do teach. But some of the stuff you get, they're going to err on the side of giving a little too much detail, something I'm pretty sure medical school students have been fighting for a long time.

How does medical school compare to undergrad?

In undergrad for an exam, I felt I could walk into the exam and you'd see a question and you say, that sounds like the third page of that lecture. You'd walk in with the expectations of, Well, I'm going to get well above a 90 and I should be getting closer to a hundred on an exam.

When you get into medical school, there's a lot more detail. You need to figure out how to learn as much material and it's a real shock in the beginning. My brain just wasn't used to memorizing such a large amount of material. That changes as time goes on. I felt like my brain's capacity had increased, somehow. I could sit down and study longer and I could learn more material. You also get a lot better at deciding what's important and what's not important.

When I was studying for my first set of exams and I was going through it at the usual pace that I would go through studying for an undergrad course, I would look at the clock and I'm a third of the way through the notes. I've used up two-thirds of the study time that I allotted for this exam. Then, you just start to realize that you can't do it, can't study the exact same way. You gotta change.

Even though you're competing for residencies, it just doesn't feel like life or death. You're going to become a doctor. I think 97-98-99% of students graduate from medical school and become a doctor.

At the Medical College of Wisconsin and several other schools, they have a system of honors, high pass, pass, low pass. As long as you are passing your classes, you're going to be a doctor. And I know that a lot of people who will say, okay that's what I'm going to study for. If I get a pass, that's fine. I'm not going into a competitive specialty, so what's the big difference whether I pass or honor?

It's not that same kind of pressure—if you're not at the top, then you're not going to become a doctor. You've already passed that hurdle. There's just that decreased level of stress.

What do you go for? High pass or do you just want to pass?

There's the term "gunner." Some people will use the term for anybody who goes for the highest grades. But there's also a connotation with gunner. When people tease you about being a gunner, that tends to be just a person who's known for the high grades.

But the people who make the malicious connotation of gunner, that's the person who will steal notes, not share material with other people, try to sabotage other students, which I haven't seen very frequently.

You'll see people who get some high yield stuff, maybe an old exam that other people haven't seen. Even though they haven't obtained the old exam in some sort of unethical way, they just don't share it with people. You're going through this with everybody, why are you going to hold out?

A great example is in the anatomy labs. Let's say some person dissected out this tiny nerve that is really hard to dissect out and they call over one of the doctors and say, "Isn't this that nerve?"

The doctor says, "Great dissection. You found that nerve. Make sure you show all your classmates. It just might be on the exam."

Then, you'll see other people who don't tell other people about that. It's just kind of selfish and that's why there are people who earn the term, certainly. But for the most part, from what I've seen, "gunner" is used more often for the student who's going for the higher grade.

Are you a gunner?

I have gunner tendencies. I like to shoot for the honors grade. It's one of those things where you kind of go for what you can get, and you try to balance school with everything else and come out with the grades you get. And if it's honors, that's great. You enjoy that.

But I've always made sure that no matter how well I do, I would never become the type of student who would sacrifice others' performances in school so that I can further my own cause.

How are you treated by faculty?

There are a lot of PhDs, and some of them get frustrated with us. You can get some really grumpy faculty in that respect who are frustrated with the medical students, {who say}, "Why do I need to know that?"

But for the most part, they want to teach us. A lot of them are very outgoing. They try to get a lot of feedback from the students. "How's this going? Is this a worthwhile presentation of the material?" And they try to bring in clinical faculty to help augment their presentation to bring on basic science concepts. I don't think it's been too bad at all.

When you get into the third and fourth years, it's a lot different because you have faculty who are all MDs, so they all know what it's like to be a medical student, and I found that to be very pleasant.

Some are still belittling. A classic example is the surgeons who are very short and to the point and if you don't know something, they get very angry. But you have to look at the fact that a lot is competing for the faculty's time. They're teaching, yeah, but they're also seeing patients and doing their research.

Have you ever been the victim of one of the surgeon's tirades?

Oh, definitely. It's like a rite of passage. You wonder if it's just kind of a modeling thing, where it was done to them. It's only a couple instances, and usually a situation where you know they want to teach you something and they're tired, been on call all night and so their delivery of their critique in teaching is a little abrupt, a little ruthless.

There was a situation where I was actually on my internal medicine rotation at the time and there was a patient who had some peripheral arterial disease. He was a diabetic. And when you don't get as much blood flow to the extremities you can't fight off infection as well. When you get sores, you don't have as much blood supply to heal the tissue. He had an infected sore on one of his toes. This wasn't even one of my patients—but I was talking to an intern about the patient. I just stopped in and was talking about him to one of the other third year medical students. She had just examined the patient shortly before. I mentioned that I didn't look at the foot at that time and one of the surgeons who was just listening from a corner, who was also following the patient, just exploded on me.

"You didn't unwrap the patient's foot! Do you understand that if his toe becomes necrotic, it can fall off and disease could spread?"

I just sat there and let him go off for a while. Inside, I'm just kind of laughing. He had wrapped the foot ten minutes before I was in there. I wasn't going in there to check the foot. I was checking on something else, and this guy just went on and on. He was probably tired. I was well rested and I was able to take it with a sense of humor.

So you didn't explain your side of the situation?
Explaining is not worth it. It just further irritates them.

Okay, you've gone from dead bodies to live bodies. How is that experience, taking all that you've learned, at least thus far, and now applying it to living, breathing human beings?
It's fantastic. To finally start to put it together is great and it's an incredible task to do so. I did research in the summer between my first and second year. I had some practice on histories and physicals on some patients, but completely different to be in the hospital for a full day taking care of patients. You have to get adjusted to the computer systems, the filing systems, the flow of care, contacting other specialists, and you have to get used to writing notes in the patients' charts, and what questions to ask, based on certain answers that you get.

It's a huge change and for me, it took a little time for me to catch my stride, to understand how the whole system works. But I'm really happy to be taking care of patients because it really is more of what I expected. I tell all of the students in the first and second years that it's going to get better. That thing that you learned in pathology class, you can finally tie in with a patient.

Now you can put a face and a name to a certain illness and how it presents. In surgery, more than a name and a face. Somebody's got a cancer of their colon, you're cutting people open. You're holding retractors to hold the skin flaps, the abdomen open, and you go in there and you use the x-rays that were taken and the CT scan, and now you're pulling off parts of the colon and you're tying off little sections. Now, you're cutting out where the cancer is. It's amazing that now you can put all that together, and that's such a more effective way to learn and not forget something. Do it. Those are the things that make the third and fourth years really exciting.

The terms rotation and clerkship seem to be interchangeable terms. There's a great variety in how they structure it. But for me, they start it off with what they call the big three: internal medicine, surgery, and pediatrics. And so the second half is all the OB/GYN and psychiatry, family practice, anesthesia, and then we get an elective.

I did a surgical rotation. I got to do one at a private hospital. I did a trauma surgery rotation, which was really something else. To see patients come in with gunshot wounds and stab wounds, or big falls that they may have had, or car crashes. It's just unbelievable what you see.

There was one patient who had his whole leg opened up from an accident and skin not on the leg at all or someone whose ankle was ripped out of the socket and pushed back in.

You're expected to be at the surgeries. You can't do anything too exciting, but they try to let you help out as much as you can, whether it be holding retractors so that you can pull skin flaps back or hold maybe an artery back, so they can then go in and work behind that. But some will let you do more than others, and the more you do, the more exciting it is. A lot of times, you're watching.

Another thing is to guide a laparoscopic camera, which is fun. It's amazing to see around the body with a little scope, seeing all the things you learned about in anatomy. To see the anatomy live is so much more amazing than to see it in the cadaver. It's incredible because I remember when I went through the cadaver, thinking how exciting that was. But you're there. Sometimes you get preference over interns and actually sit in on the surgeries, to see someone's kidney taken out or spleen taken out.

Have you experienced death of a patient yet?

Yes, I have. It's one of those things I've come to grips with a long time ago. It's part of the process. No one's ever happy to see anybody die. You love to be able to fix people and tell them everything's going to be okay. Certainly, medicine gets closer and closer to that over time, but there are still things you just can't take care of.

When an infection spreads too much, you can't do anything about it. If an antibiotic's not working, you can't do anything about it. If somebody's heart has been put through too much through a lifetime—the person's overweight, there are some clogged arteries. It's very sad.

The hardest thing is to see the families, especially if it's a younger patient or if the patient has a wife and three little kids. It's very sad to think about what they're going to have to go through.

As a doctor, you need to be able to understand what they're going through. But the important role for you is to be there for them. You need to keep it together and explain how things are going to happen, give them appropriate expectations, and answer any questions that they might have. I've been happy just to be in the room to see what that's like, to see what I can learn from others how best to go about that.

During all this training, do you ever get so tired that just want to be done with it?

When you're a fourth year, you want to be an intern. When you're an intern, you want to be a resident. And then when you're a resident, you want to be an attending. I think attendings just want to retire at that point. {Laughs}

I definitely had a good idea of what I was getting into. I saw my brother going to medical school and I know that was difficult. There are always times when you get worn out after a very stressful period.

This is really exciting for me because I'm in the heart of training. I learn about certain illnesses or how to talk to patients, how to get the most important information and what to do next for a patient. That really feels like you're mastering your craft. Medicine is such a dynamic field that it can be like that for a very long period of time.

I can see at some point how it will be nice not to go home at night and read about stuff because you already know it. Somebody who's been in practice for 20 years, they walk in and they know things. They've seen it a hundred times and they really know exactly how to treat a patient. You have to enjoy it for what it is, as you go along.

How do you relax?

It can be a pretty cruel schedule. We just go out socially and have fun, whether it be going to a bar, on a ski trip or to a Brewers game. I wrote a song about one of our professors. His name is Doctor Marvin Wagner. I think he's been teaching for 50 years plus. He knew my grandfather. They were friends. But he taught both of my parents. Doctor Wagner is just one of the guys you never forget, and students love him. He's very laid back. He still teaches anatomy and he'll say, "Remember this for the rest of your life." If he ever says that, you know that's going to be on the test.

I believe he's over 80, and he's still teaching med students. That just shows his passion for medicine, and he's always joking around with people. I wrote a song about him. It's called, *"None Can Compare."* Last year, we did a repeat of the song and he came on stage with us. The name of our band was Tenacious MD, making fun of Jack Black and his band Tenacious D. It's just so fun to have that kind of outlet.

He just gives such hilarious lectures. One of them is titled "Tits and Pits," which is about the axilla and the pectoral region. He also does one known as the "Nuts and Balls" lecture, which is all about the lower abdominal region.

> *He'll give you a lecture on tits and pits*
> *Doctor Wagner, he's sure a hit.*
> *He'll give you a lecture on nuts and balls*
> *Doctor Wagner's the best of all.*

He always hands out candy in his lecture and he still uses the chalkboard. He uses this neon colored-chalk and he draws all these pictures. He does them all by memory and I bet he can do it in his sleep.

> *He'll give candy to please your sweet tooth*
> *Doctor Wagner's the best and that's the truth.*
> *Using bright colored chalk is his style*
> *You better keep teaching for a long, long while.*

You're really going to have something to sing about because medical school will be over soon. Have you decided on a specialty yet?

I'm finishing up the big three right now. If I *had* to do any one of the given fields, that would be fine. I'd do it. People are out there doing jobs that may not be their dream. A lot of people have to work because they have to do a job. If I had to choose today, I would go into surgery. I'm not exactly sure what type of surgery. Of course, my dad: "Maybe orthopedic surgery, huh?"

Editor's note: Anderson Bauer graduated from the Medical College of Wisconsin in spring, 2007.

CHAPTER TWO

BACK TO MED SCHOOL

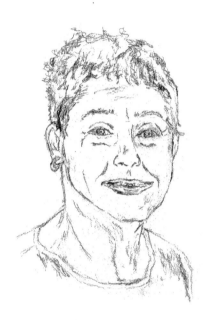

"People ask me if I'm retired and I say, no, I am not retired! I'm never going to retire. I then went to medical school {again} and that became my medical career."

Sandra Osborn, MD
Pediatrician, Madison

We can fancifully ask ourselves if we'd do certain things over again in life. Well, Sandra Osborn, MD, did more than just ponder the thought. She actually went back to medical school 32 years after she graduated the first time! For another four years, she attended the lectures each day, though she wasn't masochistic enough to take the exams.

May 12 was graduation day in Madison for the 2006 class of the University of Wisconsin School of Medicine and Public Health. The hall was filled with the graduates' friends and family, and each seemed to be wielding a camera, as their stellar student accepted his or her medical degree. As class mentor, Dr. Osborn, clad in a black cap and gown, gave her much younger fellow classmates some parting advice.

"You have chosen one of the most demanding, and yet also one of the

most rewarding areas of endeavor that exist. Think of your colleagues and patients as the type of family that they are and you will not only do the correct thing for them, but you'll also do the right thing. When you need support and encouragement, we are all here to walk at your side."

Doctor Osborn was the first of 10 Wisconsin Medical Society presidents with whom I would work closely. I've come to know her well and have marveled at how involved she has become in volunteer leadership work in the medical community since her formal retirement–a word she refuses to use to describe her life after three decades of pediatric practice.

Osborn is not the type of doctor to spend her free time out on the golf course, although in high school, she claims to have a gotten her first "birdie" when her ball hit a crow sitting on the green.

You'd have to be a real devotee to hit the links on the steamy day I spoke with Dr. Osborn, as the temperature already was close to 100 degrees before 10 a.m. But it was quite comfortable for a conversation, sitting in the shade of her belvedere, overlooking a pond and extensive flower and vegetable gardens in front of her home. Gardening is among her passions, as is knitting, counted cross stitch and needlepoint.

"I often thought that if I hadn't been a pediatrician, I could have been a good plastic surgeon because I'm good with my hands," she says.

Do you remember your first day in medical school, round two?

I was in the same room where, 32 years ago, we had been told our brains were deteriorating pretty fast. One of the things that turned off a lot of my classmates was an instructor who said we'd better work hard and learn fast, because our brain cells were diminishing rapidly, every minute he was talking. We were getting dumber all the time.

The building had changed somewhat in passageways and trying to picture where it was that such and such a thing had happened when I was a student. One of the places that we had to pass between the hospital and the teaching area of the medical school was the waiting area of the eye clinic. One day, Governor {Warren P.} Knowles* was sitting there in his bathrobe waiting for his eye exam. Things have become a little bit more private for people now.

My first day was at a meeting with the students. I needed to greet them, and tell them how they could connect with me, how I anticipated attending all of the lectures. I wasn't sure what I was going to do either, because the job description was fairly minimal.

My superior was Dr. Mikel Snow, and he said there were things that they wanted to be sure that the class mentor did. One was to be present at

* Knowles served as Governor of Wisconsin from 1965-1971.

the White Coat Ceremony; another was to be there for Match Day, for the hooding ceremony and graduation. Beyond that, one sort of created your own way of dealing with the students and how you interacted.

So how did it compare, going through medical school the second time?

It was easier and harder. The details of information had become much smaller, more molecular kinds of things. The detail that the students had to learn, the processes, were much greater than we had to learn, because there was more information available.

But clinical experiences that I had were helpful to the basic science instructors. I learned, later, they really welcomed physician class mentors because we could frequently provide examples of how what they were teaching was useful, eventually.

The medical school brings in patients, and they would tell their stories. One was of a child who had a disorder of metabolism, meaning some enzyme in the body didn't work properly and therefore, a product did not get made or a product accumulated, that could've eventually been harmful. This mother was telling about the effort that was gone through to diagnose her child, and eventually a proper diagnosis was made and they had information from the physician that they could take to emergency rooms and help the care of the child. It was very critical that the right thing was done.

They had a second child and it turned out that child had the same thing, so that it was much easier for them to diagnose. But the mother had the most unfortunate experience. The second child had a crisis, an acute situation that occurred in that disease. She took the child to an emergency room, had the information from the previous physician, and the emergency room physician chose to ignore it, and the child died. The students sat there stunned.

Always believe the mom or whoever the caretaker is. If that turns out not to be so, and you know better, fine. But first you have to go on that basis. In some ways, especially the first year, I was able to share things that I learned and hopefully, help them skip a few years of not understanding something like that.

In medicine, not everything always goes well. How did you deal with that, emotionally, throughout your long career?

I recall a case where the child had meningitis. It was very severe. While we did all of the right things, it wasn't enough and not immediately, but into the treatment, the child's heart and lungs stopped. We worked very hard trying to resuscitate the child without succeeding. I was really devastated afterwards that this happened to one of my patients. I was sitting at the nurses' station. I had my head in my hands.

Someone, a nurse or a nun, came and put her hand on my shoulder and said, "Don't you think you should tell the parents?" Of course, that was the right thing to do, but it was hard, really hard when you were feeling so bad yourself.

Physicians always must have the awareness that they have to minister to the family, whether it's the parents or the children. Unfortunately, that's where lawsuits come. The outcome probably couldn't have been any different than what it was, but how you address that makes a difference.

You practiced for almost 30 years. How did you ever get the notion of going back to medical school and doing it all over again?

I was on a committee at St. Mary's Hospital that was chaired by a colleague, Dr. Bill Scheckler. I enjoyed working on it, so I got reappointed every year. Other people came and went, but Bill and I developed a relationship out of that.

He'd take me around and show me things, so he really helped me get started. It was a "create your own program" kind of thing. He told me one day that he'd accepted an opportunity to become a class mentor at UW Medical School. It was something I had never heard of before. I said that sounds like a great thing to do and I'd really like to do that some day. He got really excited about the fact that I, in a sense, volunteered, and at that point, he kind of became my agent.

"I know who makes these appointments. I'll go and talk to them." He came back and said, "They'd like to have you do that. Do you want to do it next year?"

"I don't think so. It's too soon and there are too many other things to get arranged before getting into doing that."

I accepted being the class mentor for the following year, which was the class that started in 2002 and graduated in 2006.

What was it about this that appealed to you?

Only about 20 people have had the opportunity to be a class mentor, and only one other was a woman. I just knew that I wanted to do it. Bill described the fact that he went to the classes, how he had the opportunity to make comments and develop relationships with some of the students. As a pediatrician, you keep up on the things that you need to use, but you don't know about other things. For example, there were all kinds of drugs in the cardiac field, which I had heard the names of, but really didn't know how they worked or why they worked. It seemed like an opportunity to catch up on information that I either had forgotten or never learned because it wasn't available at the time that I was in school.

Why was that important, given you weren't going to practice any more?

I like to know things. I probably wasn't going to practice, but I made the decision in becoming the class mentor that I only wanted to do one thing: I didn't want to be a practicing pediatrician with an office to care for and try to be a class mentor at another site and try to coordinate them.

I had done a part-time practice for about a year and a half during the time that I was president of the medical society, and that was 75% practice. As it turned out, the practice always inserts itself into the rest of your life, and I knew that since I wasn't able to keep it at 75%, I wouldn't be able to do it again. That helped me make the decision about when to leave and resign from the clinic.

People ask me if I'm retired and I say, no, I am not retired! I'm never going to retire. I then went to the medical school and that became my medical career.

Here you are an experienced person, going to school with all these kids, probably in their 20s. What was that like?

It was a lot of fun. It changed as the years went by. Most of them were right out of college, and were very bright people. At the beginning, they knew they wanted to be physicians, but many of them really had not had much experience, either from observation or personal experience, because they'd all been pretty healthy. They were growing up. They still needed to grow into a professional.

The things that they would ask me varied each year with their own education experience. The first year, there were a number of times when somebody would approach me between lectures and ask personal health questions.

One thing that's been obvious to me in writing this book is that physicians who've gone through medical school together develop some very close relationships. It seems almost like boot camp, where you survived something rather extraordinary together. Did that happen the second time around, too?

The friendships I developed in the first round were much stronger because we had more experiences together. The main experiences I had the second time, involved sitting around in lectures and talking. But I didn't have any of the critical experiences during the third and fourth years, which are the clinical years, where the students go to clinics and offices.

Probably the best thing that Wisconsin does for students—it happened then and it happens now—was that during your fourth year, there's an externship kind of situation, where you actually go out and work in an office with a practitioner.

Most of the students had to go out around the state to various places where they would not be able to get home at night. That was probably the best experience I had for knowing what it was going to be like to work in an office because even then, and especially now, the hospital situation is quite different from an office practice. Hospital care now tends to be much more chronic, with some acute care, too.

How did you develop your interest in becoming a doctor? There couldn't have been many girls interested in medicine when you were growing up.

Actually, the main counselor in the high school that I went to, advised everybody, mainly the guys, who wanted to be a physician, "You don't want to do that. It takes so long before you get to do anything you really want to do."

But the moment you get to medical school, you are doing what you want to do. You're studying the things you want to study. But she prevailed for a lot of people. There was one boy, maybe two at most, from my high school, who went to medical school. What she thought people should do is become a teacher.

I persisted with my thoughts of being a nurse. What I really wanted to do was to go to the nursing school in Iowa City. But my parents said, no way. Iowa City is basically an evil place. Things happen there. They heard a lot of rumors. It was like Madison, at Wisconsin,[†] I suspect.

You can go to the nursing school here in town, but there was no way I was going to do that. I was eligible for scholarships at the state schools and had I known more about that, I might have chosen a different path. But I used the scholarship at what was known as the Teachers College, which is now the University of Northern Iowa, and went there.

After my first year, my parents said it wasn't costing as much as they thought and I was allowed to go to the four-year college and got a teacher's degree. I did well. I took all kinds of science courses. I took the chemistry courses that I had been warned against taking in high school because it was too hard.

With my degree in education, I probably would have been able to teach math, physics, chemistry, English, biology. As it turned out, because I thought it would be fun to see what it was like, I went to summer school during my third and fourth year and I graduated in January.

I was offered a junior position on the faculty at the college. These days, it would be more like a teaching assistant. I had a three-quarter position and I taught a couple basic math classes.

I did two things: I applied for a fellowship that would allow me to continue into a graduate degree program and applied for teaching positions. I was offered a teaching position in Madison at one of the high schools. I did not sign the contract until I heard about the fellowship, and I did receive a fellowship. I chose to take that.

I was in mathematics; not in education. I ended up with a master's degree in mathematics. The first year that I was in that program, I met my first husband.

After two years, the first of two children was born and another two and a half years for the second. I enjoyed taking care of the kids, but I didn't like staying home. Finally, I decided, it probably would be a good

† The University of Wisconsin has a long history of being known as a party {drinking} school.

idea to get something else to do and I decided now's the time if there's any way to complete the courses I hadn't taken for medical school because I still yearned to do that.

I figured they'd say, "Too bad, you don't fit the criteria. Sorry."

Then, I would do the second option, which was to do part-time teaching. So I spent a couple of years finishing the courses. I applied for medical school and after three interviews, which was three more than some people had, and certainly two more than most people had, they interviewed me in three manners: one was quite friendly, pleasant and optimistic; one was just a very middle of the road kind of person; the third was with a nasty psychiatrist. I don't know whether this was planned or it was just his personality.

What do you think they were trying to figure out?

I really don't know. The main thing that I recall from that was my third interview and it was toward the end of the day. He was asking a variety of things. What did I plan to do about my children if I went to medical school? I already had an arrangement with the woman who had helped me during the time that I was pursuing the few courses that I needed. I sort of explained all of that. I'd either made it or not at that point, so it wasn't going to matter what I said. I looked him straight in the face and said, "I really do care about my kids and it's really important to me that they get good care."

I left and waited a while and got a letter that said, "We'd like you to be a member of the class that starts in the fall." Actually, one of the hardest things I had to do was to make the decision and sign that letter. It was not the outcome I expected, and I realized it was going to have a significant effect on the rest of my life, the life of my husband and my children. While I had always been very optimistic about what I could do, I wasn't quite sure I could do it. You're older. You're a woman. You have kids. You won't be a productive person. As it turned out, I practiced for almost 30 years, after finishing residency.

What was the medical school experience like?

I would go home, as soon as I was done in the daytime and I didn't participate in a lot of the extra things, although there were many fewer extra things than there are now. There were only a few people who were married and there may have been one other person or so who had any children.

The women in the class—13 of us at graduation—which was about 10, 12 percent of the class, always got together and were a wonderful support group, telling how things happened, how you got through that. We were the largest number of women in any medical class in Wisconsin, at that point.

Maybe it was because I had been married, and sort of doing my own thing, but there were limitations of where you could go, how you act, and they were probably all perfectly reasonable things, but it felt restrictive to me. In some ways, it was almost like going back to high school. One of the things that was different was how the faculty overall, supported the students, which was in no way the kind of support that they give them now.

I went full-time. These days, exceptions are made more regularly for people to go part-time, when that's better for their academic process. It was a sharp curve at first because I hadn't been doing that kind of studying. I had done a few of the courses I needed to take, chemistry and genetics and things like that, but I only did one or two of them at a time each semester and in the summer. This was really intense. In addition to the studying, which I felt I needed to do after my children were in bed, I needed to be their mother and not a student. I burned the midnight oil and beyond, frequently, and that was probably, bar any other time, including residency and being on call, the time that I was more tired than I ever remember.

I would sit between my children on one of their beds to read them a bedtime story. I would read a page of the story, and then as was part of our way of doing things, the kids would kind of talk about what was on the page and after a page or two, I would read the story and fall asleep. When they were done talking, one of them would kind of elbow me and say, "Mom, wake up. Read the next page, please." It was the only time the story went like that, but that's how tired I was.

In organic chemistry, we were creating ether—the anesthetic. Of course, we were supposed to take precautions, so we wouldn't get it in the air. But inevitably, the air was full of ether, which we did not realize until after the first two hours of the morning, when we were in lab.

The day we made ether, we had an hour exam after the lab. It wasn't until I was almost finished with the exam and about to walk out of the class that I realized I had been somewhat under the effect of the ether. I suspect almost all of the class was. I had been anesthetized and had just taken an exam! It was the very last thing I needed.

I have young kids now and I can't imagine going to medical school. How did you do it?

I really don't know. But people even now work terribly hard and put in many hours toward things, besides their medical learning. Now, there are students who work basically full-time the first couple of years. I'm aware of people who've been police officers in Madison, people who are EMTs, a woman in my class who was an intensive care cardiac nurse and she would go home to Janesville.[‡] She commuted and would work a full weekend, usually.

We worked hard, but the detail these days is so much more than it was then. I'm not sure I would have passed, but one does what one has to do when you're in the middle of something like that.

‡ Janesville is 45-minutes from Madison.

What prepared you to take on medical school?

My parents both worked very hard. My mother, who also graduated from high school, had no further education, although she had hoped to be a nurse. I think she brainwashed me to think that I wanted to be a nurse. I did say that for a while, but actually, by the time I was in third or fourth grade, I really thought that I wanted to be a doctor.

I did all the things that would help me be a nurse. I took Latin and I took a dietetics course and things like that. I never told anybody about wanting to be a doctor because there just didn't seem to be any reason to think that that was a likely possibility for me.

What was your upbringing like?

For the first couple of years, I lived on a farm in Iowa. My father worked for a dairy, delivering bottles of milk and things like that. Because of that, we did get some additional food from the farm. My parents were very poor. It was the time of the Depression. The money that had been put aside for my mother by an uncle, who had some money, disappeared.

My father was in a situation where his mother had died when he was four years old. He was the youngest of six or seven children and by and large, the family sort of fell apart.

When I was a couple years old, we moved into Davenport, a bigger community. My father ended up working for the United States Post Office. Despite his lack of parenting, he got through high school and did very well. I've always been really sad that he didn't get to go to college, because I think he would have made a terrific lawyer. He was a very good poker player. He could keep a straight face, and had a very good mind.

As a matter of fact, when I was in high school, the physics teacher that I had, had been my father's physics teacher. My father had told me over the years, "When I graduated from high school, that teacher did not give me my workbook back. I think he kept it because it was such a good one and he used it."

When I was a senior in high school and took physics, this teacher approached me, "I have something of your father's I'd like to give back to you." It was my father's physics workbook.

How long before you started thinking about becoming a pediatrician?

That's why I became a physician! I wanted to be a pediatrician. That's why I was willing to go to a teacher's school. Since my undergraduate education was different from that of many of the students at that time—everybody was in pre-med—an education background was a very good background for being a pediatrician. As a pediatrician, one is teaching kids and parents all of the time—or should be—as part of helping them to do a better job of taking care of their own health or their children's health.

As I progressed through medical school into internship and residency, you just kind of learn how it was done.

What is it like to treat children?

The biggest problem was developing a relationship with the child. There were many kids who had bad experiences and that was very easy to recognize when you first met them because they were pretty negative about how they felt. The first goal was to give good medical care. But the second was to do it in such a way that the children either enjoyed the process or at least they didn't hate it, to do it in such a way that they understood what was going on, and to not hurt them. If something had to hurt, it was important to tell them that. There was no other way of doing it. I tried to make it so it didn't hurt, but sometimes it hurt.

Now, we have better medications to reduce some of that pain. One of the things that I'm proud of was that that process did work with the kids. I'm really happy when parents would say, "Johnny said, 'I don't feel good. I want to see Dr. Osborn.'" That meant they weren't afraid to come in.

I created some little devices that I thought would keep their attention away from what they were worried about. For example, one of the really bad experiences that many children have was having their ears looked into. Usually, that happened when they hurt already, but even on physical exam the kids were very apprehensive about it. One of the things that I tried to do when I was looking into the ear was to talk to the ear. For example, if it was the left ear, I'd say, "Hello Ms. Left Ear. How are you today? Suzie tells me that you hurt. I want to see what's going on down in there." By doing that, I think it did draw the attention of the child away from exactly what I was doing. I still had to do it. To be a pediatrician, you have to be part clown and not be afraid to do something silly or amusing for the child.

Is it hard to give a kid a shot? They're so unsuspecting and then, boom.

I made my nurses do it. There was a good reason for that. First of all, they were probably better at giving shots because they gave a great many more than I did. But I felt that if I did that, I don't think it was really possible to explain to a child about the pain from a shot. When the child saw me the next time, they didn't worry that I had a syringe in my pocket that I was going to pull out and stick into them. It was a way of creating some trust that allowed me to deal with them with other things.

Do any patients stand out over all the years?

One of my patients, a young girl, was out with her dad walking on the farm and all of a sudden she was attacked from behind by what turned out to be a rabid fox. Her dad killed it, so its brain was available for examination.

We treated the wound, made the arrangements for the animal to be examined. The assumption was that it was rabid and we began the treatment for rabies. That was when rabies treatment was very painful. You had to have an injection every day and it was really terrible. I saw this girl every day for two weeks. She survived.

Another situation that I had, which was funny, involved a family. The mother delivered two identical girls. Both were over eight pounds and they both had this mischievous look at life. At a young age, they realized very few people could tell them apart. One time they would say one name. Another time, they'd say another name. The parents, at this age, were not really sure that they would remember who they were if they did this enough, so they got identification bracelets for their ankles that the kids could not take off, so the parents would know for sure which one is which.

They used other devices too, for other people. They got them shoes that had their names on the bottom and so these kids were always fun to see, and see if I could figure out which one was which.

Could you?

No.

After all of these experiences, did you feel more like a teacher or student going through medical school the second time?

I felt more like a teacher. I tried very hard to read the assignments for the lectures because I felt I would understand them better. During the evenings when I was at home trying to read, unlike the experience with my children, when I began feeling sleepy, I quit.

Some class mentors wanted to challenge themselves and took exams. I decided that was not for me. I wanted to learn the stuff, become acquainted with it, be aware of it, but I didn't need to know it in detail. If I were to take the exams, I would need to study in a different way.

You've completed medical school twice now. What does it take to be an excellent physician?

The person who becomes a physician has to have a basic set of information that they can begin working with, even more than when I graduated the first time. They have to know the next step, which is, how do I find more information? I've made kind of a preliminary decision of what's going on and now I have to be certain about what I think is going on. These days, it's the Internet. Most physicians really don't have big shelves of books like I did. One of the icons of medical practice was the PDR,[§] the drug book, {but} most people don't use that anymore.

There are other ways about learning about the drugs you want to use, especially if there's an HMO and they have their list of accepted drugs. For those things where the physician needs a basic sense of knowledge and needs to know how to enhance that knowledge and improve upon it, they always have to have some feeling of care for the patient. In some ways, that's harder today because so much more of the work with the patient is done with machines or by other people. But a critical thing in developing a

§ Physician's Desk Reference

relationship with patients is to have some sort of personal involvement, and that's the hardest thing to do.

To be a doctor, you have to have an inquiring mind, knowing new information as it comes and remembering the old information. You have to have compassion to deal with the patients.

When you look at the students in medical school today, did you compare your original class to them?

For both groups of people, they went to medical school because they felt it was a way they could help other people. They were idealistic and thought they could help make the world a better place.

There is a difference in the basic class characteristics in that when I went to medical school, more or less, if you were smart enough and wanted to do it, you were accepted. Now, in order to be chosen, at least at some medical schools, which include the University of Wisconsin Medical School, one has to have an incredible background. Most of the people who are accepted into the medical school are very bright, have very high grade point averages, their M-CAT scores are above the average, most of them have spent a fair amount of time doing community work. They've worked in hospitals. They've done things in emergency rooms, to transport patients around. They've done all kinds of things that have a background in medical experiences.

Some people have had other careers, especially in medical areas. They've been nurses, EMTs, technicians. It's probably fortunate they have such backgrounds because the studying is so intense and exams are taken in different ways than they used to be. The students have to train each other or train themselves more than we had to. That's good.

When I was in school, everything was lecture and you sat there and tried to absorb it. Now, people, instead of being taught, they learn. They work on it together. They do it in groups. They learn how to get along with other areas of medical expertise.

A lot of instruction is done on the Internet. They look up a lot of information. They're at their computers regularly, both in learning and in communicating with each other. I get a lot of the e-mails that the students sent to each other and they do their social stuff that way. They exchange books. They convey information about the courses. They have websites, in which you can go look up the lecture from that day. All of the lectures are basically videoed and they can see them again on their computers, so that's totally different from what it was when I was in school.

When I was in school, one of the students brought a tape recorder to one of our lectures. We all found that not acceptable because somehow you were not supposed to hear it again. But that was a bright thing to do. More of us should have noticed it and done the same thing. Some do better listening; some do better reading, underlining. They have many modes of learning now that I think enables them to get more of the information because they can do it different ways and find the way that works best for them.

The crop of doctors coming out of school today is more sophisticated?

Yes, they are, but the patients are more sophisticated, too. Patients would come in, either after diagnosis had been made or when they came to have something diagnosed, with a stack of information from the Internet.

I attended your second graduation ceremony. What was going through your mind then?

It was kind of a sad day for me. While I was thrilled that so many people who started in the class had completed it, some of them weren't there because they had chosen to do other things. Some of them had taken time out to get a PhD or a law degree.

While I hope I will see many of these people again through the alumni association, I told them I wanted to be invited to their fifth year reunion.

I know there are people whom I never will see again or will never hear about again, which is kind of the way of life in medicine. I became aware of that when I was a resident, when the residents a year ahead of me left and they were gone. I thought it must be really hard for people who run residency programs to keep having people come and go. I'm sure there are ones that they'd like to know longer, but it just doesn't happen.

Any parting advice for medical students?

When you get out, get people to do stuff for you. You're earning enough money, even though at first it may not seem like a lot when you have bills to pay. It's more important for you to spend time with your family than to do the grass cutting or dusting. That's good advice, though I don't always take it. I grew up in a situation where we didn't have people come in and help. For many years, it was my children, my practice and myself. I did most of the work at home, sure, because it just wasn't built in for me to do it otherwise.

What are you going to do now that you've "graduated" again?

I'm also a member of the Medical Examining Board.

What's that like?

It's really quite misunderstood by most physicians. Most of what we do is deal with physicians who've had problems. Anybody can report a physician for what they consider to be poor care or doing something really wrong. The objective of the Board is to protect the people of Wisconsin. We're to try to help doctors recover from the problems they have, to rehabilitate them, to help them understand how they can be better physicians, and occasionally, there are some who have done such egregious things that we really feel that they can no longer be capable physicians, given their past.

They've gone through a great deal to become physicians and some of the things are unfortunate. Most of them are so intense about wanting to continue as physicians that they will do a great many things to make themselves capable of continuing.

You'll continue to mentor medical students in some way, right?

There are no longer class mentors. Each class, while they're still unique, is divided into five groups. It's another kind of mentoring system. It's based on the learning community; at Wisconsin, we call them houses, and I am a physician mentor for one of the houses.

They do much more mentoring of each other, such as explaining what happened to them during their year as a third year student, as other students are just going into that, so they are better prepared.

Even though the mentoring venue has changed, the students are just like my class. It's interesting to see them interact with each other a little bit more and help each other become doctors. That's the goal. We try to help the students with new experiences, as they're ready for them and launch them off and hope that we've done well because they're going to be taking care of us.

CHAPTER THREE

ADJUSTING TO MEDICINE

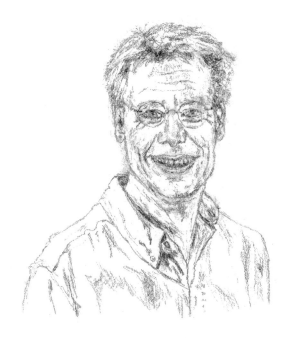

"I was white. I was male. I was over 30. And, I was a chiropractor—all against me."

Daniel Wik, DC, MD
Physical medicine & rehabilitation, Madison

Doctor Daniel Wik, now in his late 40s, made more than his share of sacrifices to become a physician, not the least of which was abandoning his thriving practice as a chiropractor. "I never wanted to be a chiropractor, ever, my entire life," says Dr. Wik, whose passion had always been medicine. Why he did become a chiropractor is rooted in the fact that he had so much difficulty getting into medical school. "I was a medical school failure," he states bluntly. But once he got in and graduated, Wik had to endure the medical profession's contempt for his chiropractic past.

When I interviewed Dr. Wik, he had just taken a break from packing his bags for a new job in Nebraska. Fresh out of residency training, he was about to begin a new life in medicine, a professional life far different from the one he had known as a chiropractor.

Tell me about your chiropractic practice.

I earned my first six figure income when I was 28 years old. I had eight associate doctors. I was one of the first to get the right to refer for an MRI or a CT scan at Longmont United Hospital, without a medical doctor to co-sign.

My practice got so busy that I only had time to really see patients three days a week. The other time I was just bogged down in paperwork and politics. I was so angry about not getting into medical school that I was willing to do whatever it took to be better than the medical profession at whatever they were doing.

When I was in chiropractic about five years, I was climbing to the top of the profession, but very frustrated. I told my wife at the time, "I really want to go to medical school. This has been my dream all along. I want to quit."

She said, "You're earning a huge amount of money. You have a family. You're at the pinnacle. Look at all the potential that you've got?"

She was right. "You are starting to climb in the political arena, as well—in the Colorado Chiropractic Association. You're gone at least two weekends every single month to seminars. You're constantly educating yourself. If you go to medical school, you're going to be even more in demand. You're going to be gone even more and you are going to be addicted even more to the education, to the success, to the power. And quite frankly, if you go to medical school, I'm going to divorce you."

I stayed in chiropractic another five years because of that and became the statewide at-large director for the Colorado Chiropractic Association. I became very politically involved. I got to know a lot of the politicians and was even asked at the end to run by the Republican Party for the House of Representatives. I would have done it, had I not gotten into medical school.

I was at the top of the game. Everybody thought that I was the practice to have. Inside, I was miserable, absolutely miserable. I took the Princeton review course for the Medical College Admissions Test, which, at that point, was 14 years after college. My wife said, "You'll probably fail and then we'll be done with this cockamamie idea."

I actually took it twice because I had no time to study. I took it again. Scored disappointingly for me for what I wanted to score. But looking back, I guess competitively enough to get in and I got 21 letters of rejection and one acceptance at St. George's. At 38-years old, I gave up everything that I had worked for, for a pair of t-shirts and shorts.

All but two or three of my colleagues felt betrayed. I had a lot of people call and say, "Why are you jumping to the other side?" Even my parents said, "You really shouldn't be doing this." And coming from my father, somebody who's a very aggressive person who said, "Shoot for the moon, whenever you can," to have him, as well, basically try to discourage me from it. I had to overcome just about everybody and listen to what was inside.

When did you first start thinking about becoming a physician?

From the time I was in eighth grade, I knew exactly what I wanted to do with my life. It was my passion. It was my dream. The doctor part was from the Indian reservation. I grew up on the White Earth Indian Reservation in Northern Minnesota. My dad went up there because, as a teacher, could make a little bit more money as an administrator.

There were two general practitioners who delivered babies, set broken bones; they were in the hospital all the time. They were the pillars of the community. The few times that I went, I thought it was the most fantastic thing in the world. The National Health Service's healthcare trailers would come on to the Indian reservation, twice a year. I was never a part of it, but all the Indian students got to go and get their free medical and free dental. I thought it was kind of neat that doctors would come from, I don't know where, onto the Indian reservation to serve that population. I really admired what they did.

Did your parents influence your career interest?

My dad was very much a proponent of education, being a guidance counselor and having seen a lot of people on the Indian reservation who never went beyond high school.

He was a tremendous businessman. He started a drive-in restaurant when everybody said he couldn't do it. He was a tremendous politician, though he never ran for politics. Whenever he walked into the room, by the time he walked out he would know every little tidbit about you.

He was a workaholic. He was never home. I grew up, basically, with a father who slept in the house, but that was it. He was always dreaming, scheming. I inherited all that from him, and admire him for that. My dad always pushed me beyond my limits. He was not one who believed I should be the one to decide what I wanted to do. He was extremely pushy. He had extremely high standards. He also gave me the parental blessing or curse that said he did better than his father and he expected me to do much better than he ever would. I had to live up to that, no matter what.

Mom was completely the opposite. She stayed at home. She wanted to be a secretary, did not want to have any of the high social life. She wanted her husband home at all times and it was a great conflict that the two had for a very long time. She had those homespun values, but at the same time, was not a very expressive person.

I have one sister. I grew up in the '70s, a white student growing up in the poorest county in the entire State of Minnesota. I had to work construction and work as an orderly. I went to Concordia College in Morehead, Minnesota because it was a spoiled little rich kids' school and I knew that it was a pre-med mill. That's exactly what I wanted. But with an extremely poor, at best, preparatory education, it was very difficult for me the first couple of years at a private college. I didn't do that well, but in my second, third, and fourth year, I got extremely high grades. Unfortunately, not high enough, so I was just missing the cut-off two years in a row interviewing for medical school, and had to do something—dentistry, optometry, or podiatry.

I decided to teach high school for a year without a teaching certificate. In the middle of North Dakota, you could do that. My wife, at the time, got into a car accident and went to a chiropractor, against my judgment. She got better and said, "Why don't you think about going to chiropractic college?"

I said, "Why don't you think about jumping in the lake?"

However, I was unemployed. I was young. My dreams were shattered. I applied to one chiropractic college, which was Northwestern. I got in because of my GPA. I would just go for a year, take the basic anatomy courses, do science courses and then transfer to medical school. There was never a time when I really wanted to be there, nor was my heart really in it. But I did it anyway, and I finished what I started. I got through a five-year academic program in three and two-thirds years.

I questioned everything that chiropractic did and everything chiropractic stood for. I questioned everything they taught me, with a medical model in mind. I argued with many professors, especially with the philosophy that just did not make sense to me. But the basic premise of the chiropractic adjustment started to intrigue me because people got better and nobody could really explain why.

There were a lot of half truths. They claimed to have some studies, but when you really looked at 'em, they weren't that good and didn't prove what they said that they were going to prove. But people got better anyway. I learned much later on that medicine is much the same way as chiropractic is in that there are a lot of drugs and a lot of procedures that don't have a lot of proof, but the outcomes are there. People get better.

With chiropractic, there is a flow of energy from above that comes down through the spine, through the body and out. You move a bone off of a pinched nerve, that energy flows through that nerve and that makes the body better. Whether that's true or not is not the point. It's an antiquated type of an explanation, but it's one that makes sense.

A chiropractic adjustment is the same as an osteopathic manipulation, even though when I say that, my chiropractic colleagues are gonna cringe. It's cracking your back or cracking your neck. That's the bottom line. The chiropractic adjustment goes into what's called the periphysiological space. In other words, if you moved your fingers so far that there's a little bit of a wiggle to it, you get this little pop. That's what a chiropractic adjustment is—taking a joint into that extreme of its motion, giving a slight amount of a high velocity, low force move that makes that joint pop. When it makes that joint pop, something happens.

Some people say the pop is nitric oxides.* Some people say it's the barometric pressure. We don't know. When you get that immediate feeling of relief and that feeling that lasts—we don't know what that is, either. We don't know if it's a bone moving back into place, taking pressure off of a nerve. We don't know if it's a change in barometric pressure in the joint that changes how that joint feels. We don't know if it then changes the way the bone moves so that it moves normally, so that it doesn't irritate nerves. We don't know if there are chemicals that are released, which then go not only within the spinal chord but within the entire body.

We don't know, even to this day, exactly what happens with the manipulation. Whether it is chemical, neurochemical, physiological, mechanical, we know that people get better.

There were all kinds of extremes in chiropractic college, and even more so when I got into practice in Boulder, Colorado, because it was anything goes, from adjusting auras, to magnets. But when I adjusted people and really got busy seeing 20, then 30 and 40 people a day and up to my busiest day—I saw 93 patients in one day—every single one of them got better. They paid. They returned. You don't have to explain why when you're getting results.

I do know that when I've done adjustments, I've had heart rates that have immediately lowered. I've had people break out into sweats. I've had immediate relaxation of muscles. I've had pain immediately go away. I've had asthma suddenly stop—all kinds of things that I can't explain.

I have had people's glasses prescription change and get better. I have had their hearing become more acute. I've had women who have had chronic pelvic pain and could not get pregnant, all of a sudden have their chronic pelvic pain go away when I adjusted their sacroiliac joints. They all of a sudden became pregnant.

Could it be placebo effect and have absolutely nothing to do with the actual procedure?

Yeah, it could. It could be a placebo effect with anything. In medicine, does the medication really do what it's supposed to do, or is it a placebo effect because people want it to work? You take credit for it anyway.

A neurologist challenged me, "I see chiropractic patients all the time and they all claim that their headaches are getting better. I think it is just a multiple placebo effect."

I said, "Sir, that's fantastic. Would you write a letter that says your observation is that there is a precedent of multiple cases of placebo effect

---

* Nitric oxide is a gas that facilitates oxygen transport to the tissues, the transmission of nerve impulses, and other physiological activities.

of headaches being gotten rid of with chiropractic adjustments that you've seen on a multiplicity of occasions?"

Well, of course he knew what was going to happen, that that precedent was going to be established and when it happens over a long period of time, it's not a placebo; it's actually what's happening.

If you ask most chiropractors, they will tell you that they've done chiropractic care on dogs, cats, horses; a lot of different animals. When I was in practice, I couldn't do it legally because it was practicing veterinary medicine without a license. I couldn't charge for it. But I got lots of pecan pies and chocolate cakes and other wonderful items when people would bring in their dogs, mainly after hours, and I would do chiropractic care on their dogs. And all of a sudden, they'd jump up and down. You can't do power of suggestion on a dog or a cat.

I've also done it on little kids and on very small infants. You can't do the power of suggestion on a little kid because they'll tell you like it is. I would adjust both of my sons whenever they had colic and it quit within two or three minutes. That was after I had rocked them, burped them, changed their diapers, and fed them.

I'm comfortable sometimes not knowing, and I'm comfortable admitting to my medical colleagues that I don't know. I'm also comfortable in challenging them that we have to find out. When you admit that and you're honest about it, rather than trying to cover it up or argue, you gain a great deal of respect. Something has to be happening. If we could really figure it out, maybe that's a Nobel.

Ask any chiropractor and they will tell you amazing stories of things that have happened that they can't explain that have happened with patients.

Why don't chiropractors conduct research to explain it?

In medicine, the research is done by the National Institutes of Health. It's done by pharmaceutical companies on a profit-driven basis. Well, with chiropractic, there's no pharmaceutical company, and for the most part, you cannot get funds from the National Institutes of Health, because they're controlled by the medical profession. The only research that you can get is that which is privately endowed, and it takes a ton of money. Then, when you do the research on yourself, you are not a disinterested third party, so whatever you find is going to be labeled biased.

Now, what do you do? There is no solution because in order to do research on chiropractic, you have to have the skill of doing the chiropractic adjustment, which means you would have chiropractors doing the research. You can't put it in a medical model of a double blind, placebo-controlled study because it doesn't work.

Who's going to do the research? Ironically, the only people who can do it are people who have both a medical degree and a chiropractic degree. There aren't too many of us.

Even if it does work, aren't you exposing the patient to risks by such manipulations?

There's a risk to every single medical procedure that's done, period. There are adverse outcomes to every single drug that's given, surgery that's done, procedure that's performed, and chiropractic adjustment. The better your skill is, the less chance there is of an unforeseen outcome, but it's there.

The problem is that in chiropractic, the number of really bad adverse outcomes is one per three to five million, which is so rare that the malpractice insurance for chiropractors is extremely low compared to medicine. An insurance company is not going to take a risk of a high amount of adverse outcomes because they don't care whether you have an MD or DC after your name. All they care about is profit and risk, period.

But when there are adverse outcomes in chiropractic, they are always amplified to a very great degree. You have to deal with it. You have to explain to people what the possibility is for the bad outcome. It's called informed consent and we do it in medicine all the time. Is it a scare tactic? No, it's actually the truth because you have the right to know what you're getting. You have the right to know what the alternatives are, as well.

But if a chiropractic adjustment can avoid an injection or avoid a surgery, do you have the right to know that, as well? Yes. But in the United States, the answer is no. That's not the standard.

How does one become a successful chiropractor?

It's much different than in the medical community. The way that you get accepted into medicine is to get accepted into medical school and survive internship and residency, and you are considered a colleague. In chiropractic, it's not that difficult to get in and it's not that difficult to get through academically. The rite of passage in chiropractic is surviving five to seven years in practice because it is so cut-throat. You're not collegial. You're competitors.

Nevertheless, medicine is something that I couldn't ever get out of my mind. I consider myself to be a Christian person. I prayed about it relentlessly. It was as though it haunted me and I couldn't get rid of it, no matter how hard I worked, no matter how successful I was, no matter how much people praised me, no matter how much money I made, no matter how successful I was with my patients.

Many chiropractic patients were very disappointed with my leaving, as well. I had to do it for myself and I did it. Not because of the money. I had lots of money. I didn't do it because of the power. I didn't do it because of the prestige. I did it because there was something inside that I knew I had to sacrifice much more than most people coming out of college, in order to get that medical degree.

St. George's is in Grenada, which is six degrees from the equator. It is a school that was started in the mid-70s. It has two thousand five hundred plus graduates. You spend two years in the Caribbean and 99% of my colleagues were people like myself who got wait listed in medical school who had very high GPAs from United States undergraduate colleges, many with masters degrees, many with PhDs, many with a plethora of research and a lot of life experience behind them—a very mature type of person for the most part, extremely motivated.

At most of the medical schools in the United States, once you get in, they will do whatever they possibly can to help you. St. George's is just the opposite. They create stress. They try to make sure that unless you are a top performer that you drop out. They do not support a lot of anything other than hard work grade gunning. It's a British type of system—a great deal of memorization, a great deal of regurgitation.

You're in a foreign country, so you're out of your comfort zone, out of your element completely, and they preach high M-CAT scores and high GPAs, so that you can get into your third and fourth year and do very well, basically to prove that you were as good as the Americans. It was a mistake that you were not accepted somewhere in the United States. That's what they want and that's exactly what you get.

Did your wife come along then? Did she come to accept this?

{long pause} We're divorced.

I'm sorry. Because you switched careers?

Yes. She was extremely unhappy and said she wanted me to quit medical school on a daily basis. When I got into St. George's I was absolutely thrilled. But it was very difficult for me because most of my colleagues were single, and didn't have kids. I studied with an eight-week old on my lap for anatomy. Every single thing that I did, I also had to play with my eight-year old. I had to try to keep my wife content, who was an extremely unhappy person about the fact that I was in medical school. I had to overcome all of those things and at the same time try to study and maintain my grade point average, competing with everybody else who was single. I'm not going to say they didn't have a care in the world, but they had less onus of responsibility.

During my third and fourth years, I was older than most medical students. I was more mature. I had already been successful. And I was rounding with some people who were ten, fifteen years younger than me. I had the burden of making sure that their ego wasn't stepped on, constantly. I had to make sure that at all times, nobody was upset with me for any reason, and a lot of the attendings were younger. A lot of the attendings were not as successful as I had been in the chiropractic profession. I had to really keep a very close watch on what I said, how I said it, how I acted. I had to take a very, extremely humble role and I tried to do that. But with a personality as aggressive as mine, it still came out.

I had to take some time off after my second year of medical school to work again for nine months to support this expensive habit. Then, I went to the East Coast and trained. It's a different type of an environment than the Midwest for training. It's an environment of extreme intimidation and degradation in medical school and in residency.

I spent a year in New Jersey, and I was in the gang hospitals. Then, I went to the gang hospitals in Oakland, California, and in Phoenix. I went all over the place and really traveled. I spent a lot of time getting my hands bloody, rather than learning about blood—all the same time, trying to see my kids, trying to keep my, at that time, wife satisfied. She refused to go with me to any of the places that I went, so I was essentially alone for two and a half years.

You are considered a second class tier on the medical hierarchy by going to a foreign school. If you go to a prestigious East Coast school or an Ivy league medical school, obviously that's something that you have more credence than if you go to a state school in the Midwest.

If you go to an osteopathic school, that's looked on, in some circles, as less than. If you're a United States citizen and go to a foreign medical school, that's another level. If you are a foreign medical graduate coming into the United States, that's another level yet.

You have to pass the United States Medical Licensing Exam by a higher amount of points. You're forced to take more tests than the Americans, or were at first. Many times, you're prejudiced against in the hospitals you train in. And a lot of times when you're applying for residencies, the residency places will automatically delete all computerized foreign medical school applicants, so you don't even get looked at.

I applied the first time in 1976, which was at that time, was the highest number of medical school applicants ever. I should have listened to myself at that five year mark and applied because it was a low number of applicants. When I applied again in 1995, it was an extremely high number of medical school applicants. Affirmative action was certainly there. I was white. I was male. I was over 30. And, I was a chiropractor—all against me.

There were many times that I would lay awake at night, going, *How can I ever get through this? How can I ever find the money to get through this? How can I ever pass all these tests?*

When you're 24, 25 years old, you can survive on a lot less sleep. It seems like you have a lot better memory for memorization and regurgitation. After being in practice for 10-years, some of the things that you have to do are just so impractical compared to real life practice. You think to yourself, *This is crap. I don't need to know this stuff. This is just about passing a test.* You just had to come to a point where you said, *It's about passing tests. It's about the process. Try to make sure that you get through every single rotation. Make sure that you do the best you possibly can.*

Did you ever consider dropping out?

Absolutely not. Never. Not even once. I knew what I wanted. The other thing is that if I would have dropped out at any time, think of what I would have had to have faced from all of my colleagues, who now thought that I had deserted them. From my wife, who would have said, "See, I told you you couldn't do it. You really just didn't have what it took to be a medical doctor all along." I couldn't turn back. The social shame, the professional shame and the personal shame—there's no way that I could have ever done it.

When I got through medical school, I did not pass part two of the United States Medical Licensing Exam. As a United States graduate, you could still enter what's called the United States Residency Match. As a foreign medical graduate, I was thrown out, so I could not even enter the match. I was completely devastated. I had to go back and study again. The reason that I didn't is because the family decided to move from Denver to Phoenix, at the time I was going to spend studying for part two. I had to actually pack moving vans and move.

I failed. I went through something called the scramble and matched at a program in North Carolina. I finished medical school. I took a test over the entirety, over the four years of medical school in order to graduate from St. George's, because I did not pass part two. I was told a couple of days after I had finished my medical school that I could not start my residency that year.

I went into a very deep depression. I went to a six-week course in Los Angeles. I took the review course. I studied from seven in the morning until 11 at night for six entire weeks, doing nothing but wanting to pass one test because I knew that if I didn't, my career was over. I was over $200,000 in debt and it was all on the line.

I passed and then went back into practice as a chiropractor in a medical office in the white mountains of Arizona. I did very well. The medical doctor said, "Why don't you just stay on with me? We're doing great financially. Everybody thinks you're a fantastic doctor." But a medical doctor with a medical degree, without a license, is a piece of paper and that's it. I said, "Absolutely not. I can't."

I got a residency in one of the toughest states to get one in, which was Colorado, and I did family practice for a year. I delivered lots of babies. I did a lot of emergency room work, intensive care work, and that's what I was going to do for the rest of my life. I was going to be a family practice doctor.

But as much as I tried, a lot of the people there thought I was haughty, arrogant, proud. I wasn't. I was just trying to do a good job and go back to managing patients the way I was used to managing patients, which was by taking charge. The only thing you want to do is sleep, especially during your internship year. You live to sleep. Before the 80-hour work week, I was working a hundred-twenty, a hundred-thirty hours a week. Where I was an intern, there were supposed to be eight interns that year. They only funded and matched five, so we were on call every third or fourth night. Most nights, I didn't get any sleep. The adage was if you got an hour and a shower, you had nothing to worry about. You were supposed to go home after 24 hours. You were absolutely supposed to go home after 30 hours. That didn't happen. You were supposed to have a least a full 24 hours off or one day off per week.

Medicine eats their young, and it's done because the volume of the cases that you see make you good at what you do. You don't have a lot of time to learn everything that you need to know before people's lives are in your hands.

That first night when I was on call as a resident, people were calling me—right out of medical school!—and asking me critical life questions, and I had no idea what I was doing and I was scared! That's the same with every single resident. They'll always say, "I was up all night. I was reading. I was just hoping somebody wouldn't ask me something that I didn't know." Well, within two months of that immersion and that kind of stress, you learn real quickly.

As an intern, it was not uncommon for me to deliver one or two babies a night, to have three or four other women in labor or checking for labor. I would be in the emergency room two or three times managing somebody with chest pain. I would be in charge of the entire intensive care ward, so if somebody had pulmonary problems, or was in a very acute illness, I had to manage that. I had five floors, with five wings each, that had all kinds of miscellaneous problems come up. You had to run all over the place, and that was a nightly occurrence.

Then, the next day, if you made a mistake, you would get chastisement for the one or two things you did wrong. You had gotten no sleep, you were on morning rounds at seven o'clock that day and you probably weren't going to go home until six or seven o'clock that evening, so it wasn't 30 hours, it was 36 hours. Many times you couldn't sleep. Sometimes you fell asleep at the wheel going home. There are many times I don't remember ever getting home. I don't remember conversations I had post-call.

The next morning, you get up, you feel like a Mack truck has run over you and you have to do it all over again.

Considering all that stress, was it difficult to pick your specialty?

I wanted to go into rehabilitation medicine in the first place. I had no intention of becoming a family medicine doctor, but I did. One of the rehab doctors said, "Dan, what are you doing in family practice? You're a chiropractor. Rehabilitation medicine is the perfect thing for you, if you're not going to go into orthopedic surgery." I applied to five different rehabilitation medicine programs, got interviews at two and there was no question that I wanted to come to Wisconsin.

Finally, I hit the big time in a major university at the University of Wisconsin. I came here, just like everywhere else, without my family. We tried to get back together for a year. My wife absolutely refused to move with me after we had lived apart for a number of years. I came alone in a Honda Prelude with no place to stay, slept in the car, got a hotel room and started my residency.

You've given up so much to do this. Has it been worth it?

Everything. Every ounce. Never, ever, a regret about medicine. If the world is a microcosm and each person is a world unto themselves, and you take away the hurdles that are there with each individual, to allow them to reach their full potential in life, you've changed the world one person at a time, and you do it many times a day. That's the most powerful thing you can ever do. That's why you do it. And you realize that some people thank you, some people don't. Some people swear by you, some people swear at you.

That inner peace that I got from that medical degree—I don't know if it's a curse or if it's a blessing, but it's a drive. I came to Wisconsin, thinking that I would strike it up with a number of my chiropractic colleagues. I would help the chiropractic profession a bit in Wisconsin, and that's it. Again, God had another plan for me, totally different than what I thought would ever happen.

I got involved in politics again, much to the chagrin of most of my residency. Within the university system, politics is not popular. It's actually looked down upon. But it's all about taking care of patients, whether it's inside the office or outside the office.

I got the opportunity to go to the Dane County Medical Society meetings. When anybody ever asked me about chiropractic, I was very honest with them. I never hid that fact from anybody in the medical profession at all, and I took a lot of ribbing about it. I would say absolutely it works, no matter what. I've done it for 10 years and I wouldn't have duped the public for ten years, if it wouldn't have worked.

Being that simple, forthright and honest with my medical colleagues, I won a ton of respect. Got to know a lot of people in national politics, wrote national resolutions. One was just passed in Chicago, which is probably going to be just as big as the 80-hour work week is and it's on resident abuse, which is rampant—physical abuse, emotional abuse.

Rampant?

In many programs, there's personal degradation, there is professional degradation, there's prejudice based upon age, race, sex, where you went to medical school, when you graduated from medical school. I haven't personally had it, but because I was in national politics, I've had many people call me and say, "Dan, you're the aggressive one. If I ever wanted to have somebody on my side, it would be you. Let me tell you what happened to me."

If you ask every single resident, "What was the worst single thing that happened to you?" they'd name five. There have been head buttings in surgery suites. There have been gropings. There have been threats, asking for personal favors, sexual favors, having to cover up for obvious flaws. That's why I wrote the national resolution that I did—the horror stories. These are the top people in the United States, the most educated, the brightest of our society, and we are treating them like this?

The 80-hour work week had to be passed. You can't fly an airplane or drive a school bus without so many hours of sleep, but you can save a life if you have been up for 36 to 40 hours. If you forget one thing, you'll be sued.

I had to write a law that said that we have to define what abuse is. We have to have a central reporting agency for it, and we have to have it anonymous, because you will lose your residency over reporting something like that.

If I would have reported some of the things that happened to me, I would have given up the entirety of my four years of medical school. I would have given up all of the time that I spent, all of the sacrifice. You keep it to yourself, very close to your heart and you may tell one or two of your colleagues.

Tell me something that happened to you.

When I was an intern, I was in the intensive care unit. It was an attending who was extremely verbally abusive. We were both interns in the intensive care ward, trying desperately to learn everything we possibly could and in no way could you ever do anything right for this guy. He threatened me one time in front of the entire intensive care unit, probably 15 or 20 people, at the top of his voice, saying, "You are the shittiest resident I have ever had. By the time you get done, I'm going to report you to the board and the only thing you're going to be able to do is practice on rubber dog shit. I'm going to make sure you never practice ever in your life."

One time when he was supposed to put an intravenous fluid at 50 ccs an hour, he did it at 500 ccs an hour, which is lethal. I called him to change it and he chastised me, for who would ever do something like that? The other attendings would not even turn down that IV because he had written for it. Nobody wanted to face him or challenge him at all in anything. But you do it, knowing you are going to pay for it later on. Every medical doctor has had this; some to more or less degrees than others.

When I was a fourth year medical student, I was in surgery. It was with the head of the department of surgery. I had stayed. It was 11 o'clock at night. I was first assistant on a surgery with him and the gang section of Newark, and he was very appreciative of the fact that I helped him with the surgery. Then, he turned to me and said, "You guys who are foreign medical graduates just should admit to the fact that you're complete, utter failures and do something else with your life."

And I said, "Sir, the great thing about the United States is, number one, you have the right to express your own opinion, and I respect your opinion greatly." He was from Harvard. "Second, the other great thing is that if you're willing to pay any price possible and give up everything, you have the potential opportunity to succeed in this great country. That's what I did."

You never, ever retort or retaliate at all. Every single resident learns that you have to say, "Thank you sir, may I have another?" You do that all the time. It's a changing personality, most certainly, with more women, more foreign medical graduates. But it's something that changes slowly, and something that most people never, ever talk about because you don't want to. You want to forget about that crap and go on with your dream.

It's not just abuse of residents, but abuse of nurses, one medical doctor to another medical doctor—that happens a lot, as well. It's what allows you to handle stress, and you never crack. It works, because now I can hear just about anything from a patient. I can see blood and guts spilled all over the place. I can see chaos happening all around me and you just focus and you concentrate.

You have gotten such a self education in getting rid of the emotion and focusing on what needs to be done, whether you're insulted, whether you're threatened, whether you are scared, you just become what you need to be.

Is there a better way, a different way? Perhaps, but it's something that when you come out the other end, you realize that you have been changed somehow and you can go on. Now, do you become less of a human being? A lot of time patients complain about their doctors, that they're not as personable as they could be. Well, take somebody who has gone through all the stress of medical school, internship, residency, their humanity has completely been destroyed and then you ask that person, all of a sudden, to be a wonderful human being.

Through all of it, however, most people still maintain an incredible amount of humanity and I don't know more than a handful of doctors who don't deeply care about the people they treat and are deeply affected by the outcomes of those people, and wouldn't do anything for them or sacrifice anything for them. That's why obstetricians in their 50s and 60s still stay up all night long, and surgeons stay up all night long.

People just expect that when they get sick in the middle of the night and you're going to get out of bed, you're going to be happy to see them and you're not going to say one thing about the fact that perhaps you, as a human being, were a bit put out, as well, and you'd been doing this every third night for your entire life. You just don't realize it.

You've just finished the marathon. How do you feel?

Phenomenal. Awesome. If God took me tonight, I would have achieved two doctorates in life. I would have helped tons of patients and now I have the ability to give back to society. Because I've got a chiropractic doctorate, I've got the ability to help people with the chiropractic adjustments. I've got the primary care as a family practice doctor. I could deliver a baby today if I needed to. I can still set a broken bone. I can still manage a heart attack. I've got the training in an acute brain and spinal cord injury unit at one of the best hospitals. I can manage all kinds of muscular-skeletal problems. I can treat the entire patient and I feel humbled to be able to do that.

With that business background that I've gotten through the hard knocks of life, and through my political background, I was head-hunted by over 20 different head hunters. I turned down many more interviews than I ever went on.

I got hired as a medical director of an inpatient, regional medical center in Nebraska. You just don't get hired as a medical director right out of residency. It does not happen. God blessed me.

I have a supervisory role over physical therapy departments, occupational therapy departments, and in patient nursing departments. I've been given a wonderful amount of responsibility. I'm going to be the only physical medicine doctor in a 150-mile radius in any direction. It just excites me to no end.

I will be on call 24/7, 365. There's nobody else who can take call for me. Now, when I take vacation, somebody's going to have to manage the acute cases, like a heart attack or something like that. But otherwise, I'll have my telephone all the time. It's service to humanity.

In medicine, you need to have a combination of business acumen and scientific knowledge, as well as the ability to communicate and motivate people. The difference between chiropractic and medicine—one of the biggest differences—is that for the most part, medical doctors are horrendously poor business people.

Chiropractors are unabashedly unashamed of the fact that medicine is business. Because when you are not number two, but when you are the dung of the medical profession, you learn how to survive and you learn how to communicate. You learn business. You learn advertising. You learn people skills. You learn management skills. That's what brought the salary that very few residents get, is that business acumen, that ability to handle people that needs to be taught in medical school, as well. But it's an art, it's not a science.

I can go on the chiropractic speaking circuit now, with my credentials, and hopefully, all over the world. I hope, as well, to be on the medical lecture circuit, not only talking about pain management and rehabilitation medicine, but also as a medical doctor, I have a unique ability, and perhaps the onus of a responsibility to talk to my medical colleagues about chiropractic, as well, from the point of a medical doctor. All the things that worked against me, all of sudden, are now things that my colleagues in the medical profession are admiring. That's the irony.

Besides the practice that I have, I hope that I can be of some help in bringing the two professions to greater understanding and respect of each other. If there can be progress made in the world because I've paid both prices, then I'm willing to serve. I don't know how to do that yet, but I didn't know how to do any of this. I just did it, and I learned. I learned more from my mistakes than I did from my successes, and so we'll see what happens.

Things are changing. Yes, while some medical doctors are working with some chiropractors, and it's on a very personal relationship level, definitely, the medical profession has not in any way, shape, form, or size, embraced the chiropractic profession at all. They may have changed from when a patient mentioned they went to a chiropractor the patient was absolutely chastised to a position of neutrality or not saying anything. If that's progress, so be it. I think it is.

But there is no understanding. There is no synergy between the two. What is perceived is that the two are in competition with each other. Drugs do what drugs do. The chiropractic adjustment does what the chiropractic adjustment does. They're not the same thing. They don't do the same thing. They're not in competition with each other at all. They are much more cooperative and synergistic than they are adverse.

Can the two come together? As time goes on, perhaps. But both have a lot of memories from the past and there is the rite of initiation. That rite is so different for the medical profession than it is for the chiropractic profession, and somehow or other that has to be resolved and rectified. The best way to do it is for the educational achievements of the chiropractic profession be understood and recognized by the medical profession.

The absolute best thing I think could ever happen to the chiropractic profession is if they started physician assistant programs just for chiropractors who already had a doctorate degree in chiropractic. They'd have had all the background, all the science, and then went through a set of the multi-year physician assistant program, an additional one to one and a half years to become a physicians assistant, to have the ability to write for a certain amount of medications, to then earn respect of medical doctors, to work together in the same office.

They can't be across the hall. It's got to be rubbing shoulders in the hallway, one to the other. You will then have a person in a combination of doctor of chiropractic who is an independent physician, yet as the ability to operate as a physician assistant, is a great way to give back and serve society. Now that, to a significant number of my chiropractic colleagues, is going to be bastardizing the philosophy of independence of chiropractic and what it stands for, which is absolute drugless, absolute anti-medicine in any form or fashion. But that's selfish thinking. That's not thinking about patients. It's not thinking about what is best to serve people. It's what's best to serve the profession. The chiropractors do it. The medical doctors do it. But patients have told me, many times, "I just wish the two of you guys would get together." You really can't say anything to me that I haven't heard before, or been insulted by.

You're starting the first leg of your medical career. You're a chiropractor and you're a medical doctor, so which one will you be?

There's no difference. I'm me. I have a lot of skills and you don't have to separate one from the other because they don't compete with each other. You can give the best of everything.

Physical therapy is not the same as giving a drug. Giving them a drug is not the same as surgery. Doing surgery is not the same as doing an injection. Doing an injection is not the same as psychotherapy. But everything that I've mentioned are sub specialties of medicine. They're all individual and they are all under the auspices of medicine, so they're all considered the same.

I don't see any difference between that and one extra skill, which is the ability to give a chiropractic adjustment. It's a learning curve just like everything else. But if you feel that it can help somebody, then you have the ability to be as complete as you possibly can, and there's probably a lot more things that I need to learn that I don't know.

If I ever quit learning, that's a bad thing. If I ever become satisfied with where I'm at, that's a bad thing. If I don't at least step 10% out of my comfort zone every single day, then I'm not challenging myself. That's what you learn to do. I'll use every single technique all of my medical colleagues use. I was taught to think like a medical doctor, to act like a medical doctor, to treat like a medical doctor. I've been doing that through four years of medical school. I have a unique advantage in that I can do everything that a physical medicine rehabilitation doctor can do, plus I have the ability to do the chiropractic adjustment.

Nothing about my medical training has made me a better chiropractor, but both have made me a better doctor. There've been so many times through my medical training and my residency that I knew through my chiropractic successes with patients with headaches, neck pain, mid-back pain, low back pain, I could have given them between one to 12 adjustments and gotten better right away. I had to bite my tongue, and I had to give them drugs, and I had to send them to physical therapy, and I had to give them injections. I wanted so desperately to just say, "Let me just give you an adjustment, not just because I have this philosophical bent, but because I have ten years of experience."

I saw all the people who went to medical doctors first. That's what people did. When it didn't get better, then I was the caboose doctor, as a chiropractor. If I didn't get 'em better, I got all the blame.

So, because of that, I know that there are a lot of times when low back pain, neck pain, headaches, mid-back pain, shoulders, elbows, knees, joints, could be just simply helped with some chiropractic adjustments. Now, if you combine that with a little bit of medication, or some injections or something else, boy, you've got an even more powerful tool.

Part of my entire training has been a training of restraint, that now I'm free to be able to do whatever I want to do. I just wish that there were more patients that could walk into a family practice doctor's office, or an internal medicine doctor's office, and see a chiropractic doctor in that office. If they tried chiropractic care as one of their primary interventions, my prediction is that there would be a lot of people that would get a lot better, a lot faster.

Being that medical doctors don't like treating that stuff anyway, it really wouldn't make that much difference. They wouldn't be taking any business away from the family practice doctor or the internist. They would be adding to it.

Do physicians see chiropractors as stealing their patients?

I don't think it's financial. It's ignorance and it's prejudice; it's ramped, it's deep, and it's ingrained. At the same time, most of the comments that I hear from medical doctors are that chiropractors see tons of people and make a ton of money.

The ones that the medical doctors hear about are those few cases, about 10%, that are interesting enough to hear about. The rest of the people who do a good job and go home and make a good living, but not a phenomenal, ultra rich living, you never hear about.

Is there a little bit of jealousy? Perhaps, sometimes. Most of the time, the medical profession really just doesn't care. It's just that we're too busy. They don't know. They don't have time to know. I don't blame the medical profession for that. Perhaps, the onus of the burden is on the chiropractic profession. But when something happens that the medical profession is threatened, or they feel that their territory is being infringed on, then they're going to fight back.

What do you anticipate your new life to be? Are you going to have a real life?

Real life is only what you define it to be. For me, it's going to be seven to seven, Monday through Friday, rounding out Saturday and Sunday. If there's any kind of emergency, I'm going to have to be in for those, as well. Medicine is not a job. Medicine is a lifestyle and you live it 24 hours a day. You live to serve. You don't live for yourself. You live for others.

In all of that, hopefully, you can find a spouse who cares enough about you to also recognize your humanity and also try to put some balance in your life, as well, so you also have some very fun times. But they have to be scheduled. It's not spontaneous. When medical doctors go on vacation, they have to go somewhere their cell phones don't reach. You do that because it's necessary, because you can't get out of that mode.

You give back to society in any way that you possibly can. But that's what makes it fun. I don't work for a living. I get up every morning and I have fun. Then, I go to bed.

What about real fun? What are your hobbies outside of medicine?

I don't do a lot of anything real well because I don't have the time. I love to mountain bike. I try to run three, four, five times per week. When I was in the Caribbean, I learned how to snorkel. When I lived in Colorado for 10 years, I learned how to downhill ski. Do I have the time to do most of it? No. Many times I have to get up at 4:30 or 5 o'clock in the morning, if I want to do a run.

But you learn to have a very high quality life, and one of the keys to that is you don't watch much TV. It's amazing the amount of things you can do when you don't watch TV. I like to watch the news. That's it. Most of the rest of it, quite frankly, bores me.

You have a fiancé. How did you manage that, given your chaotic schedule?

I was honest and said I'm a workaholic. I'm gone all the time. I love what I do and I need to have someone who understands that. Medicine is worse than any other kind of jealous lover because it consumes you, and you cannot compete, and it is extremely selfish. A spouse has to be available when you are and you cannot reciprocate. When you're off, your spouse has to be there. When you're on vacation, your spouse has to be able to go on vacation with you.

You have to say up front that it is unfortunately, many times a one way street. And when you do that and say, I'm also a human being, a pretty nice person. I'm aggressive. I'm honest.

It takes a very special person to be married to a medical doctor—male or female. It takes an extremely unselfish person to do that. I was blessed enough to meet someone who was that unselfish, so I consider myself incredibly lucky.

I met her actually over the Internet because I don't have the time. I just put out exactly who I was and who I was looking for and I didn't waste my time with any of the other social dances that you do with meeting, greeting and I talked to her many times over the Internet, talked to her by telephone. I tell her I had to search far and wide to find the gem of the East and the ruby of the Nile, and she was in Central Illinois.

Now that you're a medical doctor, how do your parents feel about that?

My mom still tells me I shouldn't be doing it because I don't take care of myself. She's giving me medical advice all the time. She says, "I know you're a doctor, but I'm your mother and I need to take care of you."

My dad is extremely proud. He just came to my graduation and gave me the proverbial parental blessing, which, even as an adult, really makes a difference. Now, he calls me with his cholesterol level. I don't know if they're more thrilled about the chiropractic doctorate or the medical doctorate.

I hope that I go into the office in the morning and I change the world. If I change the world for two or three people that day, then I can die that afternoon and somebody can say, "Job well done."

You love what you do so much that you're willing to get up every single morning and say, *This is unbelievable. I get paid for this. This is totally awesome and fantastic. I can't wait to get to the office. I can't wait to help people.*

One of the worst things that has ever happened is that when people are at the pinnacle of their ability to give back to society, they are all of a sudden reduced to playing shuffleboard. I don't ever have to retire. I can serve until the day that I die. It's worth all of it. Now, all of those voices that I was haunted with are gone and I've achieved my goal.

CHAPTER FOUR

YOUNG AT ART

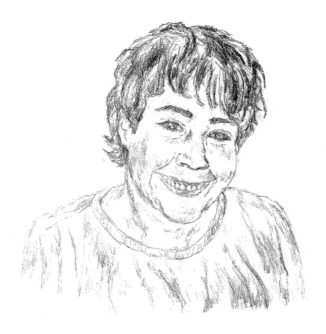

"Of the people who did anything to help me through school, on the top of that list, would be that person who gave me their physical being to go figure stuff out so I didn't go screw it up on other people."

LuAnn Moraski, DO
Internal Medicine and Pediatrics, Milwaukee

Doctor LuAnn Moraski, a residency director, states flatly that she once killed a patient. Not on purpose, of course, and she's making damn sure her residents don't make that same mistake.

It's the hottest day of the year in Milwaukee, with the temperature in the mid 90s, when I drop by her house for our conversation. Doctor Moraski, who is in her mid 30s, opens the front door dressed in shorts and a t-shirt, the only attire that makes sense on a day like this.

She has a perky, fun personality, in addition to an earnestness I've always admired. When Moraski isn't engaged with all of her medical responsibilities, she spends most of her free time with her young kids. She also enjoys kayaking and reading. "We only get three newspapers," she says sarcastically.

Doctor Moraski sinks into a comfortable chair in her family room and begins to tell me what it's like to go through the arduous educational process of learning to be a physician, as opposed to just graduating from medical school. Pain is involved, and it's not exclusive to the patients, especially during training.

Residency is where you learn what you were made of. We admitted a gentleman. His wife brought him in for a headache. It was a progressive headache, and it was a bit worrisome.

On the CT* there was this orange where one of the lobes of his brain should have been. Your gut sinks. This would be the medical emergency they talked about. He's having all these danger signs that go with increased intracranial pressure, so I call the neurosurgery resident.

He says, "I'm sorry, but I'm doing an emergency procedure at the other hospital. "If he needs a burr hole"—an actual hole in his head to relieve the pressure— "I need to know how chronic this is." I'm pretty hip with a needle, but I'm not drilling holes in people's heads without authorization.

The resident says, "Unless he has papilledema," which is a change in the retina that you see with intracranial pressure, meaning it had been going on for a while, "I'm not going to be able to come over right away."

Well, at the time, the only way to tell if there was a papilledema was with an instrument called an ophthalmoscope. At 11 o'clock at night, you're not going to find an ophthalmoscope. One of the guys who cleaned the rooms where the medical teams work, says, "LuAnn, you're a wreck. You need to go home."

"I am, but I don't understand. I'm just going to check this one more time." It was before all the computers. I was there with my nose buried in a book.

"LuAnn, go home. The book will be here in the morning."

You're trying not to cry. That whole girl thing kicks in. "I'm trying to figure it out because if I'm wrong, this guy's going to die and if I'm not wrong, he might die anyway. I don't know what to do."

"LuAnn, I've got keys. Let's go down to the ophthalmology offices."

He took me down and we got an ophthalmoscope, and he did have papilledema. The neurosurgery resident was over in 45 minutes, he was in the OR, and we saved his life. I didn't save that man's life. A janitor did.

---

* CT {computed tomography} a.k.a. CAT scan, uses different imaging angles around the body with help from a computer to show a cross-section of body tissues and organs.

When you're trying to think about who's going to help you? Who is part of your world? Everybody's part of your world.

How does stress affect you during training?

It's very hard, and you have to learn how to deal with it appropriately because it can be very consuming. I was a second year resident the first time I actually, knowingly, killed somebody. He was a wonderful gentleman who had end stage prostate cancer, who came in for a routine chemo appointment. He was working with a junior medical student who said, "Would you mind just reviewing this stuff with me?" His kidney numbers didn't look right and we did some interventions, but they didn't work because he was really sick. We knew he was sick, but it was one of those communications things where the fellow on call didn't think so.

Rather than calling the attending physician, the fellow said, "No, you're wrong. You're not looking at it the right way." He coded† the next morning and he died from hyperkalemia‡ {high potassium}—one of the first things you learn. It's page 37 in the *"Washington Manual."* It's something you learn every day, how to manage it and what to do about it. Yet, he still passed because we didn't do it.

When the attending read the notes, she's like, "You did everything right, except the most important thing. When somebody was telling you, 'You don't know what you're talking about,' you should have called me. What would have happened? You woke me up. What would I have done? Yell at you? Did anybody ever die from being yelled at?"

Medicine is hierarchical, so you have to be a little careful. But again, if you state your case, justify it and have the evidence, you're gonna usually do pretty well.

Why didn't you call the attending physician?

I don't know if it was self-confidence or following chain of command. Now, the students and residents going through are a lot more understanding of the rules. They're more afraid of the litigiousness. Interestingly enough, this family deliberately decided not to sue because they knew how hard we had tried. He had terminal cancer.

If you're worried about being sued, it has a lot to do with {poor} communication. But it weighs on you horribly. There is not a resident here who doesn't understand the treatment of hyperkalemia to this day because of that.

He needed emergent dialysis. Your heart requires a very narrow balance of potassium, and once that's out of control, you can't control a heart rhythm.

---

† Breathing, pulse or both stopped.

‡ Hyperkalemia refers to an abnormally large amount of potassium ions in the circulating blood.

It changed my view of medicine in terms of what is really selfless. What was I afraid of? If I would have picked up the phone, something different would have happened. I was afraid I was going to get in trouble, so it changed me in terms of what it means to be an advocate for your patient.

The selfless part of medicine isn't as much about time, anymore. You don't have to be the doc who works 24/7 and stays until all the patients are seen. It really means being an advocate for your patients, regardless of what it takes to do that.

That's one of the things that residency really does for you. When do I call? How do I get help? What do I do when I'm in a situation where I'm in over my head? If you can make hard decisions in the middle of the night, you're going to be able to make hard decisions in the middle of the day.

You develop a confidence and you develop ability. It's easy to get paralyzed by indecision—I'm not going to do anything or I'm going to call somebody else. Sometimes you can't call a specialist. If you call a specialist, it's going to cost the patient another thousand dollars. Do you really need a specialist or do you know it's a benign murmur?

I tell every single group of medical school students that in a couple of years, this is going to happen to them: You walk into the room and the person has already passed. Four o'clock in the morning is the last time the nurses checked, and now it's 6:30. Your first impulse is to absolutely run away, sneak out of the room. Close the door. I was never here. Not call for help. I'm not sure what occurred here. {Laughs} Those are the scary ones.

You're in a business where sometimes there are bad outcomes, despite the best efforts. How do you go about breaking the news of death to families?

Oh, I hate it. A lot of physicians see a patient's death as a personal failure. I missed something. I should have done something differently. It's like, no, they're 90. That's one of the things I've learned as a practitioner. My role as their physician can be just as important and just as powerful helping them die as it is helping them live. What matters to the patient? Is their life meaningful to them?

Helping people live their lives the way they want to also means helping them die the way they want to, and for some people it's very different. You struggle so much, but not with people who have terminal cancer.

But what about the people who don't have terminal cancer, but they still don't want to do anything? Maybe we could do this major surgery that you would have a good chance of coming through, and they say no.

You're like, "But we could make a difference." Not to that patient. You have to respect what patients want, and the same thing with families. If you have good communication going into it, if you have good relationships and good rapport, you mourn with 'em.

How often do you lose a patient?

It always happens in threes. When we have two, we're nervous. It's fits and spurts. Maybe it's one every month or couple months. It's always unpredictable, like the 24-year old who had the heart attack. The people with the terminal cancer, they surprise you just as well, because they're going to do things their way. You let me know.

There are things that we can do, but that doesn't mean we should do them. We can treat virtually any kind of pain that's out there. We can treat almost any symptom people have, if we identify them and create a safe environment for that to happen. We can put together resources, recognizing what resources a family has, what their insurance has, what Medicare has.

In many ways, palliative care is every bit as intense in an intensive care unit, but your focus is different. Your focus isn't on curing a disease process. It's on maintaining patient comfort, so it can be very different for every family. For some, it might be managing pain, for others, it might be managing fear. It might be doing everything.

My grandfather—he was in his mid-80s—had a horrific heart attack. It was one of those where you need five bypasses. My parents were all impressed because the head of heart surgery came down all the way from Loyola. Well, that's because nobody else will touch him. It doesn't necessarily mean good things, family. We were deciding what to do. He's in the intensive care unit and tubed, and on a ventilator.

"Don't do the surgery," I said. "This is crazy. If he pulls through it, what's he going to be like? He could stroke."

My mom said, "But he'd want to go down fighting." If he would have died, he would have much rather died on the table. He lived another seven years, moved twice, and really wasn't sick again until the last six months of his life.

There's no right answer to it. Oh, my gosh! If there's a rulebook, dude, tell me. I'm buying. You try to prognosticate. People go, how long? The weatherman's doing better than we are.

One of my absolutely dear patients, every time she comes to the office she brings a present for my son. She's cute as a button and she probably has an underlying malignancy. She's had life threatening bleeds. She doesn't want anything done. The output from her heart to the rest of her body, that opening, is 8 millimeters—about a half of an inch.

We sat down with the family 18 months or two years ago and said, "It could be any day." She keeps bringing in presents for my son. I don't know how she does it. She's happy as anything. She lives in an assisted living facility.

Other people, it's just amazing, their reserve. I had one woman with stage four lung cancer and she was told at her initial diagnosis, maybe three months. Spread everywhere. Nightmare. Two small kids. She said that's not acceptable. She was one of those patients who was referred to me and they said you're probably only going to see her once, but we need some help monitoring these symptoms. She was one of those patients who had the most phenomenal response through her chemotherapy and radiation and was almost tumor-free for 18 months. She had every side effect from her treatment, so she also had other health problems to deal with.

But for 18 months, she went to Vegas, she went camping, she did all the stuff with her family. Then, she gave herself as long as she could and what they said was going to happen 18 months ago, kicked in and she died in three weeks. The mind's control over health is very powerful.

Whenever they're not supposed to happen, those are the hardest. I was, oh gosh, 33-weeks pregnant with my son when we lost an infant in the practice. None of us is perfect parents. I could write a whole book about all the things I've done wrong with my own kids, but these were the perfect parents! There wasn't a book they hadn't read. They were as careful and deliberate as parents could be. The baby was strong as anything and she was able to pull herself up in her Pack 'n Play. Mom went to change some laundry and she was able to pull a bag on her head. But, three minutes... Ones like that—they're never right.

You have to be honest with people. You tell people what happened, to the best of your ability. The other thing is not to try to tell them that you understand, because I don't. That's a club—knock on wood—I hope I never belong to. You have to do what you have to do to get the family through the best way that they can. Not necessarily that it's an emotional way, but keeping focused on the fact that it's not about your grief or how you feel about what happened, or how ticked off you are that doctors at St. Elsewhere didn't know what you knew, or how so and so's uncle could be so stupid and not watch him by the pool. Put that all away and focus on what these people need.

Let's talk about what you needed, professionally speaking. When do you first start thinking about medicine as a career?

My parents bought that entire *"Worldbook Encyclopedia"* when I was five or six years old. I was always interested in the body and how things worked.

A lot of what I do, both as a physician, and in my job as a residency director, is education, because it's actually teaching people and helping them to make change in ways that benefit them. My mother was my seventh grade English teacher, and she had this huge impact on people. My dad was a mechanical engineer, so he was very analytical.

I grew up in a small town outside of Chicago called Channahon. There were four of us. One of my dad's cousins was a pediatrician when I was growing up. And my grandmother was a nurse.

My first major at the University of Illinois was pre-med. I had several other iterations after that. But it was always on the list of things to do. I always liked science. I always like the communication aspect of it. I sort of went to college with pre-med as my token major—found out what an interesting world the rest of the universe is. Funny, after going through all that and all those processes, I came back to medicine. But it was at the end, when I really realized this is what I have to do.

How hard was it to get into medical school?

I didn't get in my first time, which was actually, one of the greatest things that ever happened to me. Discouraged? Sure. There are a lot of nights of bawling your eyes out. There, there. They said no, but what are you gonna do? It really clarifies the issue for you. It really forced me to dial down about what you're doing, why you're doing it, and how bad you want something.

And it also made me revisit what I wanted out of medical school, where I wanted to go, what I wanted to do, what I was going to spend four years doing that was going to allow me to have this career for a lifetime. It really changed the direction of where I was going to go to school and how I was going to learn.

I took a year off and actually, worked in a business office of a hospital organization. That was fantastic. Then, I really learned about the business of medicine and I learned about how that organization was losing money on every pap smear they did. How do we keep the doors open? It was one of the biggest years of my life.

Physicians are high achieving individuals. I coasted through undergrad. If I tried hard, I did exceptionally well. If I didn't try hard, I did pretty darn well.

I knew medical school would be hard, but I thought it would be hard like tough courses in undergrad, just a lot of them. You finished this one, great. Here's the next one, and then the next one. It was a grind. Average has an entirely different meaning.

But I did it with such wonderful people in an organization, in a school where they basically had made some decisions about how people are going to get through. It was a pass/fail system, and at the same time, we fought for every point. You pass every course or you didn't move on, which was a real hoot with our nutrition instructor when people weren't attending his class. He gave us a final that 74% of the class failed. I've never been happier with a 71% in my life. Sixty-nine percent equaled F. *I will not be remediating. Thank you, Jesus.*

The first two years, the bookwork part, were challenging and hard, but at the same time, fun. There was not a single thing in medical school that was new—not the memorization. I had taken harder tests before. I had done harder material before. Medical school doesn't kill you in a couple weeks. It's a grind and it doesn't stop. And you get behind and the wheels keep turning, so you have to keep up. There's no getting off the wagon. There's no easy semester. There's no, *I'll just take 10 hours this time and make sure I do well in this course.* There's the curriculum. You do it or you don't do it.

Medical school was a ball in that second fascinating way, where it can be one of the hardest things you ever did and one of the most wonderful things you've ever done. I had the privilege of going to a school in Des Moines, Iowa, which was fantastic for my grades because there wasn't a lot else to do in Des Moines. I went to school with some of the most down to earth, high-powered, intelligent, rock star, wow—I would work for you anywhere in the universe—individuals.

Basically, there are two ways to get through medical school in the United States. There's osteopathic, or DO, or allopathic, which is MD. They used to be again, philosophically, very diverse. Allopathic medicine was about the treatment of diseases. Osteopathic medicine was more holistic, if you will. The body heals itself. How do you put your body in an environment that heals itself? I was in an osteopathic medical school right at the time when the two worlds really came together.

While I was doing an out rotation, I was laughed out of rounds one day. We were talking about a patient who had an ulcer, and were talking about this new drug on the market called Zantac that was saving lives, and ulcer therapy. "We haven't found out why he got his ulcer, so until we do that…" This was a person who almost died from a GI bleed. I'm like, "We have to figure out why he got the ulcer in the first place. Until we fix that, he's not going to get better." It was the funniest thing they had ever heard.

Now, to say that, wow, stress management and the appropriate environment and adequate rest and all of those things that are quote, unquote, holistic, are, in fact, completely hip and cool and part of absolutely every part of mainstream medicine.

Especially when I went to school, which was in the early 90s, there clearly was a difference. It wasn't just about the diseases. It wasn't just about the pathology. It was about how that manifested in a real person. In many ways, it's very analogous to the outcome-driven things that we talk about now. It doesn't matter. What change did you make? The cholesterol is lower, but did they have a heart attack or didn't they?

Let the body heal itself. Do everything you can to allow that to happen. But when you consider diseases and their impact on health, you have to consider the whole person. That was the core of my osteopathic training that served me very well, especially in primary care.

The first two years of medical school, they were hard. But there was no question of finishing.

Even when you had to dissect a cadaver?

The first time you look at a human being from the inside out, it's strange and magical, and disgusting and wonderful. You walk in the room and it's, *Oh my goodness. This smells terrible.* You get home at night and you're cooking dinner and you smell your hands, even though you washed twice. *Oh, maybe we're not going to have chicken tonight. Maybe a little vegetarian stir fry would be okay.*

The respect you have—that's the part that I just didn't anticipate. Of the people in the world who did anything to help me through school—whether it was financially, personally, supportive of anything, on the top of that list—would be that person who actually gave me their physical being to go figure stuff out, so I didn't go screw it up on other people. Somebody made that sacrifice, and they didn't know who I was. There was almost a reverence to it. Then, you just got in and got messy and you learned stuff. It's like looking at the most phenomenally engineered thing in the universe and just how breathtakingly efficient, and how you can do bad things to it.

You're trying to dissect a heart, but you have to take off three quarters of an inch of fat layered around it. You're trying to look for things in the abdominal cavity and you have to take stuff out. You open up an artery and it actually feels like a pump hose because it's so stiff with atherosclerosis. It was a very strange and wonderful, and still, pretty darn creepy.

A picture is not worth a thousand words. Get your hands dirty. Have the book. Have the person. There really is nothing else like it because you can look at pictures, but when you finally see it, and it was reaffirmed the first time I ever watched a surgery, let alone participate in one. You're seeing something that God never intended us to see. This ain't natural, yet at the same time, strange and beautiful, and perfect, and very smelly.

But then, when there are real people sitting across from you and you are examining them, and you're actually laying hands on them. That was much more what medicine was. All of a sudden, it wasn't an intellectual science. You're interacting with a person. The clinical years are when that happens.

We had to do these canned histories and physicals before they would let us work on real patients. They would set up at the local hospital these patients who had volunteered and we would go do histories and physicals. These poor people were saints, because you know as a first and second year medical student, you could have them locked up for four or five hours. And you're asking them questions off your card, and they're like, "Come on. No, I really don't have any of those kind of headaches, either. No, my vision hasn't changed that way."

It's not a book, or it's not about former questions on test reviews. It's about a real person, and you're tired. We did this before the 80/30[§] rules that are in effect now. For students, it was not uncommon to work a lot of hours. When you're dealing with real people and real diseases and you're watching people die for the first time, you're making mistakes for the first time, those are the days when you come home and say, "I'm done."

§ Residents may not work more than 80 hours per week and no more than 30 hours in a shift.

You grow, because you're learning the ability to work with people from all walks of life. In order to do what you need to do when you're in the room for them, you've got to learn. You've gotta experience stuff and you've gotta be open minded because you just can't make any assumptions.

Now, I see the full spectrum of ages, the newest of the newborns to the oldest of the elderly. But I also see people who are rich and who are poor, and who are from all different cultures. It's so fun. If I had to deal with people just like me all day, I would not be here. I'd be in a loony bin.

If part of my job is to go in and communicate with them and help make them better in a way that matters to them. I also have to learn a lot about where they are and where they're from.

We have to be very careful not to think people can only handle information filtered through us. That's very wrong. My patients continue to impress me. I'm talking about patients who may not even have a high school education. They may not speak well or have more than a 100-word vocabulary, but they continue to impress me that they understand the medical information that is necessary to make good decisions in their lives. The Internet's the best thing that's happened to all of us in many, many ways.

Patients have a much better ability to understand and synthesize data. How we help patients process information is very important. It's really making people understand what is truly safe, and in your child's best interest. Parents want to do everything right for their kids. But as much as they want to do everything right, they don't want to do anything wrong. Nobody wants to take risks.

I saw my last case of chicken pox, two, three years ago. It was part and parcel of what we did. But how scared are you of German Measles? Do you even know what they are? What's diphtheria look like in your world?

Now, people at least understand pertussis because we've had outbreaks. You've got this lack of information about how bad these diseases are. You can't think about kids like, "I'll let everybody else get immunized and I won't do mine."

Varicella¶ is probably the most controversial of the vaccines because most people don't die of varicella. Why did I give my kid varicella? Because when I was at Children's Hospital, I saw five children in four years who didn't leave the hospital because of chicken pox. They left the hospital in a ventilator—never to be normal kids again. It's only one city, one town, but five kids in four years. That's one hundred percent preventable by giving the shot.

Your practice becomes what you're good at and what people want to see you for. But there are some guys who actually prefer a female physician and there's other guys who are like, "I'm going to see you, but I'll see

¶ Chicken pox

a urologist if I have to because my pants are coming off." Dude, all good. {Laughs} It's not breakin' my heart. Oh, they're funny.

My practice is probably 75% women. That's partially because women are comfortable with me. There are gender issues. There are age issues—you have to interact with somebody. If you can't walk in the door and tell me what you need to tell me, then you shouldn't be seeing me. It doesn't matter whether your best friend thinks I'm a great doc. If you can't talk to me, you need to see somebody else because I'm not going to be a great doc for you.

A lot of times, that really doesn't break down as much over gender lines, as over professional lines or personal lines. "I can't talk to you because it's too much like talking to my wife."

I try really hard not to get insulted because people either think I'm 10 years younger or 10 years older than I am. "Uh, I am not 50, thank you. I know you meant it in a great way, but I don't want to look great for 50 when I'm 38."

People will treat you with the respect you deserve, and it breaks down not necessarily on gender or even age lines. People will come in and say I want x, y, and z. Sometimes, my job is not to order x, y, and z. It's to say, you need P, D, Q, and a treadmill.

People will tell you when you do things wrong. You will do things wrong, and you'll say things wrong. And, in many ways, medical school's just a foreign language course. Take simple concepts, put them in Latin and make them so nobody understands you unless they're doctors. But you're talking to real people. You're trying to extract information from them.

That old adage that 90% of the time the patient will walk in, tell you what's wrong and tell you what to do about it, is completely true. If you're pretty darn good at listening and asking the right questions, you're a pretty darn good physician. But learning how to do that and—at the same time trying to keep your intellectual curiosity under wraps, you'll walk in, you'll examine a child. *Wow. Cool murmur.* {Laughs} No. Not so much sharing. {Parents} hear murmur and think the child has a hole in heart. Think before you talk.

It's being willing to accept the fact that you do things wrong. I've been in the room with people and say, "This isn't going well. What's wrong? What am I doing? What can we do differently? And 99 times out of a 100, they'll say so.

You have no idea. "I know what you're saying, but you need to understand that I'm not going to do that right now." And you can move on to a plane where you can be more productive.

You're in a room and a three-year old is absolutely tearing the place up and the parents are there because they're very worried that he has a learning disability. They want medical testing done because he's obviously hyperthyroid, this and that. He doesn't sleep at night because he has obstructive sleep apnea and he needs to have his tonsils out immediately.

And it's like, no. "You've got to stop getting up with him. He's smarter than you are and he's running the show right now. If I could get up every night, two or three times and have somebody who I love, who smells really good, pop a snickers bar in my mouth, I'd do it, too. That's a good gig if you're three. You have to put him to bed. It's not his problem. It's your problem." But it's a serious problem if you haven't had a good night's sleep in three months, and any kind of behavior change is hard.

I bet you relate well to kids.

I have an innate ability in that I never learned to talk like an adult. I'm sort of trapped, somewhere between 12 and 13, which makes me sound really ridiculous when I use bad slang. But kids will tell you what's wrong with them if you put them in an environment where they're safe to tell you. They don't always have words.

One of the things you learn in pediatric residency is that you walk in the door and you know whether that baby is sick or not sick. It's the look. The way they breathe. Are they eating? Can they be comforted? It's just a different language. Ask the parents of a two-month old whether that baby has a language. At two months old, those parents know what every cry means. I'm hungry. I'm wet. I'm bored. And how is that possible? Well, they only have one word. It's crying.

It's no different whether they're ten. The older the child gets, the more they have the ability to use spoken language to tell you what's wrong.

You get clues. If there's a fever, a lot of what we do is pattern recognition. If someone has belly pain, what are the three things that usually cause belly pain? What are those three things you have to make sure it isn't, because disaster could strike. That's the art of pediatrics. That's where pediatrics and medicine are a little bit different because not only do you have to be the same diagnostician, but be able to do it quickly and do it when the patient can't tell you what's wrong.

But you usually have to do it on a very short time frame. Will they let you push on their belly? Based on what you see when you walk in the room, based on what the parents tell you, you're forming lists of what's going on, what could it be, what do I have to make sure it isn't? To examine a child usually confirms one list and rules out the other. And then you use diagnostic testing to confirm or deny what your top one or two things are from each list.

People aren't going to come in and say, "I'm relatively certain my appendix is bursting." But they're going to come in and they're not going to want to move and they're not going to want you to touch them. They haven't eaten and barf all over you. You figure it out.

In medical school, I actually worked in a family medicine clinic. I worked with some of the most amazing physicians I've ever worked with at a clinic in rural Iowa. They did everything. Even though they were in family medicine, they were the foundation for me going into internal medicine and pediatrics.

Medicine is so much fun because when something goes wrong, it's usually because one thing out of these 12 complex variables—one thing tipped. You pick the right thing, tweak it back just a few percentage points, they go back to feeling great. But again, understanding that complex environment—lots of balls in the air. Lots of intellectual juggling, if you will, is internal medicine. It is just phenomenally fun and challenging, plus you get to deal with real people talking back to you.

Then, there's pediatrics, which is almost the opposite. They're completely fine until they're not fine. And when they're not fine, you've got a very short window of time to figure out why or they're going to be not fine, forever.

With adults, you've got time to sort of ponder this and consider that and make changes. In both arenas, you have to be an expert diagnostician, but be able to deal with the emergent, be able to deal with the chronic, and then how those two things interweave. I love pediatrics. I loved families. I knew people who said, "I hate dealing with adolescents." They're so fun. No, they're not obnoxious. You were a kid, too.

Being a pediatrician, they said, "You have to deal with all those parents." The parents are just like us. I knew my crew was going to include pediatrics and yet I loved medicine. I couldn't separate away from it and I didn't like the idea that I would have to hand my patients over to somebody else when they crossed some magic threshold.

At the same time, I loved delivering babies. But I'm a terrible surgeon—not cut out for that at all. That sort of took the whole OB realm out of it and I was left with, how do I do this? How do I take care of families? I can't do everything that a family practice doc can do. I can't be sure I'd be good enough at it.

I look back at things I did as an intern and if you asked me today, could I do that? I'd tell you no. I could not do that. It's another one of those moments when you know you're in trouble. You worked hard. It was crazy. I distinctly recall procedures that I did working with people all night, multiple codes. Doing stuff like that, if you asked me now, I'd say, I couldn't do it. And I know I did. I was there. I can't imagine a time of such growth. You're in the thick of it. You do what you're supposed to do.

You take all these things that you learned and you apply them, and you dial them down on one person and they get better. There's no rush like that. There's no bank balance or stock ticker that comes up to somebody saying, I feel pretty good because of the order you wrote, because the thing you found. I mean, that's slick.

I remember after graduation, I had started my new job. It had been five or six weeks and I rolled over. It was one of those brilliant moments you have at 2:30 in the morning that you make your spouse participate in.

"Kevin." {whispers}

"What?"

"I get two days off every single week."

He's like, "Uh, huh. They're called weekends."

"No. You don't understand. Two days of every week I don't have to work."

"Go to bed."

I don't begrudge any of the time I did. Was it hard on my family? Yeah, it was hard on my family. But I'm fortunate enough to be surrounded by people who supported me, and who sacrificed with me, and understood and allowed me to become what I could be. It was as much their gift, as my ability.

Were you with Kevin during medical school?

You betcha.

That had to be hard on your relationship.

Oh yeah. It was great! {Sarcastically} I started medical school and then he started business school when I was in my third year of medical school. Of course, they weren't in the same towns. Then, we got married in my third year of medical school, so that was our life for a while.

The first two years that I was a resident, he actually worked in Chicago, and went to school in Chicago two nights a week while we lived in Milwaukee. We were pretty hard on cars. We had to be pretty independent. But at the same time, we were both busy together and we both knew what we were doing. It was worth it. We freaked out the neighbors a little bit. We didn't shovel our walk very regularly. We would roll in at all hours of the day and night.

As you look at your career now, is it as you imagined it?

Lord no. Nothing like I imagined. I was going to take care of families. That was my gig. I was all impressed with myself. I figured out I was going to medical school. I figured out what I was going to do after medical school and then met with my program director for the first time when I started in Milwaukee. He said, "What are you going to be when you grow up?"

I said, "I'm going to be a doctor. I'm going to take care of families."

He said, "What else?"

"Uh, excuse me. I'm done. This is my 10-year plan."

"Na, na, na. You're going to do other things. All of a sudden he's talking about teaching and education and leadership. I'm like, okay. Ride the wave.

It's really schizophrenic, but really fun. I do about 50% practice time, which means I do 4-5 half days per week of time in clinic. My sessions in clinic—anybody can walk in the door. They can be any age, for any reason. There's always a theme. I'm working with the residents, because they're like, "Okay, we've had eight people today that have had headache {laughs}. One was a four year old. One was an 80-year old. Lots of different differentials, but everybody had a headache today."

Clinically, I also do a month in the hospital, working with people who are admitted to the hospital who as a rule, are not my own patients, but patients of my practice partners. That's a lot of teaching, as well as direct patient care.

Then, I also run a residency program, which takes a large chunk of my time. We have 24 spots training other med-peds residents in the same program that I was trained. That's very slick, very fun. And the residents are amazing. As much as the patients jazz me about what I do, the residents do just as much.

It's amazing to see. Residency is that period of growth—watching other people go through it and being able to help shape it and help them avoid some of the pitfalls and get successes that you never even attained.

One of my colleagues says the way that you tell a good resident is you make sure they worked in food service, because if you've ever been a waiter or waitress, you understand customer service, communication, and working with unhappy people. Good wait staff make great doctors. It's his theory. It's not a bad one.

But when future residents come in the room—and I usually only have about a 30 minute interview to figure out what I think. Will I want to work with them, be on call with them, have their kids play with my kids, go out for a beer with them? Then, I know I've got somebody who's going to really work in our program and really be something because they're all that.

Feast or famine. In busy times, it can be a lot. A hundred hour week is not unheard of. But there are also a lot of 40 and 50 hour weeks. Average probably—I'd like to say 60, but probably closer to 70. When I have a grant due—and I also do some research on the side—I try to stay really involved with fantastic organizations like the Wisconsin Medical Society and the American Academy of Pediatrics, which also take time away.

I have amazing kids. They'll tell me straight up when I haven't been around enough. That and I'm married to a wonderful man who's very supportive. I say, "This is what I need to do," it's not questioned. It's not discussed. It's how do we make that happen?

With extraordinarily flexible scheduling, we've both decided that we made a commitment that we don't let our jobs interfere with what we need to do as a family. So if there's more work I have to do, it happens when they're in bed. If I've got a grant I have to write, I'm not staying late at the office to do it.

One of us is always here till 7:30 in the morning. Somebody else is always home by 5:30, six o'clock every night. But that doesn't mean we're both here. We make sure that we cover each other. You know when it's match time or it's interview season. You may not be able to do anything about it—but you know it's coming.

It's really hard because I've got friends who stay at home with their kids. I have great friends who work, but work fewer hours. There are a lot of days when I certainly would like to work less, be a little bit more balanced.

It's going to be harder when the kids get a little older. At the same time, the kids know if I had to spend all day with them, they would kill me. It's respecting what you're not wired for. At about four days, they're like, "Don't you have somewhere you have to go, mommy? Do you have to spend your vacation home with us? Don't you have friends?" {laughs} I'm very blessed with some intuitive kids. It's like flipping a switch. When I'm not here enough, they're acting up. They're sassing back.

So what's your plan for the future, professionally?

I'm still surfing the same wave I picked up on 10 years ago and I have no idea where the beach is. I'm having fun. But it's really hard sometimes. I get really tired. And at other times, the view is really impeccable. The one thing I'm certain of is I probably won't be doing what I'm doing now in 10 years. What I'll be doing, I have no idea.

There's a ton of interesting things. When you look at health, what can you do on a population level? If I'm great in the office and I see 12 patients, I did a perfect job and everybody bought all the crap I sold 'em. And they're on their treadmills the next day. They stop smoking and everything else, and they're not spanking their kids. The babies are all sleeping on their backs. Wonderful. But I still only impacted 12 people, maybe their families.

I go to Grace's {her daughter} school and talk to all the first graders about safety. Now, I've impacted 150 families. You change laws. You get people to fund different things. You make people understand the priorities—that if more kids have access to dental care, they'll actually be healthier, overall. Those are big, powerful things.

Just in terms of the business. Health care is eating up a huge chunk of money. I'd really like to see how we could deliver health care more efficiently. I'm a bit of a process wonk. Get things down so they're well-oiled machines. It's not what I imagined. It's been a lot harder than I imagined. But I have rewards coming out of my eyeballs.

Is being called "doctor" one of those rewards?

I wouldn't know. Nobody calls me doctor. My patients don't call me doctor. People I work with don't call me doctor.

What do your patients call you?

LuAnn.

And you're okay with that?

Absolutely. What am I going to call them? The vast majority of people just call me LuAnn. And Dr. Moraski—yeah, it is an honored thing. It's certainly a title of respect that goes toward something being earned, but at the same time, it needs to be all the good and not the bad. It can't be about the power struggles. We work together or nobody works.

Why is it when I write an instruction, it's called an "order?" We're the only profession that gives orders that have to be followed without question. What the heck is that? Yeah, I'm probably least described as Dr. Moraski.

Chapter Five

Blood, Sweat and Fears

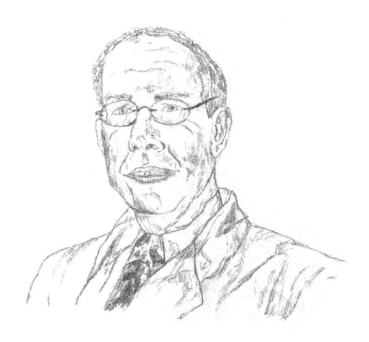

"I gave blood once in my life. Now, I do operations that let quite a bit of blood. It doesn't bother me one bit. But if somebody puts a needle in my arm—that's an interesting phenomenon."

Layton "Bing" Rikkers, MD
Surgeon, pancreas and liver, Madison

Layton Rikkers has always been uncomfortable with being on the sharp end of a needle. It's so uncomfortable, he can't give blood for fear of passing out. Yet Rikkers not only is a physician, he's a surgeon, and not just any surgeon. In his early 60s, he's the chairman of the Department of Surgery at University of Wisconsin Hospital. On top of that, Rikkers is editor of a prestigious and influential surgical journal.

How did he rise to this level in the profession, given his fears? If passing out was a likely possibility every time a needle pricked your skin, would surgery be a career choice?

For all his accomplishments, I had never heard of Layton Rikkers be-

fore. A physician friend was not just effusive in his praise for Dr. Rikkers, but described him as a surgical giant on an international scale. "Amazingly, people in Madison don't even know who he is!"

Okay, I was hooked. Of all the doctors I interviewed, most in their homes, but some in their cramped, sterile offices, Rikkers had by far the best, largest and snazziest office I had seen–complete with rich, luxurious woodwork, leather couches and a receptionist!

Although I had never met him or even talked to him on the phone before this day, Dr. Rikkers struck me as rather down to Earth. With a nickname like "Bing," maybe that shouldn't have been such a surprise. He says nobody has called him Layton since his older brother coined the nickname after repeatedly failing to pronounce his real name.

One of "Bing" Rikkers' real interests outside of medicine is photography. Before we started the interview, he shared some beautiful digital images he captured while on safari, including a giraffe's head peaking out of a tree. He not only must have good hands, as surgeons would say, but a good eye, too.

During our conversation, one of the first things he revealed was his fear of needles and blood. Only a doctor comfortable in his own skin could nonchalantly discuss this with somebody he just met, especially when that somebody was holding a microphone.

I always had a tremendous fear of blood. Even as an undergraduate student, when I saw blood I would get very light headed. It really concerned me about going into medicine at all.

In fact, I courageously went down once to give blood, and my girlfriend went with me to bolster my confidence. I really thought I pulled this off, but when I came down to finally give blood, the nurse told me that I was ashen and white and had a low blood pressure and therefore, couldn't give blood. Eventually, I did accomplish giving blood. I gave blood once in my life. Now, I do operations that let quite a bit of blood. It doesn't bother me one bit. But if somebody puts a needle in my arm—that's an interesting phenomenon.

Given this fear, why in the world did you select surgery as a specialty?

At Stanford, we all had to buy our own microscope, so I was looking for a good used microscope. Someone said, "Gee, there's this guy that's working in Dr. Norman Shumway's laboratory." He's the great heart transplanter, and one of the medical students in his research laboratory had a microscope. I peeked in, and here are all these people in greens operating on a dog, doing a heart transplant.

I said, "Hey, I heard you have a microscope for sale."

He said, "Yeah, I do."

I said, "What are you all doing?"

He said, "Well, put on some greens and come on in and look."

The following morning, I was working for Dr. Norm Shumway and getting up at 5:30 every morning as a first year medical student and doing dog surgery—valves and heart transplants, and so forth. I did that all the way through medical school and that just got me going on the surgical edge of things. The first morning I worked in Shumway's laboratory, I almost fainted, but that was the last time that that's ever happened to me.

What did you do to overcome it?

I don't know. I guess it's just adaptation. Even now, when I go to have my annual or bi-annual check and I need to have my cholesterol checked, I lie down when I have my blood drawn to make sure that I don't faint.

The serendipity of dropping by that office led to your becoming a surgeon?

It's unbelievable. What stands out in my mind are the first procedures that I did on animals. The first operation I personally did myself was a mitral valve replacement in a dog, followed by a heart transplant in a dog. Both of them survived, but I had a lot of help.

How long did you work with Shumway before you realized, "Surgery is for me?"

During those first three years, I worked half-time and actually did a lot of dog surgery myself. Then it turned out, I was doing reasonably well in what was then a five-year medical school and they said, "Gee, if you have enough credits, we'll let you go a year early." I was nervous about that because it gave me just one clinical year in medical school.

My mentors then were the chairman of the department of surgery, Dr. Bob Chase, and Dr. Shumway. I discussed it with them and they said, "Save the year now and take off. You can use it later." I still wasn't positive about surgery as a career. I enjoyed caring for the whole patient. I thought maybe internal medicine was where I ought to be.

What I eventually learned was, as a surgeon, you could be as much of an internist, as far as taking care of the whole patient, as you wanted to be, but the reverse didn't work. I ended up doing a mixed medicine-surgery internship at the University of Utah, reflecting some of my indecision.

We were very busy one night and I was working with my chief resident. I went off to the operating room, where I did my first really big operation, a splenectomy in a trauma patient, and at that moment I knew I would become a surgeon.

What led you to medical school in the first place?

I wasn't sure I was interested in medicine. I really enjoyed science, as I took my courses at the University of Wisconsin. I was a zoology major, yet really enjoyed my interactions with people, and thought that by putting those together, medicine would be a good career.

My brother was a stimulus for me as well, in that he was very interested in medicine. He ended up not going into it. But he had a lot to do with starting a premed club that I got involved in. I went to the meetings and that stimulated my interest in medicine.

The only other medical doctors in our family were one uncle, and my grandfather, whom I never met. He died before I was born. I grew up in Waupun, Wisconsin. I have a brother and two half sisters who have passed away. My father was a small town lawyer, and when I was about a junior in high school, he took a job in Fond du Lac, as the head of a savings and loan. I remained in Waupun to finish high school and then came to the University of Wisconsin as an undergraduate. One summer, I worked as an orderly at the old University Hospital, and that further stimulated my interest in medicine.

I met my wife as an undergraduate. We graduated from the University of Wisconsin in the summer of 1966, and decided we wanted to be really independent, so the medical school I chose was Stanford University. We honeymooned on the way out to California.

My wife worked all the way through medical school. We had our first child when I was a senior in medical school. She was absolutely supportive through this whole thing. When I was in surgical residency, we had another child. My wife was the iron person taking care of the family, because I was gone so much.

My plan had been to return to Stanford and be a cardiothoracic surgeon. My second year at Utah, a new surgery chair came to the University of Utah and became my next mentor. He was just a very stimulating guy and he got me very interested in the physiology and surgery of the liver.

I decided to go off into the research laboratory and spend a year with him, where I got involved in animal surgery again, but continued in a direction toward an academic career.

We also had an interesting visiting professor, from London, England, that year, a person who founded the specialty of hepatology in medicine. I became convinced, as my wife did, that it would be great to do a second year of research, but do it in London.

So we packed up our one and three-year olds, and hopped on a plane and went to London for a year. It was a real eye-opening experience for both of us as we had always lived in relatively small towns. Now, all of a sudden, we were in London. I was having a very good medical experience, but it was also a great cultural experience, as well as a growing up experience for both of us. That year's experience got me firmly involved in the area of liver surgery, which I've pursued throughout most of my professional career. My life gets split up among a number of things. I have my own surgical practice, which tends to be complex liver, bile duct, and pancreatic problems.

I'm also chairman of the Department of Surgery, which has a faculty of about 90. We cover six divisions of surgery—not all of the sub-specialties of surgery are within the department, but most of them are. There's a large administrative workload in running the department, but I've got a lot of people who help me with that. I'm always working with my patients, medical students, and with surgical residents, so I'm involved with teaching as I care for my patients. Then, finally, I'm very involved with a journal that takes a fair amount of my time as well, plus my own academic pursuits.

How did you develop that managerial side?
I don't really know. My first job out of residency, after I completed some fellowships, was to join my mentor, Dr. Moody, and I spent seven years on the University of Utah faculty with him. The last year, he went to another institution to be Chairman of Surgery, and I then served as acting chief of the general surgeons.

At the same time, the University of Nebraska was looking for a chairman. I went and looked at that job and had no idea that that was what my career would be oriented towards. Again, I talked to my mentors.

Nebraska wanted somebody to come in and start a liver transplant program and grow their department of surgery. My mentors both thought, as I did, that it was a good opportunity for me. So we packed up, decided to become Cornhuskers and went off to Omaha. That was in 1984.

The most satisfying part of surgical administration is mentoring people, be they the young faculty, residents, or students. I'd had some wonderful mentors who helped get me to the point in my career that I was at, and it gave me an opportunity to pay back and develop young people.

Over the past 23 years, I've had the wonderful opportunity to serve as chair of surgery for Nebraska for 12 years, and now for the past 11 years at Wisconsin. I've had the opportunity to mentor many young people.

I've recruited a large number of faculty, most of them quite young and enthusiastic. It's also a special thrill to see a neophyte surgical resident come in at the first year level and finish five years later as a complete general surgeon. Mentoring students, residents, and young faculty as well as taking care of patients has provided me with a very satisfying career.

Why the decision to come back to Wisconsin?
You can stimulate a place for just so long. If I had decided to stay at Nebraska and finish my whole career there, I would have been the chair of surgery there for 25 years. But I think it's better for people to have an exposure to a place for ten or twelve years. Then, they should reinvent themselves and allow the unit they developed an opportunity for new stimulation.

When Wisconsin was looking for a chair, it was very difficult to leave Nebraska. We loved our department. Our family was there. Both kids were out of the house, but they were living in Omaha.

The first time I was asked to look at Wisconsin, I declined to visit, but they came back at us about six months later and we decided to take a peek. Actually, they recruited me here by some very tricky means, knowing what my weaknesses were. I'm a big sports fan, and a life-long lover of the Packers. My first interview at Wisconsin was in the summer. One of the reasons I arranged it for that time was that the Packers were playing a pre-season game in Madison.

I was going through my interviews and the head of sports medicine sauntered by and said, "Bing, would you like to go to the game on Saturday night?"

"Thanks a lot, Ben. But I already have tickets."

"Well, would you like to be on the sideline with me and interact with the Packers and be in the locker room?"

"Well, that doesn't sound too bad!"

I watched the game standing next to Reggie White and actually talked with Bret Favre in the locker room. It was unbelievable. That enticed me to come back for a second visit.

On the second visit, while we were still making up our minds, they said they had a secret interview for me. They drove me to the stadium where I had an interview with Barry Alvarez, the head football coach. At the end of the interview, I said, "Coach, you've got more important things to do than talk to a surgeon."

He said, "Wait just a minute." He went to the back of his office and got a Badger jersey, number 11, with Rikkers on the back.

"Bing," he says. "We've retired your number. We want you to come to Wisconsin."

That was it. That did it for me. I said, "Okay." Of course, I had to discuss it with my wife. We'd been away from Madison for 30 years, but we had fond memories from our undergraduate days when we met.

What really attracted me was a department of surgery that was on the verge of greatness. My predecessor, Fred Belzer, did a marvelous job of developing this department and left some very good resources. It was in a position to develop into one of the elite academic surgery centers in the country, and that's what I've been trying to work on with my very good colleagues over the past 10 years.

How do you get there? Is it the recruitment of people who can get you there?

Some things were the best in the world when I got here, namely the transplant activity. Doctor Belzer was a transplant surgeon himself and had fully developed a marvelous vision of transplantation surgery that I used as a model for the other divisions to develop, hopefully to similar levels of excellence. We're still working on that, but a lot of those divisions are well on their way.

It's about recruiting the best people you can from around the country. You need to develop all three missions of a department: superior tertiary care while doing innovative surgery, the very best educational programs for students and residents, and finally, the whole new knowledge game—good research laboratories.

We are now almost in the top 10 departments of surgery in the country in the amount of research funding. We have as many good surgical residencies and training programs as can be found anywhere in the country. It's not because of me, because much of it existed before I arrived.

You need great surgeons to be a great department. But what does it take to be a great surgeon?

You need to be a little obsessive-compulsive, pay a lot of attention to detail, and have genuine concern and empathy for others. Hopefully, that's the reason one takes care of patients.

As you look back over your career, how much has surgery advanced?

There have been major advances in surgery. When I came into surgery, the big growth area was cardiac surgery and I got involved in the heart transplant program while a student at Stanford.

Over the past 15 or 20 years, it's been minimally invasive surgery and robotic surgery. We just bought a robot for our Department of Surgery, and we are frequently utilizing it. The complete spectrum of robotic surgery is yet to be defined; however, there are certain areas where the robot already has proved its usefulness. One major area is in resections for prostate cancer. The robot is a device where the arms of the robot are placed through tiny incisions in a patient's abdomen or chest, and the surgeon sits at the controls of the robot and manipulates instruments with very fine movements with no tremor, and does it in three dimensions. The robot is expensive and the tools that the robot uses are expensive, so one needs to develop those areas that can be done better by a robot than by laparoscopic or open surgery.

General surgery has been stimulated by the development of minimally invasive surgery. We are doing big operations through tiny incisions. The advantage to the patient is usually less pain, a quicker recovery, more rapid time back to work and a shorter hospitalization. Almost all of the gallbladders we take out are done by laparoscopic means and 95 plus percent of these are done as outpatient operations.

The other operations we do by minimally invasive techniques include anti-reflux surgery on the esophagus, thoracic surgery, endocrine surgery, and colorectal surgery. Using minimally invasive techniques allows patients to go home the day of the operation, or a day or two later.

I learned minimally invasive surgery late in my career. Now, I see our residents rapidly learning minimally invasive surgery, as they've sat many years in front of the TV, and playing with their Ataris. They take to it very naturally.

With all this, how did you find time to get involved with the "Annals of Surgery"?

Like any academician, I've been involved in writing a good part of my career. As one moves along through an academic career, you are asked to review papers for journals. If you do that reasonably well, you're invited to serve on editorial boards. I was on the editorial board of several surgical journals, and the editor-in-chief of the *"Annals of Surgery,"* who was chairman of surgery for years at Duke University, was giving up his editorship. For some reason, I was invited to interview to replace him.

It was just after I had moved to Wisconsin, and I was hesitant to do the interview because if selected, I knew it would be a big job in addition to my Chair of Surgery responsibilities, but I decided to go ahead with the interview. They offered me the job. I consulted with a lot of people, including my own faculty, and everyone thought it would be a real plus to have what is the finest surgical journal based at the University of Wisconsin. It has been a positive thing for our department. Several of my faculty review for the *Journal.*

The *Annals* receives a thousand manuscripts a year. The entire review process is on-line now, so it can all be done on my computer. My job is to ensure that now the manuscripts we receive are reviewed in a fair and even manner, so I send them out to experts in the field. Then I make my judgment on whether they should be accepted, revised, or rejected, based on those reviews.

It's a very time-consuming job, but an important job. The *"Annals of Surgery"* is the most highly cited surgical journal in the world, so it's one of the more popular surgical journals among general surgeons internationally. Playing a major role in determining the contents of that journal has a major impact on the field of surgery.

I don't have time to read all of the manuscripts that come through, but I do read all of the abstracts. I suspect I will continue doing this close to the time that I retire as chairman.

It's tiring, but it's very fulfilling. I'm doing what I like to do and I'm usually able to watch a few sports events. It's common for me to be watching a good football game with my computer running and also get some of my editing work done.

My children told me that they did not admire my lifestyle. When we were in Nebraska and they were in high school, I would go downstairs on a Saturday night to say hi to them and their friends, with my coat on. They would ask, "Dad, what are you doing?"

I would say, "I'm going in to the hospital."

Starting work at 11 o'clock on Saturday night isn't exactly what they thought was a good lifestyle. Now my daughter does it herself for sick babies. She is a pediatrician and has two children of her own. My son has become a superb graphic artist.

It was fun to be on the faculty of the University of Nebraska while my daughter was a medical student. One of the great disappointments of my life is that I would've had an opportunity to have her on my own surgical service in her third year, but that was the time that I left Nebraska to come to Wisconsin.

What do you consider your more important accomplishments?

I've been given a lot of opportunities, including editing the *"Annals of Surgery"* and leading two departments of surgery. I'm a fairly good organizer in getting these things done and helping to make them happen, but many other people contribute.

If I looked at my whole career in the order of what I'd be most proud of, number one would be the two departments of surgery that I've had the privilege of being chair of the University of Nebraska and the University of Wisconsin.

The *Annals* might come in second. Also near the top of the list would be my time on the American Board of Surgery, and the privilege of being Chair of that Board during my final year on it. That's a very important organization that determines the course of general surgery in this country.

My surgical practice mainly consists of liver and pancreatic resections. They tend to be long operations, sometimes with a fair amount of blood loss. Fascinating to me is that, when I make rounds that evening, the patients are often sitting up in bed watching television. In the not too distant past, they were lying in an ICU attached to a breathing machine. A lot has happened in surgical care over the past decade or two that has markedly improved outcomes.

How much does the patient have to do with recovery?

Having a positive attitude is a stimulus to the immune system, and I have no doubt that there's a whole spiritual component that plays a major role in the recovery of people from surgical illness.

I've been surprised how many doctors have mentioned spirituality as an important factor in their own lives and work.

Packing off some bleeding, closing your eyes, saying a quick prayer and asking for a little bit of help to get bailed out of a difficult situation, has happened to me on more than one occasion. I don't pretend to understand all of this, but certainly there are forces much greater than ourselves that must be at work.

When you're not working, how do you spend your free time?

A major hobby is photography. Every time I think of something I would like to do, but I don't have time to do now, I write it down in my Palm Pilot. Those are things to do when I am semi-retired or fully retired. Right now, I have 46 items, everything from taking university history courses to learning how to sail.

A lot of people work and do those things now. Do you feel that you've given up a lot to be a doctor?

Not at all, and I do some of those things now. If I were a better manager of time, I could probably do more of them. But I've had so many rewards for what I do, it's incredible.

If I regretted not having enough time, it would be mostly with respect to when my kids were growing up. That only happens once and then it's gone. In the early years, I was a very busy surgical resident—and there wasn't an 80-hour work week then. I had limited time to spend with my children. When I'm not working, I'm usually with my wife. My best friend has always been my wife, so I've never been one to go off golfing with the guys or go fishing. She loves to ski and golf, so we do those things together. We're both very interested in nature.

I've learned some of her interests and gotten involved in them, and she's learned some of mine. Sometimes I come home and she's watching a basketball game. That never used to happen!

What are your plans for the future?

I play things year to year. Retirement from surgery presents an opportunity to do other things, to learn some things that you haven't had a chance to learn during your busy professional career.

On the other hand, it's scary, because I've enjoyed being a surgeon. I hope our department is better now than when I started. But before too long—two, three years—it'll be time for somebody else to come in and take the reins and bring this Department of Surgery to the next level. I see fascinating things every day, and the heroes of the story are usually the patients. People survive who you didn't think would survive. For a surgeon, every day is like Christmas. You try to sort out what's going on inside and then, you open the package and find out.

Chapter Six

Operating Without a Scalpel

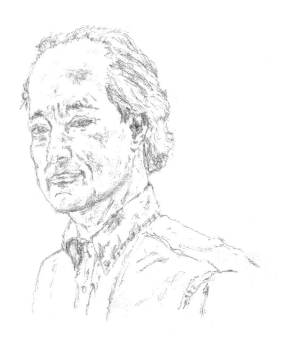

"I was physically toasted. I'm not going to be able to operate. Being able to accept that, mentally, was almost impossible because I had no other life."

Mark Aschliman, MD
Orthopedic Surgeon, Milwaukee

Right when a man's doin' all that he planned
And he thinks he got just what he needs
Life will deliver a shock that will shiver
And driving him down to his knees[*]

I don't know whether Mark Aschliman, MD, cares for country music, but he sure won't argue with Kenny Rogers on that philosophical point. Midway through his medical career, Aschliman was forced to confront the unthinkable after having devoted so much of his life to honing skills as an

[*] "Love Will Turn Your Around," by Kenny Rogers

orthopedic surgeon. But then something terrible and unthinkable happened just minutes from his home.

I would soon hear about it as I arrived at his doorstep, not knowing there was much more to his life than I was aware of during our nine-year acquaintance. In his mid 50s, Aschliman has four young kids, and lives just a few blocks from Lake Michigan, in a wealthy suburb just north of Milwaukee.

I know this doctor well, but midway through our interview he lets loose with startling revelations, such as the fact that he grew up Mennonite, with Amish grandparents who drove a horse and buggy. There can't be many kids with that background who became surgeons. But that isn't the story that blew me away.

It got icky when I broke my neck in the car accident a few years ago. I was driving at low speed. It was a beautiful day. The sun was out. A girl who had her driver's license for two or three weeks, was screwing around with the radio, turned into the south bound lane while she was headed north, and I whacked into her at 30 miles an hour. Boom! I had my seatbelt on or I probably would have been quaded out. I had a real low car. My head went up; hit the ceiling—compression load on my head. I exploded C-5—a vertebrae in my neck.

When it's cold, it hurts a lot. I'm getting very weary of the winter, and particularly now, with my neck and my arm. Sometimes I just wish I weren't here. But this is where my life is.

You don't appear to have any physical disability.

It's pain and weakness. Two of the nerves in my neck don't work, so my left hand is very uncoordinated and has little endurance. If I try to manipulate things, I drop them. I've got an area of loss of sensation in my fingers, so if you touch it, I can't tell where things are. If you're a surgeon, those are critical skills. You need to know where your hands are. You need to coordinate movement to manipulate instruments. You need to be able to tie. I can't tie very well. My hands just don't do it. That kind of puts the lid on being a good surgeon. My left arm went kablooey, and didn't work after that. I couldn't work for several months. I lost the ability to operate. That was extremely unsettling. My job was a surgeon and my identity was a surgeon. The two were inseparable.

I worked every day, all day, all the time. I went one eight-year period without a vacation. That's not healthy. I didn't want to be famous. I didn't necessarily want to be wealthy. When people would say, "Who's the best orthopedic surgeon in town?" I wanted it to be me.

You're always worried, *Gee, if I don't show up, or if I don't do this extra case, if I don't work this extra hour, somebody else might supplant me.* There's a bit of fear and a lack of confidence. It's really dichotomous. I was always very confident, but you're always unsure.

My dad tried to tell me not to let my studies get in the way of my education, meaning, "Enjoy yourself. Have a little fun." I was not always, and still am not, fun-seeking in that way. I would get on task and lose sight of what was happening around me because I was so focused, so task oriented.

How did that level of commitment to your profession affect your home life?

Well, there wasn't much home life. My wife is a nurse. Her dad was a doc. She knew what she wanted. She liked free time, and knew things I didn't know. If you're a doctor and work real hard, you'll get paid, so she enjoyed living here and spending my money and having a few kids. She ran the show and that was that.

Now, one of the problems I've had as a physician and a surgeon, compared to being a husband and a father: You're in the office. You're in the operating room. You tell people what they're to do and they do it. Even if they don't want to or don't like it, they do it. Okay?

I come home. You tell your nine-year old kid to do something. They don't give a hoot who you are. They just do whatever they want to do. I tell my wife to do something, and it doesn't matter. Her response is, "Look, this is my place. I'm going to run it the way I want it. You've got some input, but very little." That's not cool from my point of view. I have to turn over the reins to somebody else here. With kids, it's not a matter of turning over power. It's just a matter of understanding that kids are kids.

My skill at communicating to people is really very good and perhaps better than many. I say things to people in terms they can understand and give them an opportunity to ask questions. Since I'm not operative, I schedule fewer patients and I spend more time talking.

You have to understand that when people leave the doctor, they forget about 40% of the information within an hour or two of leaving the doctor's office.

You're there. You're partially unclothed. The guy might stick a needle in you. He may tell you something you don't want to hear. People are scared when they're at the doctor, so I understand that. I try to remember that.

You have a better sense for what they're going through now?

I'm willing to cut them a little more slack, perhaps. I give them more time. I don't know if that's age, the car accident, or both, or being a dad. Maybe a little bit of everything.

In some ways, the car accident made me less compassionate because I see people coming in moaning about stuff, when I feel worse than they do. I understand more about the system. It's educated me. It's made me probably a better doctor. I just understand that life isn't perfect. People aren't going to listen to me all the time.

Compliance greatly varies from patient to patient. You can often tell ahead of time who's going to be compliant and who's not going to be compliant. Recent case in point: New mother here. Had a problem with tendonitis. Hurt her, started to bother her during her pregnancy, happens relatively commonly. And she came to me and asked me what to do and I told her, "You gotta do blah, blah, blah." A week after a visit, I call people to find out how they're doin', to see if they have any questions? And she says, "Well, I haven't seen the therapist. I haven't been wearing the splint, I haven't been taking the medicine and I'm carrying the baby, and it still hurts. Why?"

Patients tell you what they think, but they don't always think about what's going on. I ask my patients a lot of questions, one of which is, do you smoke? If they say, yes, I say you need to quit. If they say, "I've been trying," I give them the phone number to call to quit. They never do.

I ask if they drink alcohol. Almost always the answer will be a little bit, occasionally, socially. Now, 10% of Wisconsinites are alcoholics, which means that if I were to see 100 people in a week, 10 should say, "I drink myself blind all the time." I don't hear that from anybody, ever, so people simply don't tell the truth about alcohol consumption and they're deluding themselves about cigarette smoking. Those are two very big issues for every patient who walks through my door that I ask them about, that I talk about and for which, usually, I don't get an honest answer.

The trouble with most alcoholics, it's the devastating effects over time. It cooks your brain. It wrecks your heart. It wrecks your lungs. You can fall and hurt yourself.

Same with cigarette smoking. Smoking will increase your incidence of osteoporosis because it compromises bone function and metabolism. It compromises your peripheral circulation so that it can cause skin problems, extremity pain, amputation of the knee for extremities, makes for weaker muscles, can cause strokes that can lead to muscular skeletal problems. Smokers have a 50% higher incidence of back pain than non-smokers. That's staggering! And given that most people have some amount of back pain, and you increase that by 50%, that's inordinately high.

What's the best way to convince patients to change?

If you tell the truth and you do it without an edge and without being nasty, people may be mad at ya, but they can't tell you, you lied and you weren't a good doctor. I'd say a few things to people and thought, *Gee that was kind of harsh*. And it was. But it's what they needed to hear.

And we still have issues where, you tell people what the problem is and it's not your fault. They don't want to believe you, or they blame you for it or think you're a jerk for telling them what's wrong. It's just part of the practice.

I'm not here to tell people what they gotta do. I'm here to tell people what their choices are and empower them to make a good decision by giving them the information that they need to make that decision. I will certainly guide them and offer counsel. You can tell people, "If you take these choices, your leg's going to fall off."

For the most part, people really respect your opinion. And I found that by making the follow-up call, I get much greater compliance than most doctors and, as a result, better results. And, I develop a rapport with my patients that really gains their trust. They know because I really do care. I'm calling. My job, that you paid me to do, is to give you advice that will make you better. And if I can just make a simple two minute phone call and make them better, that's worth it. It's good value. And so, the patients like it.

I don't think many people can fault my clinical skills or my honesty when it comes to the practice of medicine. That's very important to me. Integrity's important—very important.

It's really nice when people come to you, and maybe in the past you've laid steel to their skin. You want those people to like you. You want them to respect you and that's a non-cash remuneration of being a doctor. That's one of the reasons I went into medicine was the respect that a physician generally gets. I get paid in ways that aren't just in dollars. I get paid in respect and honor.

Did your job satisfaction decrease after your accident?

When I suddenly couldn't be a surgeon, I had no identity. I had no other interests. I was a dad and a husband, and a suburban guy, and then I was a surgeon over here. I was the surgeon, first, last, and everything. And, oh by the way, I have a wife and a couple of kids. They're around here somewhere. That's really how it was.

I was physically toasted. And being able to accept that, mentally, was almost impossible because I had no other life. I didn't know what to do, so I made my wife and my kids crazy, and, frankly, about everybody who came into contact with me, crazy. There were some very rocky times. I was cranky. I was, frankly, depressed, and I wasn't listening to anybody. I was pissing and moaning. Finally, my wife said, "Either you get help or get out."

So I called some of my colleagues, and it turned out that one of my medical school classmates is a psychiatrist here in town. I called him and said, "Okay, my wife says I have to talk to somebody or she's going to make me move."

He said, "Why you don't make her move." Wise acre.

"You don't know her. Can I talk to you?"

"Yeah, okay."

And that has been very beneficial.

I have pain in my neck and in the left arm all the time, but I don't like medication. I exercise, and I use traction. I try to stay in shape.

Being a doctor, was it helpful to fully understand...

{Interjects} Helpful and harmful. The helpful part is I understood what was going on. The harmful part is I knew what was going on and how potentially dangerous surgery could be. I was very, very, very afraid of having an operation to fix my problem.

An orthopedic surgeon reticent about having surgery himself?

Certainly my God-like self image of, *This can't be me. I'm a surgeon.* Uh, it screwed me a little bit. I screwed myself a little bit, to some degree. My wife will tell me so.

Retrospectively, had I had the surgery in a more timely fashion, instead of waiting nearly a year to do it, I might have had a better result. But I was just paralyzed, mentally, with regard to the ability to pursue surgery. I just didn't want to do it 'cause I was afraid it would screw me up. It did! But part of it was waiting so long to get there that I had permanent dysfunction in the nerves. They just don't work and they're never going to work. I got cooked.

Did you think your career was over?

I thought it was over. *Okay, what am I going to do? Teach? Should I sit at home in front of the computer screen and day trade?* I explored all those things, and you know what I found out? I really liked being a doctor. I like going to my office. I like being able to know patients intimately, instantly. People come in and they tell me things, and I can ask them questions about their life and their being. They tell me things that are right to the core, right now.

I went into medicine because I really wanted to be my own boss. Frankly, I just love doing orthopedic surgery. I didn't listen to my dad, in that I let my studies interfere with my education.

What did your parents think of your interest in medicine?

My mom's a nurse. She revered physicians. They loved the fact that I wanted to become a doctor. I was the first of a huge family. Okay, 101 first cousins. Being a smart kid and going to school in the late 50s and into the 60s, medicine's kind of where they wanted you to go. People always thought I would be a scientist or a doctor.

My dad was an Amish man. His parents were Amish, horse and buggy, as were his grandparents, and all of his other ancestors. My father was smart and he wanted education. So when it was time to quit school, as all Amish men did when they got to high school, he didn't quit. That got him in a heap of trouble. His parents didn't disown him, but the church pretty much rousted him out.

Then, World War II happened and he was a senior in high school and he wanted to go fight the fight and nobody would let him do that because we're Amish and we don't believe in war. He went to college and then to Purdue to get a PhD.

Well, my mom came from a significantly different background. Her family was from Ireland—full of cops. Hard drinking, hard working, working class, cussin,' drinkin', smokin' people—completely different than my dad's family.

I had a sibling who died at a very young age. My mom got sick after the loss of my sister, and I spent a lot of time back with dad's family in Indiana. I started grade school in Indiana, in a one-room school house. Many of the people there were my cousins, or distant relatives. Everybody was Protestant. There was no smokin', no drinkin', no cussin'. Very straight. And I lived there off and on through my grade school years.

I always found my dad's family was a little bit more comfortable for me, probably because that's where I spent the time as a kid. I honored them. I loved them. And I lived with them off and on for many years, so I viewed them as surrogate parents many times.

I found my mom's family intimidating. They were more boisterous, more physical—just a bit rougher. My mom is a bit tighter, pretty wound up, not nearly as smart as my dad. I'm lucky enough to get his quickness, and I don't know, some people might say I'm lucky enough to get my mother's edge. From my mom, I learned to just say what's on your mind. Sometimes I shouldn't. It's cost me jobs. It's cost me acquaintances. As my best man said, "Ash, people meet you, and in five minutes they either love you or they hate ya."

My father is and was a very devout Christian, a very gentle man, patient to a fault and kind and forgiving. I'm not as nice a guy as he is. I learned from my pop—don't lie, don't cheat, don't steal, so I don't.

When I started a practice, I tithed of time and money. I would have a free clinic for half a day each week, figuring five days a week, ten half days. One of those half days, I took care of people who didn't have insurance, or didn't have the means to pay, or had some other issue. I grew up with an abiding faith.

I went to a large suburban high school, thirty-four hundred students, again in the suburbs of Chicago. Hell, I was an athlete. I was in the plays. Of our class of 950, I was voted best dressed and most likely to succeed. And I was lucky enough to be really smart. I got A's in everything. It was just the hand I was dealt.

Throughout my entire educational career, A's in everything, except on the citizenship skills. When you open your report card on the right side, your grades in Math, English, that kind of stuff—A, A, A. And on the left side is citizenship skills, which is raises the hand before speaking, respects the opinions of others, works and plays well with others, I was getting check marks in all of those for needing work. Not much has changed.

Went to Lawrence—decent college. Okay, piece of cake. I was very shy and extraordinarily naïve for my academic intelligence. And I was just more comfortable going from that big Chicago suburban high school to Lawrence—Midwestern town, kids like me, safe, comfortable. I liked it.

I looked at schools out East. I didn't really care for the people there. I applied. I looked at a lot of schools and finished applications to two and was accepted at both. The school was the big one in Cambridge, Massachusetts. When I got home from there, they said, "So are you going to go?"

"No, I don't want to go to school with those people. I just don't want to spend four years with them." I was really parochial then.

But after Lawrence, I was ready to move on. I had grown up a little bit. I had taken a year abroad. I lived in London. That really opened my eyes up. It gave me a great deal of confidence in myself. I was academically confident, but in terms of life, I really didn't have much experience or knowledge or confidence.

I went to a party with a bunch of my brothers. We were in a frat house. We got plenty to eat there, and at about one in the morning we went back to my room to type up my medical school application. I was really unfocused. I figured I could do whatever I wanted to do because I had a 4.0 in college and I had taken the M-CAT because I was kind of expected to, but I didn't really know what I was going to do. I ended up getting into some darn good schools. I went to the University of Chicago.

When I went to U of C, I thought, big city, comfortable, at least I grew up around there, got cousins or cops there in case I got in trouble, and that was the big leagues. Moving from one of the quietest, most Republican, highest income districts in the United States, where my folks live in Western Chicago; from western suburbs to the least white, lowest income, highest number of people on welfare districts in the United States, which was District 1 in Chicago. That was a very big change for me, just in terms of my surroundings.

I grew up in very insular world, so I learned a lot about academics and a lot about people. I met people from foreign countries, other parts of this country, people from the same city that I was born, who were so different than I. U of C went year round, so I got five academic years in four.

I can't speak highly enough of the University. They're some of the most liberal people in terms of accepting other thoughts. I learned a lot about liberality and liberalism, which doesn't mean leaning to the left politically and shouting down everybody who's on the right. It means listening to everybody and making your own opinion. That's really what I liked about it. There were people who just looked at it so much differently than I that weren't right or weren't wrong. I really began to understand how much more interesting the world can be.

One of my dad's friends was a dentist, actually, was the dean of the U of I dental school, who said, "You're not going to be a family practitioner. You're going to be a surgeon."

I said, "I'm not going to be a surgeon. They're assholes."

He goes, "Yep."

Med school was the first time I was challenged, academically. I thought it was pretty hot stuff. Well, half the class is valedictorians. And some of those guys are really smart and work really hard, so I was humbled. But then you pick up your racquet and you keep hitting the ball, and the next thing you know, you're playing pretty good tennis against guys who are better than you. But you can still stay in the game. I really had to study, put in the time, and I had to be very focused. And it was different.

I took a course in animal surgery, but I never thought I would be a surgeon. I loved it. I loved taking the knife, taking the tools and fixing stuff. So then a little further into the training, you rotate through different services. You learn about all kinds of stuff, orthopedic surgery, ophthalmology, and gynecology. I really like plastic surgery.

As much as I liked plastic surgery, I didn't really care for general surgery. It was just too mundane for me. People were actually sick. Orthopedics was a more immediate feedback specialty. You fix something, you see it. I really liked that. And then the guy goes home.

I go back and tell the guys, "I'm thinking of bailing out of plastic surgery. Can I do orthopedic surgery?"

The chairman said, "Orthopedic surgery is the most desired specialty in all of medicine. We have way more applicants than we can accept."

I said, "Oh well, if anything comes up, give me a call." About a week later, he said, "We've got an opening and we know you and you know us. Yeah, we got 50 guys who want the slot, but you want the job?"

Sure. I'll move back to Chicago for a year. So there I go, back to U of C for four more years of orthopedics.

I wanted to become a tumor surgeon when I went into orthopedic surgery, because I really liked the reconstructive aspects, because when you remove the tumor then you've got to rebuild the part. I did a lot of research on it. But what I realized after taking care of a lot of these people with cancerous tumors, about half of them died, even if you did a really good job and fixed it. I had no stomach for having half of my patients die. One of the reasons I went into orthopedics was because people don't die.

Even so, orthopedic surgery is in one of the highest classes for malpractice because people can see what happens. Not every result is good. Sometimes we don't do a good job, sometimes the patient doesn't do a good job, sometimes both. But in American society, somebody has to pay, and in this world that we live in, pay means malpractice. Because you have a bad result doesn't mean the doctors did a bad job.

They're non-compliant and you think they tell the truth when they're non-compliant? No. And sometimes things don't heal up or turn out like they should. But in general, we have great results. We make people's lives better. It's pretty cool.

We're toy friendly in orthopedic surgery. We do surgery on TVs, videogame type surgery—minimal incisions to fix rotator cuffs, knees, shoulders, ankles, through little incisions, while watching on TV. We can replace joints that we couldn't replace before. We're even replacing discs in the spine now that we couldn't replace before. Technology has really come a long way.

Orthopedics is a specialty that doesn't generally save your life, but it gives you a measurably better quality of life, which is a problem when it comes to malpractice issues. Because somebody comes in with a really crappy knee and your replace it and have a cruddy result and they come limping into the court room with lawyers saying, "Oh gosh, look what you've done to this guy." You should have seen him before!

Tell me about some of your early surgeries.

Cutting is a tactile skill. We had a guy named Dr. Richard Belsey, British surgeon. He came down to show these ignorant sophomore medical students how to do surgery on the chest of a dog. This is a world famous surgeon! There are procedures named after him, so this guy's high drawer. He was such a gentleman, and I thought, *Boy, I want to be like this. I was hooked.*

It was an operation on the chest. Make an incision, split the ribs, go down and take a lung out. I just really enjoyed doing it. You find the bleeders. You stop them from bleeding. You take the tissue out. You actually do something. I just liked that after years of talking. "Take this pill and maybe your blood pressure will go down."

The first {human} operation that I ever got to do from the incision, the whole operation, to closing up, to putting the bandage on, was a circumcision on an adult—a gentleman who was well endowed. Some guy who had problems with infection and bad hygiene. I was with the urology resident, who knew I had good hands. He said, "You're up." He got a picture with me holding the operative body part—a big picture of me grinning.

How did it go?

It went perfectly! As I look back, my skill wasn't necessarily hugging you and kissing you and making you like me. It was great technical ability. That was my gift. I could do it fast and as well as 99% of them in the world.

Training in the inner city of Chicago taught me a lot. I got called to the ER one night by one of the residents who said, "We have somebody down here who's got some orthopedic problems. Come on down and take a look."

I said, "What's wrong?"

And they said, "You really gotta see it."

I go down there and there's this old guy and his legs were covered with sores and maggots. You could see the bone of his tibia because the skin had all been eaten away. They were down in his calf muscle and going down and eating his foot. The guy was just sitting there smiling.

I asked, "What happened?"

And he says, "You know, my leg's been hurtin."

No kidding. And we had to amputate both of his legs because they were gangrenous and just full of bugs. That really changed my perception of people.

Was it a mental health issue?

The guy was out of his mind—just crazy.

How confident were you in your abilities as a young surgeon?

You can't go into it being a back seat person. You're in the front row, in terms of life. Yeah, I was very confident in my abilities. At no point did I think I would fail, and that's what you need. You have to understand when you're not doing it right and when you need work, but you don't think you're going to fail, because then you do. It's not arrogance; it's just...well maybe it is. Like most of our cases, at least my classmates, we all deserved to be pretty doggone confident. I had classmates that are really smart guys.

You've all heard of herpes virus, herpes simplex, the sexually transmitted form. One of my classmates is the guy who discovered that that was sexually transmitted. You have to remember, people actually have to figure out how this all happened. He figured that all out as his PhD project. How smart is that?

One of my other classmates got a young genius grant for a million dollars a year for five years from some foundation. I'm not that smart, but I was good enough to keep up. It really crushed my confidence when I got whacked. They do a good job of picking out students to stay there because they know you'll pick it up and do it.

I wasn't going to be the top of this class. You had to accept that. You had to subrogate your ego and say, *I am going to be as good as I can possibly be, and be excellent compared to the rest of the world.* And that's what happened.

I've always exuded confidence, because when I went to the University of Rochester, New York, I was on a plastic surgery service as an intern. We were doing a case and I was with the chairman of the department and somebody said some comment about something and the chairman said, "Oh, we knew when Ash showed up—gray suit, white shirt, red tie, polished shoes. This guy, nothing was going to rock him. And we rank people on 10 categories and five out of five, he got a 50."

I said, "Jesus, I never knew that." But, evidently, other people could just see that I was unflappable.

Maybe confidence is behind why the first inclination for many surgeons is to cut when there's a problem. But you're a different kind of orthopedic surgeon now.

I'm sure I did operations that might have been treated better non-operatively. But I was never knife-happy. I still have a wealth of information and knowledge about orthopedics and medicine in general, and I really like using it.

I go to the office and see people, because nine of ten people in orthopedics don't need surgery. It can be a non-operative specialty—back pain, strains, sprained ankles, you know, hurt elbows, tendonitis, bursitis, stuff like that. In the one in 10 people who needs an operation, I've got associates.

I take as many days off as I want. I work when I want. I take one week off per month, period. I don't work more than 20 hours in the office per week because if I do so, I start to feel so cruddy that I can't function. My neck and my arm start to hurt so much from the reading and the talking. I just can't do it. When I start hurting, I get real crabby and then life sucks. It's not worth it.

There's been a significant drop in income as a result, but you know what? It doesn't matter. If you feel cruddy, it doesn't matter. I've got a nice house. I've got more than I deserve, frankly. I didn't look at myself as a victim at all. Life is inherently unfair. It's not fair that I've got what I've got. But that's the way it goes. I'm not going to sit around and cry about it.

Now, I certainly sat around and cried about not being able to do what I wanted to do, but that was just because I was goofy—not necessarily because I was feeling victimized. I was disoriented because I had no other identity. Why did it happen? Don't have a clue. I don't think there was a grand plan. It's just what happens, and so you make the best of it.

With the recent passing of my mother, I realized that you work hard, you worry about a lot of stuff and then you die. Some people have said the joy is the journey. I was never the guy who enjoyed the journey. I was always looking at the next prize.

Boy, I gotta get through college and be the top of the class. I gotta get through med school and be one of the gang. Okay, I gotta get my internship done. This year residency, that year residency, finish my residency, fellowship. I gotta build it. I gotta be big. {long sigh} Why? Um, I wasn't enjoying myself, peripherally. I wasn't doing anything else.

So it gives me a chance to read other books. Look at this stuff—stuff that I haven't read before. *Birds, Zen Golf, The Limerick.* I never traveled. I didn't do anything. Now, I take off a lot. This year—San Francisco, Florida, South Carolina.

I like to hunt. I like to have the dogs outside. I like firearms. The harvesting of birds or animals is incidental to the experience of hunting. Hunting is being with your buddies outside. It's being out in the woods or in the prairie. It's messing with your stuff, your clothes, and your equipment. I like hunting, shooting, because it's very personal, like surgery. It's very powerful like surgery. You may do it in the company of others, but it's really about your own skills, which is what surgery is.

One of the guys I hunt with is a doc. Doctor Owen Royce, a guy here in town. He's 92 years old. He still takes a computer course at MATC,[†] occasionally, to tune up his computer skills. He's always studying. He can still shoot a shot gun. He is still sharp as a tack. I want to be that guy. And he's a gentleman—a southern gentleman from Mississippi. I don't think I'll be as nice as Dr. Royce, but I want to be as sharp.

Golf is similar to hunting. You're doing it with other people, but you're outside and you're walking, but it's about your own skills. The other guy can shoot a 72 and you shoot a 90, and it doesn't matter. I'm having a good time. I really love golfing.

My new thing I'm learning is Spanish, because I'm seeing one or two people per week in my office who speak Spanish as a primary language. They're not learning English. I may as well learn Spanish.

I learned French as a kid. My mom wanted me to be a diplomat. That was before she fully understood my personality, which is not necessarily diplomatic.

I grew up where the old Swiss German was the primary language. They all spoke German—old German dialect. I did have—maybe I still do have—a strong faith. And it didn't matter to me if you called me Catholic or Protestant or whatever, so I converted to Catholicism. I did the Rite of Christian Initiation for Adults and went through it. Now, I'm active in the parish. I'm on the parish council.

You're the son of an Amish man, living a life that seems to be as far away from an Amish existence as conceivable. Do you ever think about that?

Well, eventually the whole family bailed out, including my grandparents when they were very old. They're good people. They're hard working people. Come on, it's the 21st Century. You can be a good person and lead a good life and still have a Lincoln Continental. So most of my family now is Mennonite, which is an Amish man with a TV and a car. And that's fine. Frankly, as my aunt Mary, who's 87 said, "You're not Catholic. You're still Amish. You're a Mennonite boy inside."

I know who I am. Call me Mennonite. Call me Catholic. I don't care. Just know what you believe. My Aunt Mary said, "So does this mean you worship the Pope?" So my other aunt says, "What's this Mary thing? I thought Jesus was our intercessor."

I don't know! Give me a break. Come on, who really follows dogma, okay? Nobody. All I know is it's the original church of Saints Peter and Paul and it's got a long tradition and they've got a ton of troubles. But it's

† Milwaukee Area Technical College.

big and it's a nice group of people who do nice stuff and they've got a good school and they have a bar in the basement that makes my family crazy. I love that.

Do you still love being an orthopedic surgeon, even though you can't operate? Will you continue practicing like this until retirement?
I don't know what I want to do. I might want to try something political. But I don't have the stomach for that public scrutiny, or for that complete compromise of principles. Okay, I couldn't do that. Hell, I'd take an interest in it, but I'm generally an uncompromising guy. Politicians compromise themselves daily.

I really don't want to become a dinosaur. Fifty percent of the medical information we know changes every year. It may not be wrong, but it changes to some degree, so you don't necessarily know which 50% unless you're keeping up. Patients are interested in medicine, too. There is so much new stuff. Like those books. {Points to the shelf} There's stuff in there that wasn't even discovered when I was in medical school. It's exciting. Medicine can make you live longer. I'm interested in stuff like that.

Are patients becoming more informed, too?
It's diminishing. As we learn more about medicine, medicine becomes more complex. The public becomes ignorant on a relative basis. They can go to the computer and start clicking on the web and they come in and they think they know stuff that, when frankly, they don't.

In orthopedics, in residence, some guys did a project looking at information on orthopedic websites. Found that about one in three pieces of information was wrong. Okay? Now, we know what's right and what's wrong as physicians, but the public doesn't know it's wrong. And that's the trouble. It's difficult to try to dispute that because people look at information off the web as Gospel.

What I'm going to say sounds arrogant. But most doctors are smarter than most patients—just are. We just have more equipment. And it's difficult sometimes to try to explain to somebody—it's like showing a hog a wrist watch. They don't know whether to sniff it or to eat it. They don't know what it is.

Has your passion for medicine rubbed off on your kids?
I've got one who's an eighth grader at the middle school. She wants to be a psychiatrist. I said, "Forget it!" Psychiatrist? She's smart and the only one who really looks like me and she kind of acts like me, which makes life somewhat more difficult for her and for people around her. She isn't athletic or musical. I haven't figured her out yet.

I'm a very liberal man, in the University of Chicago sense, that I will give my children the opportunity. I will encourage them. Good decisions are encouraged. If they can get into a school and they can demonstrate the ability to do it, you gotta let 'em. I've got three daughters and a boy and whatever they want to do, they can do. My children are much, much more worldly. I didn't want to leave Indiana for college because I was afraid, uncomfortable with things foreign. My children have been to Europe, the Caribbean, and all over the United States and they will have much more confidence.

You sound surprisingly content with how things turned out, despite the accident.

It's not fair that I busted my neck. It's not fair that my arm doesn't work, but I have no axe to grind. I was going to leave behind a widow, four kids and a gazillion dollars at 60, if I didn't change what I was doing. Or it was going to be an ex-wife and four kids. And so, it turned out to be okay, in some ways.

How long has this been?

Seven years.

And how long did it take you to come to terms with the fact that you weren't going to be able to operate anymore?

Uh, yesterday, I think. Maybe not. We're still working on that.

II

Innovators

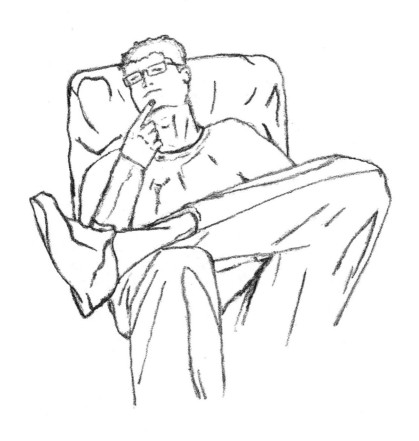

"Trust that little voice in your head that says, Wouldn't it be interesting if...; And then do it."

—Duane Michals

CHAPTER SEVEN

SEEING THE INVISIBLE LIGHT

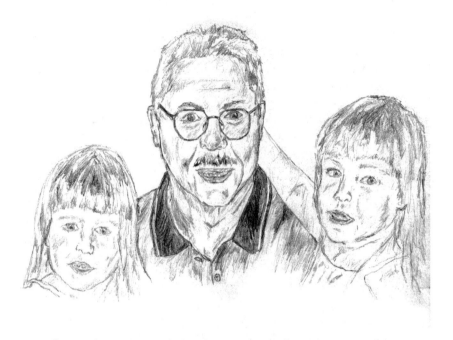

"Was it the greatest operation that was ever performed? I say, yes. What other operation can prolong life 225 years for babies who were almost certain to die or develop cerebral palsy without it?"

Julian E. De Lia, MD with twins Madeline and Julianne Claas
OB/GYN, Milwaukee

They don't have to die–perfect twin babies, that is. Although it's been almost 20 years since Julian E. De Lia, MD, pioneered an intrauterine laser surgery that saves these identical twins from a fatal condition called twin-to-twin transfusion syndrome {TTTS}, there are still doctors who recommend terminating the pregnancy. Desperately, these parents search the Internet and if they're lucky, they find their savior in Milwaukee, Wisconsin.

De Lia, who's in his early 60s, has treated patients who come to Milwaukee from all over the country and consulted for others and their physicians, from 45 states and 30 countries, via e-mail and phone.

Yesterday, I received two phone calls. One was from a patient in New York, who went to see somebody at a major hospital. "Terminate." They wanted to terminate her pregnancy because nothing could be done. "Your babies are going to have brain damage, or they're going to die."

I performed operations on Monday and Tuesday, and we got the babies disconnected. Four babies are still alive. It's something so simple. It's so intuitive. The donor* twin had no fluid. The recipient† twin had a massive amount of amniotic fluid.

All the problems associated with identical twinning—such as prematurity, growth discordance—one baby weighs more than the other, one baby has heart defects, and even death. Almost all of this occurs in those that share the same placenta. These babies can be doomed because they do not have enough placenta to survive. Eighty percent of them are normal—identical twins with one placenta. Twenty percent of them get into trouble.

By disconnecting the twins, you can save two babies, if they have enough placenta, and keep them healthy. Sometimes, you can only save one.

When I fire the laser, which is invisible to the human eye, the light beam heats the molecules in the tissue. It's like cauterizing them, but with light rather than doing it with sutures. There's no other alternative. You could use stitches, but you'd have to filet open the uterus and risk loss of the pregnancy.

I've stopped the transfusion of blood from one baby to the other, and turned a placenta that used to be shared by the twins into one that's still shared, but functionally, it's like they have separate placentas.

I performed the operation for the first time on October third, 1988. This is fetal therapy.

Tell me about your first twin to twin transfusion case.

It was in 1983. I was in Salt Lake City at the University of Utah. One day, a patient came to see me. I notice that her womb looked a bit on the large size, and I was suspicious of twins.

Ultrasound was really coming to the fore. It wasn't available back in my training. Not only did the ultrasound find the twins, but the diagnosis of twin-to-twin transfusion syndrome was made. Twin transfusion had now moved from a pediatric diagnosis or a pathology diagnosis, to an obstetric diagnosis, as a consequence of ultrasound.

I was with her when she was having her ultrasound scan. The physician doing the scan was a sub-specialist in maternal fetal medicine. He told her, "There's no way these babies are going to survive."

I began to think. The recipient twin was in heart failure. There's a donor. I had read something somewhere about giving the mother digitalis for

---

* The donor twin is deprived of most of the blood and nutrition.

† The recipient twin gets more blood and nutrition.

fetuses in heart failure from a very fast heart rate. We gave the digitalis to the mother, and it made the heart stronger to correct the heart failure in the baby.

The babies were born alive, but it was a bittersweet victory. One of the babies had cerebral palsy. The parents of those babies, who'd heard that they were going to die, were ecstatic.

It turned out that this baby with cerebral palsy is just one year behind his brother in high school and college and so on. It's a mild cerebral palsy, with mild mental retardation. For the longest time, they thought he was worse until they realized he needed glasses. As soon as he had the glasses, he would follow you when you spoke to him.

So that was an example of twin to twin transfer, but you dealt with it with medicine?

True, but when their placenta came out and I examined it with the resident, we found a one millimeter connection between the circulations of the donor and the recipient. The donor was pumping blood through this connection into the recipient baby. It was the recipient baby who had the heart failure and the cerebral palsy, because his blood was hyperviscous[‡] from a very high blood count.

One twin was bright red when he was born and the other one was pale, which typically defines TTTS. But they were born alive. It was a miracle in their parents' eyes, and I guess in our eyes, too. We tried something we had known about and it worked, but we did not know if it would work all the time.

It didn't matter, because when I saw that placenta, I recognized the role of the connections in TTTS. At the time, my chairman wanted me to use the laser for problems such as condyloma,[§] dysplasia[¶] of the cervix, and so on, but I was reluctant because there were other ways that were faster and better.

John Dixon, who was a professor of surgery and director of the laser lab, said, "We have these lasers. Try to find something useful for them."

How do these patients find you?

That's where the Internet came into play. In 1993, the TTTS Foundation in Cleveland was established and had set up its website. A father of twins we saved, who worked in IS {information systems}, became webmaster and helped save 75 percent of the twins I treated from maybe 1994 to 2004.

Unless you have this syndrome, you'd never hear of it. It happens in

---

‡ Term that describes thickened blood.

§ It's another name for venereal warts.

¶ Term for the abnormal development or growth of tissues, organs, or cells.

about five percent of identical twin pregnancies or 15 percent of identical twins that share one placenta.

Everybody knows conjoined or Siamese Twins. It seems as if there's conjoined twins born in the Amazon, they will show up on the national news because some children's hospital, with a billion dollar endowment, will separate the babies and do it for nothing.

Meanwhile, for every one of those, there are about 200 cases of twin transfusion syndrome. The babies are connected in the placenta {not in the body}, and nobody knows and nobody cares about that process because it's so damn obscure.

Then, how often are you performing laser surgery?

Maybe one every two weeks. We use comprehensive, versus single therapy. We also discovered that these mothers have poor nutrition, so we encourage programs of bed rest and nutritional therapy in mild cases. You need to make sure that a surgery is necessary. Although I operate on the placenta, it's not all I do.

For every one I operate on, I'm helping 12 that don't go to the operating room.

{Letters** to De Lia from patients confirm what he preaches}.

> *To a doctor whose middle name should be 'dedication.'*
> *A doctor who throughout—was so compassionate*
> *and caring. Who worried for my wellbeing and reiterated*
> *again and again that I should not come for a consultation—*
> *nor fly by plane.*
>
> **Judy**
> New York

> *Of all the doctors I saw through my pregnancy,*
> *I'm most grateful to the one I never met.*
>
> **Jill**
> New York

> *Thank you for helping my daughter and saving my grandsons'*
> *lives. Without you, there would be no grandsons or only one.*
> *I know this in my heart.*
>
> **Grandma Pat**
> Wisconsin

** The letters are posted on www.covhealth.org, where Dr. De Lia practices.

Why hasn't the procedure caught on, so other doctors could save their twin patients?

Early on, colleagues did not put me on their shoulders and carry me off the field. On the contrary, many tried to dig a hole and bury me, and it was that way for 20 years. My work didn't appear in the *New England Journal of Medicine*. I tried in 1990. Five years later, a group from London sent a paper there on laser, and they published it. I'm the only person in the world who had done this operation, so peer review would dictate my review of the article. It wasn't sent to me for peer review.

Is it petty jealousy, or do some surgeons just not believe this is the best way to do it?

It's all of that. You say surgeons. In reality, the power in obstetrics and gynecology is held by docs in three sub-specialties. Maternal fetal medicine or complicated obstetrics are those who care for pregnant women with diabetes and other medical disorders. They also work with fetal genetics—brilliant people whose minds are packed with information.

Others go into gynecologic oncology. They perceive themselves as surgeons, primarily, or infertility and endocrinology—those who do not want to get up in the middle of the night. Many of these doctors don't care as much if a pregnancy is lost or survives with handicaps. "It's somebody else's baby. I don't care if the baby dies." That happens often.

The maternal fetal medicine sub-specialists perform most pregnancy ultrasounds and make the TTTS diagnosis. They pounded me for years and years because, A, it was something they could not understand and B, couldn't believe it was feasible.

The lasers we were using in gynecology in '83 were not lasers that could be fired inside a uterus filled with amniotic fluid at the placental blood vessel, but they were using these lasers in bladder surgeries and in other specialties. I had to disconnect a specific pathology—abnormal connections between these babies.

The laser can fully coagulate, destroy, and ablate blood vessels, and this must be done with a scope that is small enough that you do not disrupt the continuation of the pregnancy.

I did some sheep experiments. I had to pay for the experiments personally. No NIH {National Institutes of Health}. No fellowship. No post graduate training. All I had was this idea, and when I told faculty about it, they looked at me as though I just got off a spaceship from Mars.

I just went ahead and did it. That was 1983, '84 at the latest. I went down to the animal lab and said I needed a couple of pregnant sheep. I filled out a form and I had myself three pregnant sheep. We studied the way the laser was interacting with the blood vessels with a live fetus pumping blood through its placenta. Of course, the laser could stop blood flow through the vessels.

I needed another model with a placenta similar to a human's. That's when Dr. Kurt Benirschke came to Utah from the University of California-San Diego to give a lecture. He authored the text book on placental pathology. He is professor emeritus in reproductive biology and science. I said to him, "I think I can solve this problem of twin transfusion syndrome that you wrote about in the *New England Journal of Medicine*. I can take this laser and interrupt these blood vessels that connect the twins."

He seemed very skeptical about everything, but nevertheless, he served as a go-between to get me rhesus monkey pregnancies from the California Primate Research Center.

I had four monkeys over three breeding seasons in two years. I finished that work in 1985, '86, and knew then that there was no question technically, this could be done, because I had operated on a normal monkey pregnancy at mid pregnancy. There was hair inside there and very little amniotic fluid. Now, I was going to be working in a {human} uterus, over-distended with amniotic fluid, on the placenta with a fetus that doesn't have hair, so it would be a lot easier.

The amazing thing is the people—instrumental people. I said to the veterinarians and PhDs at the California Primate Research Center, "This is what I want to do."

I had a scope. I had a laser manufacturer lend us a machine. But I didn't know what to do next. I was scared to death, thinking that they were going to turn to me and say, "Well, now what?"

But instead, they put the monkey to sleep. They performed the incision. They brought out the uterus, and said, "Okay, you can stick the scope into the uterus." They gave the monkey anti-labor medication and antibiotics routinely for surgery.

Earlier this week, I took two humans to the operating room. I gave them anti-labor medication. I gave them antibiotics. It wasn't a matter of just looking at the… {tears well up and he must regain his composure before continuing}.

An interesting part of these monkey experiments is that the mother eats the placenta after the baby is born. These {monkeys} were scheduled to have a cesarean section just before term, so we could study the placenta that I lasered at mid-pregnancy. However, if the monkeys had delivered their babies over the weekend {when fewer staff are on} they would have eaten the placenta. They would have eaten my results and I would have never been able to write a paper! I don't know whether I could have been able to take the next steps.

In 1986, back in Utah, I was convinced that this can be done, but still encountered some jealousy in my own department. I hoped to raise the level of the lakes, so all the boats went up.

By the time I was finished with those monkeys, the night I did the first human being, I was as relaxed as could be. But I could not get someone to make me the equipment that I needed, because by the mid 1980s, ultrasound had almost eliminated the need to stick a fetoscope into the uterus. You could now use ultrasound technology to accomplish any visualization you wanted.

I knew of arthroscopy for knee surgery with very small endoscopes. That's what I wanted to do. But I needed a much longer version of the scope. I contacted all of the major manufacturers at the time and I told them what I wanted, but to no avail. An independent salesman finally found me a small manufacturer in Germany, who made the fetoscope. I told this salesman, "People will be doing this surgery all over the world." I come to find out, 20 years later, that every Tom, Dick and Harry doctor who has an idea for a new device, goes to these companies and say, "People will be doing this all over the world. You guys are going to make a fortune."

After a few operations, I flew over to the company in Germany. I showed videotapes of the operations to the engineers and described what I do. I used the fetoscope for the first time in 1988, and moved to Milwaukee in 1991. They had started doing the laser operation in London, in 1993. This operation was now being embraced by people who had good intentions, but who did not know what they were doing.

Here we are in 2006, and the surgery is being done all over the world, just like I said it would. That's the good news. The bad news is that no one seems to be doing it correctly. The survival rate of babies is not as great as it could be and the babies aren't as healthy as they could be.

The first {patient} in the world to have the {laser} surgery was from Montana. She had the nerve to let me operate on her. She did, and we got the job done on October 3, 1988. One of their children survived and that baby is my Godson. After the baby was discharged from the intensive care unit, I became friends with the parents. The three of us and the surviving baby are people that they may write about in the future.

Months later, the father asked me to come up and go fishing. Sure enough, when I got out there he said, "I want you to be the godfather." I had no idea what religion they were, but I accepted.

You've been on quite an odyssey. Were you prepared for this?

I always wanted to become a doctor, although I hated to study. That may have been a reflection of the fact that I had a mind that was just too out of control, in terms of being able to see things that other people weren't seeing. This may be the reason why it was I who made this contribution.

I was born in Newark in 1944. I was the middle of three sons, born two years apart, to mother Anita and father, Emilio, who was a physician. My brothers were much better students.

My father began a private practice in our house, in the summer of '41. He didn't have any employees, and he would accept a dollar, two dollars, for visits He was very committed to taking his education and using it in a significant way.

Of course, by February of '42, the office closed and he was in the service for the duration of the war, although he stayed stateside. He was a general practitioner with an essentially blue collar practice. He took care of many Italian immigrants and others in Newark, a low to middle class, relatively poor area, because most of the people, after time went by, were moving because the industries had disappeared. It wasn't the town that it had been.

He was the son of an Italian immigrant growing up in the Italian ghetto of Newark. I grew up with my father seeing children and people of all ages, as a general practitioner.

As his kids, we went on house calls with him. We would open his office. We would take messages and answer the phone for him. He had a listed phone number! People would come to see him and ring the doorbell at odd hours. I was bathed in that environment.

But the thing that was perhaps more striking than what my father did for a living was the way he did it. He was a very humble fellow, who never flaunted anything. It was like my father was a plumber because we lived in a blue collar neighborhood. I never really thought much about another career. I found my dad's life to be very appealing. He seemed to be having fun, and he was fixing people.

What did your dad think of your interest in medicine?

He thought both my brothers would be physicians. When the Vietnam War got hot, it had the amazing ability to sober people up and get them to study. If you were about to graduate college and you did not have anything else planned, you would be sent to Vietnam.

It's not that I didn't want to go to Vietnam. I would have loved to be a pilot in the Navy, but all of a sudden, I realized it was going to be much harder to get into medical school because excellent students were afraid of not going on to graduate school. I would say that a third of my class in medical school did not share my background nor my perception of what medicine was like, so much as they wanted to keep out of Vietnam.

How hard was it to get into medical school?

It was a very easy admission. I went to St. Peter's College, in Jersey City. This was a first generation college, children of immigrants. Being a student at St. Peter's College—a significant number of St. Peter's graduates went to the state medical school.

At that time, the Medical College Admissions Test was a very important hurdle. Your grade on the test got you your first look into the medical school, so I had to go back and study all those things I didn't study when I was in high school or before I really started to get serious.

I also had a pre-med advisor at the college who was very supportive of my work. He saw something in me. He observed something very subtle in one of the science labs. I was just pouring a solution from a container that was bigger into a smaller container, using a stirring rod to guide the fluid and prevent spilling.

How long before you knew what specialty to pursue?

This may sound inane or silly, but there was one other motivation to study. That was my desire to be a brain surgeon like Ben Casey.[††] Unlike contemporary doctor shows, there was a time in the '50s and '60s when they were somewhat inspirational and probably helped guide people to choose medicine as a career. My father could tell me to study until he was blue in the face, but Ben Casey didn't have to tell me anything. I would just watch the show and found myself motivated.

I did my internship year in general surgery, and then went on to my OB/GYN residency training. I had an interest in obstetrics and gynecology, because of all of the specialties, it seemed to be the most fun. Most of the residents I met as a med student were very dynamic. That's how I was drawn to obstetrics and gynecology.

Do you recall what the first few deliveries or operations were like?

My father, who also gave obstetric anesthesia, brought me to the hospital one night when I was young, because there was nobody to watch me. While he was administering anesthesia, I poked my nose on the other side of the curtain, where they were doing the cesarean section. That was my first experience and I thought it was terrific.

I watched my father straighten bones, set dislocated fingers, and stitch this and that. Actually, as a high school student, the neighborhood kids, if they got hurt, would look at me. "Well, what should I do now?" I was the one who knew to put ice on this and wash it with soap and water. I already knew, just from observing my father, the management of some minor issues in medicine.

As a med student, I recall the first time I was really up close, watching an incision being made into someone's abdomen. My eyeballs almost popped out of my head. The fat layer sort of bulged after the skin was cut, and it was spread apart and bleeding. I thought, *This guy's in a lot of trouble now. How's he going to fix that and put it back together again?*

Doctors often say, watch one, do one, teach one. For some reason, that's the way my mind worked when I watched it. There was a certain logic to what they were doing. There were certain fine movements that I didn't notice, but basically knew what had to be done.

When I was a senior at St. Peter's and my father knew I was accepted into medical school, he started in with, "In my day..." One of his more interesting stories was how interns used to ride the ambulances.

My last half year of college, and my first two years of medical school,

†† A TV series, 1961-66.

I was an ambulance attendant in Manhattan on weekends. I was making great money, and at the same time I saw just the most amazing things in Manhattan that you could imagine. The whole palette of what my father was describing when he used to ride the ambulance.

Give me an example.

We went out on a medical call. It was spring, and this couple had gone for a walk. He was obviously having a heart attack. When we got there, the wife was trying to find his physician. I was new to the job, and the ambulance attendant working with me tried to talk the woman into getting off the phone to take this man to the hospital. The police, finally, helped out too. When we answered a call, there would always be a squad car with two policemen there.

The husband, of course, was scared to death and wanted to go to the hospital. He was in the emergency room for only about five minutes when he went into cardiac arrest. This was somebody I had been talking to just a little while ago. So the cardiac fellow started doing cardiac message, then the resident, and then the intern. Then, it was my turn, as the youngest, perhaps most vigorous person there. We couldn't pull him out. After 45 minutes or more of cardiac message and attempts at resuscitation, he died.

I could see his face—it became mottled. Then, I had to wrap him and bring him down to the morgue. It was my job to put the tag on his toe, wrap him up in plastic, put him on a stretcher and put him in the cooler.

Well, for a month, I saw every relative I had, my father, my uncles, my grandfather; they all had this mottled look on their face in my nightmares. I was pretty much watching everybody die in front of my face.

That stayed with you.

Exactly.

How did you overcome it?

I was already on my way to medical school, and there was two years of basic sciences, so I had a chance to recover. By the time I hit my clinical years, it was never as traumatic as that experience. You'd think that retrieving the body of somebody who jumped 60 stories, or the like, would be more traumatic, but it was really that cardiac arrest episode, having interacted with this person who you are now wrapping and bringing to the morgue.

What was your OB/GYN training like?

It was fun, but I still had this desire to be a neurosurgeon, so my internship before residency was in general surgery. I still wasn't certain about what to do. Then, finally, in 1972 during the earlier part of my internship, I did a rotation in OB/GYN and decided it was going to be OB/GYN.

We were treating infection after infection for septic abortions on women who had illegal abortions. They weren't cared for very well and they would come in with their septic miscarriages. You'd see one, you'd see them all. All night long, people would be coming in, poor women, infected, needing an emergency D & C,[‡‡] antibiotics, maybe a hysterectomy.

How did you transition into what you specialize in now?

I chose OB/GYN because it was a happy specialty. I was a general obstetrician and gynecologist. I began with a year and a half of private practice in fashionable suburb in New Jersey. I came into contact with patients who were very different than the people my father took care of. It wasn't the same. The people weren't as appreciative and a bit more demanding. God only knows why because they certainly had a lot to be grateful for.

On the other hand, I also found private practice, even though I was doing well, was limiting. I really wanted to teach and maybe make other contributions. I had never lived out of the New York metropolitan area. I did all my training within a 25-mile radius of Newark. However, when I was looking for an OB/GYN residency, I did drive from Newark to Atlanta, then back up through Kentucky in the Blue Ridge Mountains, where I had to pull my car over because I couldn't believe how beautiful it was.

I spent my youth playing ball on asphalt playgrounds or on the street. Nobody had any lawns. As a matter of fact, Al {McGuire} at Marquette {University} never wanted anybody playing basketball for him who had a lawn because they had too much. They couldn't be as hungry as people who came from the city. We were not poor, but my father wasn't a high roller by any means.

I made this cross-country trip because I was looking into academic positions. I liked Salt Lake City, because my nieces and nephews were getting old enough to visit their uncle and ski.

Then, I started to meet people from Wisconsin, Illinois, and Minnesota. There was something about the Midwest—it was attractive to me.

While I was at the University of Utah, of course, as a generalist in OB/GYN, I had the opportunity to run a general practice, teach students, and keep my eyes open for something to contribute. But I had not done a fellowship, nor was I a sub-specialist. I didn't spend any time at the National Institutes of Health—all the usual steps that people take who make contributions, except I walked around with my eyes open. I was always thinking about a better way of doing things.

I realized that there were some {doctors} who were limited by those who trained them. The boss said it had to be. I've seen that over and over again in my specialty, and I've seen people who were believed to be smart simply because they trained where someone else trained.

I had no mentor. I did not come from an institution that some of my fellow faculty members came from. I was the only one from New Jersey. I

---

‡‡ Dilation and Curettage is an operation to scrape out the lining of the uterus.

came from a decent medical school, but it was not one of the so-called top 10 medical schools.

I did my residency locally. I was taught by people who went to many different medical schools, so I had 80 teachers with different techniques. But you had to decide what was going to be the best way and safest way to manage a problem, and even think about doing a different way yourself. At Utah, I met people who just never believed that. I was an OB/GYN generalist with common sense.

I was having a lot of fun. I really got into what Utah had to offer—horseback riding, hiking, skiing.

I had grown up in an area where the women teased their hair, chewed gum, had foul mouths. Then, in Utah I saw a woman run after a fly ball, and she caught the ball over her head running away from home plate. I couldn't believe it. There was something really amazing about that. I had a ball there and learned that there were other people in the world.

By the time you moved to Milwaukee, what was the status of your laser surgery?

I moved to the Chicago-Milwaukee area in 1991 because of my commitment to these TTTS patients who might come from throughout the U.S. Salt Lake City was 500 miles from anywhere and you couldn't get there with direct flights.

When I came to St. Joe's {Milwaukee}, the maternal fetal medicine people here said to me, "Why don't we look at the cervix when you use the laser?" The uterus puts pressure on the cervix. Then the cervix gets short. And even though you do the laser or any other treatment, the babies fall out because there's not enough cervix to hold them in. Sometimes, you have to push the water sac back into the mother's uterus if it's in the vagina, and put a stitch there to keep the cervix closed.

When I watched this colleague do this for the first time, it was like seeing an elephant fly. Can this work?

In 2006, we noted a short cervix in 25% of the people I operated on. We find a short cervix, and one of my colleagues stitched her cervix. Throughout the 1990s, the laser surgery had resulted in at least one surviving baby 80% of the time, but I didn't know why it didn't work in the other 20%. My enemies said, "Your operation is causing the loss of the pregnancy." I knew that wasn't the case.

Now, 20-30% of the TTTS patients who come here not only have the laser surgery, but also a cervical repair. Now, more than 90% of the time, at least one of the babies survives. Now, the cerebral palsy or handicaps from those premature deliveries are rare. It isn't just the laser surgery that we've made people aware of. We also made physicians aware of malnutrition and cervical problems in TTTS, and the need to treat those. Unfortunately, many doctors don't think that cervical stitching works.

The point is the doctors did not want to stitch the cervix. Remember, these experts are not surgeons. This is a hard operation to do, putting a stitch in a cervix that is thin, open and where it is. I try to help them as an assistant surgeon, because if they succeed, just like me, we're talking about two human beings' lives, and lives without handicaps.

I'm also known throughout this country as the doctor who recommends fairly strict bed rest and drinking Ensure or Boost throughout the day, when TTTS isn't severe enough to require surgery. You see, I identified severe protein calorie malnutrition in all TTTS mothers, including two women recovering upstairs. They can't believe it. "What do you mean? I live good. I take care of myself." Sick as a dog—dangerously sick.

I was telling a friend a little bit about what you do. And his reaction, was, "What's a guy like that doing in Milwaukee?"

Tell me about it. When I had to operate on someone from Wisconsin, they look at me and I can tell from the expression on their face, because they were told, "You have to see Dr. De Lia over at St. Joe's."

I'll ask, "But are you wondering if I really know what I'm doing? What the hell am I doing in Milwaukee?"

Nine times out of 10, they say, "Yeah." Then, I tell them that I started in Salt Lake City, but knew that I would be operating on people from throughout the United States.

During that first decade, I didn't know anything about their cervix. St. Joe's is the first place I've been where anesthesiologists really understand what I'm doing, because they have full-time OB anesthesiologists here. And, finally, the maternal fetal medicine sub-specialists who assist me knew that there was something about this that probably works, and decided to quit fooling around with all these other nonsensical treatment options.

I was in here on Sunday and Monday with this couple. If these babies live to be 75, I did an operation that prolonged life 150 years. I operated on a set of triplets last summer—225 years and without cerebral palsy. And, in that case, one of my colleagues had to suture her cervix, which was already dilating from the pressure. Not only did we use the laser, we had her on nutritional therapy. Was it the greatest operation that was ever done? I say, yes. What other operation can prolong life 225 years, for babies were almost certain to die or develop cerebral palsy without it?

I tried to get March of Dimes money at the national headquarters. I begged them for money and I haven't gotten a dime. The staff who came to one of my lectures were bouncing off the walls. They could not believe what I was talking about and they had a nurse who said to me, "You're going to have to make an end-run around on some very powerful doctors in this country who influence, by their relationships, the research supported by the March of Dimes."

How many of the TTTS pregnancies are getting the proper treatment?

I don't know. It's really a condition that required a few doctors to think about nearly full-time, which I have, and the result is a whole different perception of the world than other people in my specialty.

Before you operate, they have to find you. Is the Internet still the way couples are finding you?

They do come across me on the Internet, but they also find people who are not totally honest about their capabilities. You've got to have a website that people can find when they've never heard of this before. I did not go near a computer until I was 40 and now, of course, I can't live without one.

Have you thought about your legacy? Are you mentoring anybody else?

{Doctors are} going to put their patients through their own learning curve. Why would they bother to see me?

The couples that I meet, I could probably go from one end of this country to the other and never have to pay for a motel or for dinner. I've helped the majority of couples who've contacted me with mild twin transfusion syndrome manifestations, without having them come here. I have them lie down, drink Ensure, and they get better. And if necessary, I have them get a good doctor to suture their cervix

What's it like to have that kind of job satisfaction?

It's terrific. "Oh, Dr. De Lia, thank you very much." But then, you don't hear from them for a while. How would you like to be changing three diapers, 24 hours per day? These people disappear. They're worn out. I give them a little bit of rest after the surgery, and then the babies are born, and the poop hits the fan, no pun intended. They don't have any time. They forget about me.

Once in a while, it's really a very, very lonely existence. All these people love me, but they're poor now. I make people poor. They buy two-three times as many diapers as you buy. Think about that.

Tiziana Shea

I spoke by phone with TTTS patient Tiziana Shea, of Connecticut, one day after her laser surgery with Dr. De Lia. She was still recuperating at St. Joseph's Hospital in Milwaukee, but spoke with a clear, strong voice.

I met Dr. De Lia through the Internet and also through my doctor in Connecticut. When we were diagnosed with twin-to-twin-transfusion syndrome, it was very difficult on me and my husband, so my sister looked it up to try to get more information for us. When we were first diagnosed around 17 weeks, we weren't quite sure what all of our options were, but we soon found out. I'm lying in bed recovering right now.

How did things go?

So far, it looks like it was pretty successful. I'm in a lot of pain, but other than that, there were two heartbeats this morning.

If you hadn't had this surgery, what was at stake?

One of our daughters would have had heart problems, and we might be looking at the loss of both of our babies. A lot of people were telling us to end the pregnancy, telling us that the surgery is dangerous. But we decided we have to do this for our girls. There are a lot of people who really don't understand.

My due date is October 10, but we expect them earlier than that. When we came into this, we really thought we had a chance to save both of our babies, but only time will tell.

My biggest qualm is that I would have liked my doctors to have understood the surgery and explained it better to me, and maybe not push so hard for ending the pregnancy.

Postscript: The Shea girls were born by cesarean section in Connecticut, August 15, 2005, two months premature. The recipient, Isabella was 3 lbs. 5 oz and her sister the donor, Mira was 3 lbs. 1 oz. They were both admitted into the neonatal intensive care unit, where Isabella would stay about one month before coming home. Mira stayed about six weeks, due to an intestinal disease related to prematurity. At their first birthday, they weighed around 18 pounds each. "They are in the beginning stages of walking, and are a handful! It's great," writes Tiziana in an e-mail. "I take nothing for granted with these two. They are amazing, and I can't say enough, how highly we regard Dr. De Lia."

Note: De Lia's dream is to create a Foundation in Milwaukee, for TTTS patients who lack insurance coverage, or can't afford to travel. See the link at www.whitecoatwisdom.com.

CHAPTER EIGHT

DELIVERING THE MALE

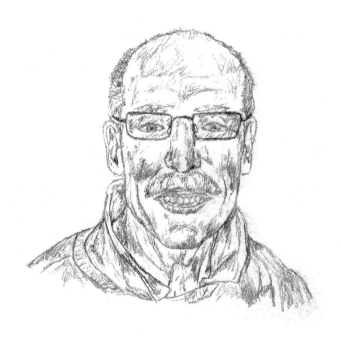

"Males are, in small part because of biology and large measure because of behavior, the more needy and weaker sex. Yet, men are taken care of, from a preventive health perspective, at a rate that's one half that of women."

Robert Alt, MD
Internist, Madison

Men take great pride in maintaining their cars, but when it comes to their own bodies, well, the wheels fall off. Doctor Robert Alt is convinced that men die younger than women largely because of self-neglect.

In his own practice, Alt systematically tries to even the odds for men by getting them into the office more regularly for preventive health check-ups, as well as employing some other rather creative strategies.

He explained how he became so impassioned about men's health, ironically, when his initial foray into medicine was in the female dominated nurs-

ing profession. Doctor Alt, who's in his early 60s, gave me an example of what he thinks is all wrong about men's health habits.

———

A married, father of two, was passing some blood with his stools. He rationalized that, thinking he had some hemorrhoids. He had not had a physical exam since high school. He was traveling, and for the first time in his adult life, he claimed, had an {extra-marital} sexual encounter. He confessed his failure to his wife, who remained loyal to him. His wife was responsible for dragging him into my room.

When I saw him, he'd suffered with intermittent rectal bleeding for a year, and was losing weight. What brought him in was his sexual indiscretion. He felt he had AIDS, so we did various tests. He did not have AIDS, but mild anemia was present in his lab.

We did a complete physical exam and arranged for him to have a colonoscopy and we found a malignant lesion in his colon, which blessedly, we were able to remove. It was against all odds and was contained. He was, apparently, cured at this time.

This case illustrates many of the characteristics of the present status of men's health. When they do have a problem, they overlook it as long as they possibly can, and the problem may well be far advanced when they're first seen.

At what stage in your career did you develop this interest in men's health?

First, I got married and watched my own partner undergo the transformations associated with the women's movement, which were very significant and advantageous. It was very dynamic, very empowering. The second thing that played a very potent role for me was the fact that, just as I entered medicine late, I married late. We had one child. I watched him go through school, and as I watched him, I recognized that to a great extent, the pendulum had swung from being unfair to women to neglecting or even disadvantaging males.

Thirty-five years ago, we assumed that everything was loaded in favor of men. For example, all the medical research studied men and didn't pay attention to women, so the whole institution of both society and medicine was kind of oriented toward being supportive of men, and to some extent to the detriment of women. In fact, what was happening was an almost Victorian gentleman's code, which did not want to subject women to the vagaries of research, did not want to subject them to potentially harm a fetus.

More chivalry than blatant discrimination, the way it evolved?

Some of the things; not all, and I don't mean to be an apologist for the way society was. There were many injustices. As I watched my son and his buddies growing up, they lacked the kind of models of excellence which young females had. The boys suffered a shift in the way that the schools educate children, that seems to value feminine ways of teaching more. We're really not paying enough attention to boys and men. As a consequence, males are really struggling. It culminates in the shorter by five years life span guys have.

If you look back in history, to say, around the 1920s, male and female life expectancy was always very close. On the other hand, there had always been more male conceptions than female conceptions.

Similarly, there are some psychological challenges which are biologically inherent in being a male, in the sense that a boy has to separate himself from a very caring, very feminine milieu that he grows up in as a child in order to become a male. However, the effect of biology is relatively small compared to the behavioral impacts that cause premature mortality and morbidity {illness}.

For example, guys visit physicians' offices for preventive health services at about half the rate of female visits. Every year in the United States, for example, males have 150 million fewer preventive health visits in doctors' offices. The balance could be corrected by every male having a once yearly preventive health check. That's something which I've been lobbying for throughout the time that I've been interested in men's health.

What typically happens to females is that about the time that menses begin, they begin to have yearly physical exams. From adolescence, girls are programmed to visit their doctor once a year for a pelvic exam, and in the course of that visit, what actually happens is a lot of primary care. There is a wide consensus about its value and its essential nature

I've done a chart review at our clinic, which concluded that in the course of the annual visit for a pelvic exam and general gynecology evaluation, more time was spent doing essentially preventive health and primary care activities than was actually spent on the pelvic exam.

What we need for men is a way to bring them into the clinic in an analogous way. At every age, there's an opportunity to talk with men about the way they're behaving: Are they practicing safe sex? Do they drive carefully, wearing seatbelts? Do they drink too much or smoke? Are they careless about eating? Are they cutting corners about their sleep? Are they having success at work? Do they have friends? Men often don't have any friends. Do they have faith? Having faith affects their resiliency as they go through their lives. Do they know their cholesterol and blood pressure?

At every stage of a male's life, he suffers higher levels of morbidity and mortality than women. Although all the statistics show that males are, in small part because of biology, and large measure because of behavior, the more needy and weaker sex, we are taken care of, from a preventive health perspective, at a rate that's half that of women.

What's required is a major educational effort to get guys to come in.

117

We need institutions to make a commitment to see men at a frequency that we're seeing women.

It would require HMOs going through their statistics, their records, and saying, "Joe, you've been paying us premiums for the last five years and you haven't seen a doctor or any other health professional in that whole time. We want to take care of you."

There's a large push for evidence-based medicine right now, and one of the weaknesses of evidence-based medicine is that it does not study the underserved well. If you ask me to scientifically prove the advantage of having a man come in to the clinic once a year for a visit, I would be hard pressed. I'm making my recommendation for an annual preventive health visit for men on the basis of common sense and the belief that preventive health interventions are valuable.

I'd also base it on the fact that in the course of my visits with both men and women, their annual visits, I almost never fail to make an intervention which may be life saving. We can't necessarily measure it, but whether I'm telling a fellow to start aspirin or to exercise more, or diet more, or sleep, it's in the nature of preventive health that this may be extraordinarily beneficial.

Plus, there's the whole area of emotions, where guys are at such a disadvantage. It's common wisdom that women suffer more from anxiety and depression. Yet, paradoxically, almost all of the suicides in the United States are from men. There's a disconnect here, and I believe it has to do with the fact that if you ask, first of all, guys are simply not forthcoming about their emotions. They will deny being sad or troubled.

I even had a man I'd seen shortly before he committed suicide, who I interrogated about his emotions, and that's not an uncommon experience. It's essential that we establish relationships with these guys who are so reticent about their emotional needs in order to build the trust that enables us to reach them.

At every one of my annual visits with guys, I'll beat the bushes trying to figure out where this fellow is emotionally. Does he have a good relationship? Is he angry? Sometimes if we really have established trust, I can talk directly with him about whether he's feeling sad or anxious. Often, that direct questioning will be a possibility only if I establish considerable rapport.

It is very much the case that guys simply don't take good care of themselves anymore. In today's paper, there was a story about a coach {who had testicular cancer}. He woke one morning and went downstairs, and the world just went blurry. He couldn't focus his eyes and he couldn't get balanced. He wasn't going to wake his wife and bother her. He was going to solve this himself. He had suffered two strokes. It took a combination of literally, blinding headaches, coughing up blood and finally, probably most persuasively, his scrotum was so swollen he couldn't get on a bike. He had a combination of all three of those excessive symptoms before he would go see a doctor. Testicular cancer is eminently treatable if it's found early. Guys think they're invincible, that this just can't happen to you. When it happens, reality sets in. You either change or you die.

If you believe in preventive health, you want to know a guy's cholesterol when he's 20; not when he's 44 and has heart disease. It just doesn't make sense to wait.

What is it about men that they don't think it's necessary to go in to see a doctor?

It's thought to be macho. The male code permits men to have only one emotion, which is anger. It generally doesn't permit us to have close male friends with whom we are truly intimate.

The tragedy of the *"Brokeback Mountain"* movie is that the suggestion for a man to have a close male friend is it will result in an erotic relationship. Two damaging principles that guys are taught are homophobia and competitiveness. For that reason, we rarely have close friends, so the male code involved being independent, being isolated, usually, being strong, being aggressive, only being able to express anger.

We're taught that big boys don't cry. If it works, don't fix it. Don't sweat the small stuff. Those are all attitudes that lead us to overlook the small symptoms of what may become major problems at a time when we could do something about it.

There are so many ads on TV today that are just amazing because they so carefully illustrate what our culture is saying to men. There's one ad for beer and these guys are pictured sitting on a sofa. They're watching a football game and they're having pizza. One guy on the end is blotting the grease off his pizza. The other two guys look at him like he's nuts and the saying is, "Be a man." A big, giant beer can comes down and whacks this guy and he just disappears.

The whole message is, again, "Don't take care of yourself." That by definition is what it is to be a man. To be a man is to be careless, to not be careful, to ignore the fact that you're having a stroke. In extreme cases, it's to ignore the fact that you're spitting up blood.

So do you recommend that all of your male patients in every age group see you every year?

Yes, I do. I start taking care of males and females when they're 18. I use the testicular exam the way gynecology uses the pelvic. I use it as a realistic preventive health intervention, which I think is evidence-based.

Every male from 15 to 35 should have an annual testicular exam by a health professional because those are the ages of the highest incidence of testicular cancer. They should also do monthly testicular self exams, which few know to do. Once I have a male there, then I can do all the other health measures which are important.

If an HMO wanted to distinguish itself to a health-purchasing group like General Motors, it would be strategic to reach out to men. We're health professionals. We believe in prevention, so that a person doesn't need to be sick to come in.

Guys die five years younger than women. A lot of that is because of bad health behaviors. We, as professional care givers, should set as a top priority that we will reach out to men. We should do anything we can to get guys to come in for medical visits at a rate that approximates women's. I'd like to say that to all the major health organizations throughout the United States.

If that were to happen, wouldn't HMOs save money by catching illness early?

Theoretically, it would be valuable for health organizations to be doing preventive health, but you have to realize that health care organizations are driven by two motivations: one is altruism, the desire to keep people well, and the other is profit.

Our organizations are financial entities just like any other financial entity. Their window is way shorter than the benefits that they may reap by taking care of somebody at an early age. In other words, my finding high cholesterol in a young man who's 23 years old, may be beneficial to someone—certainly the patient when he's 44—but that man may be in a whole different state, let alone our present health care organizations.

Health care organizations don't have the long view that is necessary, so something really needs to happen that enables us to value preventive health delivery at the time that it is delivered.

If we were in some sort of fee-for-service situation, in a competitive marketplace the health care organizations would be fighting over men because they don't have to expand their geography. They just have to get men to come in.

How difficult is it to get men to come in?

It's very difficult. I can give an example. We had an employee health fair directed just toward men at St. Mary's Hospital. We beat the bushes. We sent notices around. We had awards. There were many prizes, including Packer tickets, but the response was disappointing.

You have to realize that the forces of society, the forces of men's peer groups, are marshaled against their taking care of themselves. It really takes outreach to get them in.

I'm the director of the Men's Health Service at the clinic and our first publicity was to make two pamphlets, one directed to women and one directed to men. That was an attempt to try to help the women to help to get their guys to come in, because women play a vital role in getting their partners, or their dads or brothers, or their sons, in to the clinic, because otherwise they have to suffer their male partner's decline. They have to listen to them whine {laughs} or, they end up having to live without them for multiple years, as they grow older.

Work is another way to get guys to come in. I've worked with a few employers that do a really great job of getting their guys to attend medical services that they offer on site. Screening, they offer rewards, lower health premiums, so it's money in the guy's pocket.

Work is a primary focus of guys' lives, but I don't necessarily think it's a cause of why they don't come in, that they're busier. It is true that the times that doctors' offices are open are during the traditional work hours. As more women are in the workplace, this impacts them as well.

How important are a doctor's recommendations? If you recommend he come in, how likely is he to do so?

Very high. When I conclude my visit with a male patient, he will leave my office with a written instruction about the timing of his next visit and complete physical or a reminder of that exact date.

If I'm seeing a young man, maybe 22, and I've just done a preventive care visit, he will leave my office with an after-visit summary. I say, "Go right out to the reception desk and set it up right now." I have a high percentage of follow-up visits. Once I have a male or female engaged in the process of being connected, the success rate of maintaining that connection is extremely high.

That's extraordinary. I don't know any doctors who are doing that. Do you have a sense for whether you have a healthier population of male patients than the typical physician in Madison?

Well, that's wishful thinking. One of my other passions is the health history and I also give every one of my patients a full and wallet sized copy of their health history. It has been the most powerful thing that I have done for my patients. One of the core three or four important activities for primary care doctors to accomplish for their patients is management of their patients' health history. The reason it's so important is because the health history also includes preventive health measures that you want to maintain. Over the past nine years, I've made a New Year's resolution for my practice for every single one of those years, and they're ongoing.

One year, I will give every one of my patients a power of attorney for health care form. With the health history process in place, the fact that I've done it and the fact that the patient has completed it or not completed it, is in their health record, in their health history. So every year that they keep coming back, they haven't done their power of attorney for health care, I ask them about it. I don't nag. I just say, "Have you done it?" If they haven't done it, I say, "Do you have it? Do you still have the forms?" If they haven't, I give them a fresh copy.

Another year, my resolution was to focus on all my patients who reached the right age for gastrointestinal preventive health.

Another New Year's resolution was to change all of my patients' prescriptions to be written in language that was oriented toward their understanding. I wouldn't say "propranolol, 20 mg, BID" and give the number of refills. I would say "propranolol, 20 milligrams, twice a day to lower blood pressure and calm the heart." That was an enormous undertaking, especially if you have a patient on 15 meds, but I did that for everyone.

Giving everybody their health history is a multi-year resolution. My current New Year's resolution is to introduce all my patients to a program that allows them to access their chart electronically, and my second focus is to amplify their social history so that I know what their interests are. I've done these resolutions year after year, so I've had 10 or 12 things that are ongoing. Last year, my resolution was an aspirin analysis because a lot of patients should be taking aspirin.

Each time I've done these, all my patients who should be taking aspirin are taking aspirin. When I focus on this, I was astonished at the number of my patients who have high blood pressure or high cholesterol or diabetes who were not yet taking aspirin. It shocked me.

So when you ask me, is my population healthier than the rest of the population? I don't want to come across as boasting, but with respect to this activity in which I provide my patients with their health history, I am able to give to them a demonstrably superior product in that regard. With respect to each of these resolutions I've undertaken, I'm probably operating a practice that is superior to my colleagues.

If I was to have a head to head comparison to Dr. A, B or C on completed more power of attorneys for health care, whether more of my patients have their gastrointestinal preventive health, their mammograms, their pap smears, etc. than these other doctors, then I'm doing a pretty good job.

It is the primary care doctor's responsibility to establish and maintain the health history. In so doing, they will be giving the highest quality of care because they'll be paying attention to preventive health. Patients will know their diagnoses. They will know their family history and immunizations. They'll have it all there. If they have an emergency, they can reach into their pocket and give it to the emergency room doc.

I take their health history and I reduce it by 50%, and it becomes the size of a quarter of a piece of paper. They fold it up and put in a little plastic envelope and put it with my card in their purse or wallet and they're good to go.

I just had an elderly patient who was visiting family in Texas when he had a crisis. He has a list that's probably 15 problems long, and a medicine list that's literally 20 medicines long. He had his health history. It was very beneficial when he required hospitalization.

You're so passionate about what you do. What drew you to medicine in the first place?

I came to it late, actually. I've been practicing 20 plus years, but I didn't get into medicine until I was deep in my 30s.

I was traveling in the Far East, and I spent about 18 months traveling around the world in my late 20s. I was sort of searching for myself. It became a goal as a traveler to stay out on the road. I'd met people who'd been out for years doing various things. I felt a little uncomfortable in my role as a tourist, because I felt like a consumer. I was just taking from whatever situation I was presently in, and it felt a little bit superficial.

I was really struck by an experience that I had around Calcutta and Bangladesh, where I encountered people who were working in Save the Children. The people I met were doctors, nurses, and other health professionals. They would have a profession in their home country, but periodically they would go to crises around the world. It struck me as this would be a way to travel about the globe in a way that you weren't just a tourist. It was a way where you could contribute wherever you were.

When I finally went back to the states, after I got back on my feet, one of the first things I did was apply for medical school. They told me I was too old. I was 28. That was in Colorado, where I returned because some friends were there.

I continued what I was doing, and was actually coordinating a Denver Free University. It was that hippy time when free universities were operating. Among the classes we offered were a first aid training program and a nursing assistant program.

To coordinate this program, you talked to a bazillion people, to try to coax them into teaching at the University, helped produce the catalogue, answered the phone, and cleaned the floors.

Eventually, I jumped into a course myself and became a nursing assistant. Next, I enrolled in the community college of Denver's LPN program. They had a program that was a "ladder concept" where you could practice and go to school, so I became an LPN and eventually enrolled in and completed an RN program.

Each time I was working and going to school part-time. It took me a whole decade, in the 1970s, to finally earn an associate degree RN. I tried practicing, and was the head nurse of the first in-patient hospice unit in Denver. That was kind of the culmination of my nursing career. Then, I applied to go on to become an advanced degree nurse.

But I realized that at the end of another three or four years of school and work, I would still emerge as a nurse, which I cherish as a noble profession. But I realized that I was going to spend all this time, and at the end of it I would be exactly what I was at the beginning of it, but with a bachelor's degree.

At that point, I enrolled in premed courses, finished those, and enrolled in medical school. I was finally accepted back at Loyola University in Maywood, which is what drew me back to the Midwest from my beloved Colorado.

Before travel, nursing and medicine, I was also a teacher. As a teacher, I was a member of a religious order called the Christian Brothers. This order was dedicated to teaching the poor, young males of France. One of the vows we took was to teach the poor without being reimbursed for your work. During this time, we wore these outfits that were all black and I lived in a totally male community and taught boys.

While I was in training to become a nurse, I coordinated a nursing lab at the community college that I attended. I wore white, because I was a nurse and I was working primarily with women, because at that time, all the nurses in training were women. It was like a 180 degree polar opposite, gender-wise.

Did your nursing background enhance your ability to get into medical school? How come you weren't too old to get in the second time?

Ageism, as a prejudice, became more prevalent, and so medical schools could not exclude people because they were older. Our medical school class had a number of older students.

My nursing background did absolutely help. It lent credibility to my aspirations in medicine. By the time I got into medical school, I had a ten-year history of working in health-related areas, so folks could recognize that I had staying power and a vocation, as it were.

Going to medical school and participating in the medical training program was extremely rigorous. I related to it as almost a boot camp for the profession. There was the dichotomy between the younger students and us, the more mature people. We used to be very serious compared to them. We'd sit up in front, and we had life experience and recognized that this was a once in a lifetime opportunity. We tended to be a little bit more intense and directed as students.

There were some circumstances in which the volume of patient needs were overwhelming and really, especially as part of the residency program, threatened to just swamp one.

On the other hand, it was utterly thrilling to me that I had the opportunity to have multiple professions and multiple, almost, incarnations, in a single life. I went through decades of my life when I was a young person in school, then a teacher, then searching, then the whole nursing thing and medicine. There was enough of a change in those areas in terms of orientation and capabilities that it was a dramatic thing.

As you were going through your medical training, did you have more respect for nurses, since that was your background?

There was a natural rapport. I had made the beds. I had given the back rubs. I cleaned bottoms. I had struggled with getting IVs inserted. It made me aware that when things didn't happen the way I ordered it as a doctor, in many respects, it was because of the difficulties which the nurses encountered and the practical realities of their challenging lives.

Usually, the knowledge that I was a nurse followed me and enabled me to deal with all levels of nursing people with empathy. I could easily astonish the nursing assistants by straightening a bed linen and do some of that basic stuff every so often.

Did you have any difficulty deciding what specialty you would pursue?

I realized that there was value in some level of specialization, and that I just couldn't do it all. I'm self aware enough that I felt I needed to limit the enormous content of medical skills in order to be able to feel comfortable that I was doing some good for people.

I also liked the intellectual nature of internal medicine. As an internist, it's extremely demanding and constantly changing. I very much appreciate change and there has been so much continuous change in medicine that it's hard to keep up with it.

Previously, I would do something for five or 10 years, and then I have that tremendous need to do something different. Medicine is the one place where there is enough challenge inherent in the profession that I haven't had to burn my bridges and do something entirely different.

While changing the nuances within the profession, that was my current passion for a time, I was able to play roles in the clinic where I've been able to help coordinate and facilitate changes within the clinic. Each of those has been a major, multi-year commitment, because of the pace of changes. The pace of change in organizations is somewhat slow, so patience is essential.

Another thing that appealed to me about internal medicine was that I started out in my first profession out of high school or college, as a teacher, and I also saw, to a certain extent, that medicine, as an internist, involves a lot of teaching. I saw that as kind of completing the circle, enabling me to use all my previous skills.

My older sister became a teacher. My younger brother became a lawyer, and my younger sister was a nurse. We grew up on the west side of Chicago near Garfield Park. It was sort of a mixture of Irish Catholics, Italians, Jewish, and some early Hispanic immigrants. It was a great place to grow up.

My dad was a bridge tender for the City of Chicago. My mom worked part-time at Sears. She did that for almost all of our growing up. My folks were sort of raised on the tradition, as first and second generation folks, that to be a professional was a highly desirable aspiration. They really pushed us. The way to "make it" was to successfully have a practice or profession.

As you look back at the profession you chose, and the emphasis you've put on men's health, are you at all concerned about inadvertently creating the opposite problem, that men may come to the doctor for every little thing?

I had a quote on my bulletin board, "The less you think about your health, the better." Now, that quote is relevant to about 50% of the people—a group of folks who are the worried well. For them, that quote is pertinent. For the other 50% of folks, and many guys are in that population, they need to spend more time attending to their health needs and their ailments, and getting taken care of.

Any parting advice for men?

First is, to do as good a job of taking care of yourself as you would your car. Do the fundamental things to take care of your body and your person. You need to listen to your body. You need to respond to inexplicable events and symptoms, and bring them to someone's attention—the doc's attention. Share it with your wife or a friend. Air it out. Ideally, if it is a physical problem or emotional problem, get medical attention. Those types of problems are what we're supposed to be tracking and taking care of as health professionals.

Take heed of your feelings. You may be sad. You may be anxious. You may feel powerless. You may be frustrated. Those are all feelings that we men tend to transmute into anger, so listen to yourself and get help.

It takes courage to resist the macho, careless stereotypes. It takes courage to take care of yourself because you've been taught to not do that. After all, since we've been taught that to have courage is manly, having the courage to take care of yourself, to seek help, to seek answers about things that may be wrong with yourself, is real manliness.

CHAPTER NINE

UNCONVENTIONAL WISDOM

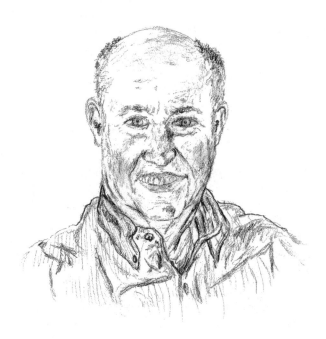

"The sublingual approach I've proven works for molds. Shots do not work, as well. We've treated 70,000 people at our clinic, and I would say as many as half had asthma."

David Morris, MD
Family Practice & Allergy, La Crosse

Who wouldn't prefer a few drops under the tongue to allergy shots, especially if they're more effective? No surprise that patients have voted with their feet to see a doctor who swears by the approach.

In the medical community, however, Dr. Dave Morris is something of an outcast. For the past several decades, he's been treating allergy patients with a therapy most of his colleagues discredit. It's known as sublingual antigen treatment. The theory is that antigens–substances that induce an allergy fighting mechanism–trigger cells under the tongue to shut down, or at least slow, an allergic reaction. Many doctors dispute the theory. When I asked a skeptical allergist why so many patients would keep coming back to Dr. Morris for an ineffective treatment, he said Morris is just a "good salesman."

Well, he must be good because patients from across the country come to his La Crosse clinic for this unconventional therapy, which Dr. Morris claims is 90% effective. So effective, apparently, that he has accumulated enough resources to create a Foundation, the largest recipient of which is the University of Wisconsin Medical School. In 2000, David and Sacia Morris donated $2 million, which was used to establish the Morris Institute for Respiratory Research.

Morris, in his late 70s, is casually dressed, soft spoken, and is quite relaxed as he discusses how he came to rely on his controversial treatment method.

I saw a woman who had spent more than a week at a {research center} in Colorado, and brought a very thick record with her. She had just spent five days at {another major allergy clinic} and was told that they couldn't help her. She didn't have allergies. It was odors and chemicals that bothered her. Over the last many years, her husband refused to quit smoking. She had spent $41,000 in the last month or so through their workup and when they got through, they had no diagnosis and no treatment.

Sublingual antigens cost no more than $3 a week for whatever inhalants we treat. Treating foods and chemicals, that costs $3.50 or $4 a week, keeping in mind that the better antihistamines are two dollars apiece a day.

How did she find you?

Somebody who was also at the clinic, told her to come to La Crosse. One of the things that I've tested and treated for 37 years is formaldehyde, because it causes a lot of trouble with dermatitis. They itch all over and any place they touch, it breaks out, easily becomes infected. We've had horrible cases. It's so heartwarming when they come back without asthma, maybe some stuffy nose and hay fever, no skin lesions. Sublingual is the only way they can be treated for the foods and inhalants.

On her skin test for that, it was a very strong positive reaction. I only started seeing her yesterday, but she'll start taking drops. On the basis of skin testing, there are a number of molds we'll be treating, and formaldehyde, sublingually. It's exciting to see patients respond with the dendritic cells under the tongue. It turns allergies off.

That's really the effect. It ends the allergy?

Well, it cuts it down. Down regulates would be the scientific word for it, and it's one of the things that has been somewhat puzzling. Doctor Walter Canonica—whom I visited a couple times in Europe, was the first one to actually show that when you give patients drops under the tongue, they actually stay under the tongue for up to 20 hours. Of course, at first we thought they were absorbed quickly like nitroglycerin. It's immediately into the bloodstream.

What we've learned over the past 10 years in our practice is that the people with very strong allergy, like to ragweed, birch, grass, dust mites, or mold, actually need a much larger dose, sublingually, to counteract it. And this last year a doctor in Germany has pointed out that the higher the person's allergy, the more dendritic cells they have under the tongue, the more they're actually coated with specific IgE *antibodies. When you put the drop in the mouth, it stimulates those.

All of our patients are treated with the very best antihistamines and the topical steroid-type things for the nose and for the lungs. But we find they do much better than on medication alone, and many after a while, don't need the medication. They all have it. If they need it, they take it.

So how many types of allergies are helped by this?

All types. We see people from all over the country with chronic sinus conditions who've had multiple sinus surgeries, who've had shots for 20 years for molds, and in a matter of a month or two, we can get a response.

I imagine patient referral is a big part of your practice.

Most is patient referral. If you have a terrible eczema and all of a sudden your skin is clear, it's pretty easy for people to say, "Where did you clear it up?"

Clinton, Iowa, is an extremely strong place for Allergy Associates. It started while I was still in West Salem {Wisconsin}. A young man who spent most of his time at the University of Iowa Hospital with his asthma saw me, and I was able to diagnose food allergy, which nobody had before. He had inhalant drops, too, but he got well. His parents and friends—everybody started coming to La Crosse, instead of Iowa City.

We must have hundreds of patients from Clinton. We still see most of the patients who are having terrible trouble, who are more apt to go to La Crosse than any place. I've been in the La Crosse area since 1957, doing family practice and allergy from '57 to 1970 and then limiting myself to allergy, starting Allergy Associates in 1970. We occupy almost the whole first floor of the Professional Arts building, and we are now five physicians, one of whom is my daughter, who has been a partner for 14 years.

My daughter, Mary, is doing her research project on the sublingual treatments on dust mites in children. Our experience is that when you catch them when they only have stuffy noses, they never get asthma. If you get rid of their dust mite allergy, they get better.

Asthma is a terrible, disruptive illness, and the incidence has gone up tremendously over the last five, 10 years. With asthma, it's usually molds that are the worst problem. The sublingual approach, I've proven, works

IgE is an abbreviation for the protein immunoglobulin gamma E.

for molds. Shots do not work, as well. We've treated 70,000 people at our clinic and as many as half had asthma. With our treatment, they do better.

The largest collection of dendritic cells in the body is right under the tongue—sublingual area. When they're stimulated, they actually down regulate allergy through the cervical lymph nodes...which is the ideal for immunotherapy.[†] Here it is, directly related to sublingual antigens.

Are the skeptics still there or have you won them over?

They're still there. The less people know about it, the more violently they speak about it. The very best allergists in the United States have a very open mind to it.

At the University of Wisconsin, their allergists, 30 years ago, were extremely negative about what I do. My wife and I decided to start giving heavily to the University of Wisconsin Medical School, where I owe a great deal of gratitude for my medical education and the influence of the doctors there. Four years ago, we had given so much more than any other person or drug company, that they wanted to name it for us. It's the Morris Institute for Respiratory Research on the ninth floor, K tower. They've done great research over the last 25 years. There were no strings attached to our gift, except that it be integrated research, that not just allergists, but pulmonologists, pediatrician experts in cystic fibrosis—they would all have access to the labs at the Morris Institute.

What kept you going, to persevere, when people said this wasn't workable?

I got my satisfaction from my patients for many, many years. We see patients on half of the Saturday mornings. They're usually people who come just once or twice a year. These are people whose whole lives have changed because they no longer have asthma. They no longer itch all over. They no longer get sinus infections, one after another.

When I was 16, they elected me president as a senior at Waukesha High School. That helped me a lot. The person I ran against was very popular, very top athlete and everything, and by golly, they chose me. I graduated from high school a few days after my 17th birthday, so the extra year worked out just fine.

At Carroll {Wisconsin College}, I had a chance to play football for four years and do track for four years. I was never real good in basketball, but I could run fast. I was on the team for freshman and sophomore years, so that helped with my attitude. I kept working. I had a double major of chemistry and biology in college.

My dad was the hardest worker I ever knew. My father had been a farmer. He had a sixth grade education. My mother had an eighth grade education, and took a correspondence or a short course in stenography.

My mother was an optimist. She always thought I should make some-

† Immunotherapy is a treatment that relies on natural substances in the body to fight infection and disease.

thing of myself, and she was pretty sure I would. They both reached the late '80s, but their brains didn't make it that long. I think they'd both be proud of their son.

What drew you to medicine?

I knew that I was smart. I was actually planning to go to Purdue, in engineering, and my cousin and I, after I worked at the foundry for six weeks, saved enough money so that we took a car to California. My mother said be sure and stop and see your cousins in Santa Barbara. When we got there, {one cousin} was a young ear, nose and throat doctor, just getting out of the service and {another} was an anesthesiologist. Instead of staying overnight, we spent almost a week with them.

During that time, they took me to see their offices and hospital, and thought that I should really think about medicine. It was the hardest thing to get into, and I realized that these cousins had a really good life. They enjoyed what they were doing and it just turned out that I wanted to give it a try.

When I came back to Waukesha, I registered at Carroll College and decided to take two years to decide what to do. At the end of the first semester, I realized that I really did want to go into medicine. The fourth year, I had interviewed with Dean Middleton {University of Wisconsin Medical School} midway through my junior year, and he told me I could come for the next year or the year after.

In those days, there weren't Med Cats[‡] and so on, but my record and my recommendations must have been very good. I was dating Sacia, who now is my wife, and realized if I didn't stay for senior year, I might lose her, so, it was very much worthwhile.

Medical school was a whole new experience. I was very impressed with the instructors and I was a serious student.

So at what point in your medical training did you start thinking about allergy?

When I was a junior, some of the good research on Farmer's Lung was being done at the University. It was a very common problem with the baling and stacking hay. It always got moldy, so it was a very brutal type illness for a farmer to get. It starts with coughing and wheezing, and ends up with systemic infection-like symptoms: chills, fever, aching, weakness, fatigue.

A young assistant professor, in smaller group discussions, really helped you think out of the box about what's going on with these people. Why should they get this pulmonary problem? I took extra allergy because I just happened to be interested in it. As a junior in medical school, actually, I knew much of what they knew about allergy in those days, because very little was known. We didn't have mold extracts that we could test or

‡ Medical College Admission Test

treat, so it was a very beginning-type knowledge we had in allergy. But it fascinated me.

When I got in the service, in the Air Force, we had a dermatologist come to the base for skin problems and I always made sure that I was with him. Why should one soldier get a tremendous dermatitis from a fungus and the next have a little athlete's foot and get over it by themselves? We had absolutely no anti-fungals, so you really saw the breadth of what molds and fungi can do.

I had been in a full-time practice of allergy for two or three years and had published two articles in peer-reviewed journals. I applied to take the boards in allergy. I had boards in family practice by examination, too. They have special courses that last a week and you study up to pass the boards. Well, I had three weeks with nothing but my brain, and it was actually one of the happiest days of my life because I knew the material and—I wasn't writing it to pass; I was writing it for an A. I knew they couldn't flunk me and they didn't. I got my boards in '73.

In the late 60s, I was able to identify a case of mucor mycosis.§ This farmer had hay bales against cement walls all the way around the barn, and they always got moldy, so he just left them there. It meant that every year he was getting the same mold back in the new hay, as well as in the old, moldy bales. I worked with him carefully and was able to get extracts of mucor and I felt I could diagnose it. When I talked about this at the Wisconsin Allergy Society, I had such horrendous criticism from one or two allergists there. They knew that mucor could not cause farmer's lung because they were taught that.

Was it considered so far off base to the medical community back then?

It was considered totally off base. And of course, for 15 years in Europe, now two-thirds of the people in southern Europe with allergies, get sublingual treatment.

Are there any more allergists in this community, or in Wisconsin, who are doing this as well?

We've had meetings once or twice a year, and we've had allergists, I think, from 45 states and four continents who have come to learn, so there will be many more. It does take a while to get started and to know how to do it. But in the years ahead, there will be more and more doctors doing it because it works on things like mold when mold shots don't work. I got a lot of sore arms and fever, and disgruntled patients, and that's where I started looking for a better way. In a matter of six or seven years, I helped farmers not with just bad sinus or with farmer's lung, but with asthma.

Do you tend to get the cases that other doctors are unable to solve?

Ah, yes. And it's kind of fun because most of them can still be helped.

§ Mucor mycosis is an infection involving an ulcer in a patient with a weakened immune system.

The traditional allergist is very limited in what he can do with allergy shots. It's really seasonal hay fever, and nowadays, with the newer medications, they're really all you need for the four to six-week hay fever season. To get shots for over a year or five, just for relief during ragweed season, is just not cost effective.

Even patients with emphysema—I've tried to treat these people all these years and it seemed like I was helping them. We've looked at it, and quite a high percentage—as many as 40, 50% actually, who, after six months or a year or two of treatment, their breathing actually improves.

Doctors from Vancouver, British Columbia very carefully dissected and studied lungs from people with COPD, and lo and behold, along the very tiniest airways, there's still marked inflammatory cells, which means there's still a very active disease process. And so it's not just giving them prednisone and oxygen, and watching them die, 10% a year. That's a place where people will do what we've been doing and see some improvement in such a difficult problem as emphysema.

Is there any down side to sublingual?
Uh, no.

If it doesn't work, it doesn't work. They're no worse off?
Right. It takes very careless dosing to aggravate an allergy symptom, and if you stay within ranges you just don't see it.

What is your typical success rate?
We've done questionnaires, and it's over 90%.

It would be hard for a more conventional allergist to beat that, wouldn't it?
I'm sure.

Have you ever considered opening clinics in other states?
We'll actually be helping a doctor open a clinic in the southern United States, the first of January. We'll help him to know how to do it. Allergists are going to have to find out that things are changing, and that another way is out there, and it's a better way.

Tell me a little about your relationships with patients. If you're able to do what others have been unable to, how do they react to you?
They love me, in the sense that if you're a physician and you treat a patient and you help 'em, there's a relationship there—in a broad sense, a love relationship. If somebody suffered terribly from allergies, and all of a sudden, they're good and they come to see me once a year, they're elated every time I see 'em. That's what has helped me maintain good attitudes and satisfaction and eagerness to keep helping people. It just feels good—just plain good. It keeps me practicing.

Sure. I've been able to think out of the box, not afraid to try new things.

One of the first new things that I did was the first cardioversion[¶] in this whole Midwest area, and perhaps one of the first outside of Boston. We had old AC defibrillators which were always in surgery if a patient had a cardiac arrest. You open the chest and shocked it.

Given your experience with allergy, could there be all kinds of examples like this in medicine, but doctors aren't pushing the envelope?

That is the case. The thinking nowadays is broader than it was when I was trained. You're trained to do certain things and this is how you do it. Now, there's more leeway to do research and explore other directions.

Do you have any advice for young people considering a career in medicine?

They should think broadly and think of applications of some of the things they see on TV everyday. A drug does this. Well, would it also help something else? Maybe I could treat something we can't treat now with some other method. There's still a long way for medicine to go. There will be tremendous advances, and maybe the sublingual approach will be awfully crude. But if it is, it's going to be something better. We've got something right now that can help up to 90% of the people. It's time to make sure doctors and patients know about it. As a physician, you treat many things off label. Any good doctor knew years before the FDA approved it, that a blood pressure pill was good for the heart.

What was your medical school experience like?

I was in medical school from 1950 to '54 and that was the time of the Korean conflict. We weren't drafted, but it was obvious that I would be, so I enlisted in the Air Force and went in right after my internship. I was on Guam, with a B-47 wing, so I lived in a Quonset with a commander and the pilots. I could better understand the problems they had. I was taking care of them with an idea that I knew more about how to help them with particular problems and flying.

They gave us three months extra training down in San Antonio, Texas—ear, nose and throat, ophthalmology, pulmonary—some things like that. The myringotomies[**] and the tubes made a lot of sense to me after I knew the function of the ears and the Eustachian tubes.

Then, there weren't ear tubes yet, so I flamed polyethylene tubing and put a tube in the ear. It would last a month or two and the surgeons—there were two ear, nose, and throat doctors at our hospital—and they called the chief of surgery, that I was doing unnecessary surgery. Over the last 10 years, that's the most common operation in the United States, and obviously, it's a good thing to do.

¶ Cardioversion is delivering an electrical shock to a person's heart to rapidly restore an abnormal heart rhythm back to normal.

** A myringotomy is a tiny incision in the ear drum.

Do you anticipate a day when you'll retire?

Uh, no.

You just plan to work up until the end.

Correct. I go to work every morning enthusiastic. Sacia and I take more time off. We've got a beautiful home and guest house in the Yellowstone Club in Montana. It's the only private ski and golf resort in the world. I'm still skiing.

We've had a chance to travel more than most anybody and we still enjoy it. We'll be going to Europe this spring, fly into London, go on the Chunnel and spend time in Paris and Southern Europe. But I'll be glad to get back and see patients again. I love tennis, travel, and golf, but not every day. Fortunately, I've had very good health, so I plan to continue.

I'm a great TV sports fan and we live, as you can see, right on the golf course. My wife and I are avid golfers. I see her on the green right now. {Points out the window} She's right down there in the blue. And when I golf, I try to walk 18 a lot of times, but in the heat, I walk nine and ride nine. I play tennis a couple times of week in the winter, especially.

I understand you're quite an astute art collector.

Well, I'm not an expert. We {commissioned} an art dealer, when the Russian paintings could be bought with powerful dollars. One of the very best investments that I'd ever made—and obviously, if we donated the Morris Institute, we've made a lot of good investments—was when I started practicing 47 years ago. They offered a lifetime subscription to the "*New England Journal of Medicine*" for $300. It's a hundred and fifty dollars a year now. Forty-seven years, I've gotten that every week.

I bet $300 back then, was a lot of money.

It was. Actually the first month that I was in practice in West Salem, I earned $300. That was 1957.

What will ultimately convince your colleagues that your life's work is legitimate?

The newest thing is evidence-based research. Actually, a hundred-year-old laboratory in North Carolina is making molds, and we've used their mold extracts for quite some time. They're going whole hog toward approving sublingual treatment, with evidence-based research, with four very prominent medical allergy centers in the country, and then to carry it on through patient studies.

How long before this treatment goes mainstream?

I'm not sure. I hope it's a short time. But whatever it is, it will happen.

III

Ounce of Publicity, Pound of Cure

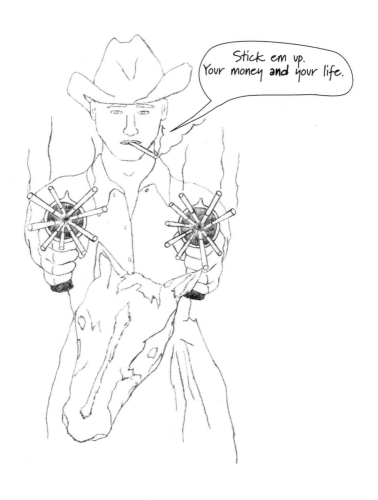

"Prevention is better than cure."

—Desiderius Erasmus

Chapter Ten

Lights, Camera, Reaction!

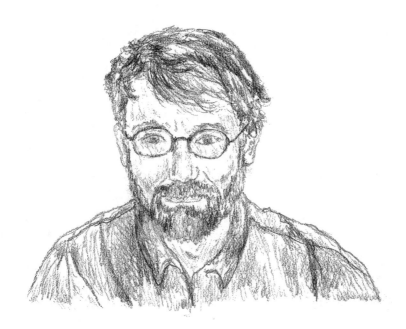

"People come up to me and the first thing they do is apologize for having a cigarette. Or I actually see them put out their cigarette and then look at me like they're 14-years old—busted again by Remington."

Patrick Remington, MD, MPH
Public Health, Madison

"We're number one!" It could have been Wisconsin's mantra back in the late 1980s, but I'm not talking about the Badgers. Having the highest obesity rate in the nation isn't anything to cheer about, but being fat made for a big news story.

Doctor Patrick Remington, who's now in his mid 50s, realized early in his medical career how effective the news media could be in getting his public health message out to a broader audience, pun very much intended.

When I was a young radio reporter, he would occasionally call and let me know about the results of a study he was about to release and inevitably, I would get a great story–like the obesity one. Doctor Remington soon became my source for just about anything public health-related.

I've continued to work with Dr. Remington through the years because he still publishes studies that are of interest to ordinary people; not just doctors. He's got this knack for investigating medical questions that laypeople and policy makers alike find difficult to ignore.

We did a simple analysis looking at rates of obesity in Wisconsin, and we found, in 1989, that Wisconsin led the nation in the prevalence of obesity. A graduate student and I wrote that paper. We published it in the *Wisconsin Medical Journal*.

We thought it would be of interest because there was, potentially, a health problem. Of course, this was prior to any media discussion or any increase in obesity in the country. In 1989, the rates had not been increasing and there was not yet an epidemic.

AP put out a report and it got on the national wires. When all was said and done, we had 85 or 90 media inquiries—National Public Radio, a couple of morning shows, and newspapers around the country.

Now, one might think that that was a success story. But the lesson learned was that despite all the media attention, the message was simply that Wisconsin is the obesity capital of the world. It was primarily a message of ridicule and humor about the sad state of the people of Wisconsin.

I've learned since that you need to think carefully about the message that you convey. When you talk about a problem like obesity, it would be very important to follow that with a recommendation for a solution. In that instance, we did not take advantage of the opportunity to talk to people about the importance of individual change, the importance of smart community design, about physician involvement in nutrition and physical activity, and counseling. None of that was addressed. It was simply a humorous story about Wisconsin—the fattest state in the nation.

The Mayor of Monona* wrote a letter, asking who paid for such a study and who cares? What difference does it make? Clearly, some people thought it was an inappropriate use of tax dollars.

I was quoted in AP as saying the reason for the obesity problem was "beer, butter, and brats." Although that's a good sound bite, it didn't settle well with the Milk Marketing Board. A few days later, a press release accused me of shoddy science. It said "Wisconsin may have high rates of obesity, but Vermont has more ice cream consumption than Wisconsin, and they don't have high rates of obesity." It really led to not only a humorous commentary, but actually, quite a bit of derogatory comments about the role of epidemiology and the role of public health.

---

* Monona is a small bedroom community that borders Madison.

Do you recall when you first realized how powerful the media could be in promoting public health messages?

I remember very specifically. There was a breakout of typhoid fever in the Fox River Valley[†] and my job, as a medical student, was to investigate the source of the outbreak. The media were very interested in this, not only from the perspective of knowing more about the disease, but concerned that it might harm other people in the community.

I was very interested in family medicine and primary care, but left clinical medicine after my internship. I went to the U.S. Centers for Disease Control, where I did an epidemiology fellowship, continued with my graduate training in public health, then went on to my career in public health.

Over the years, I learned how to "practice" public health, which is, fundamentally, looking at the health status of communities and trying to connect what we know works—the science of prevention—and putting it into practice. I discovered that the media were extremely interested in this, in particular those problems that were specifically related to Wisconsin.

It was a win-win proposition. We wanted to get information out to inform the public, and to persuade policy makers that there were things that could be done to improve the health of the public, and the media were interested in the public appeal of the message, in that they might sell more newspapers or people might be more interested in watching television. However, you have to be careful not to simply get media attention for media attention sake.

Surveillance is really the cornerstone of public health. You have to start with information. You have to assess and interpret it and communicate it to those who need to know. That's the fundamental toolkit of an epidemiologist and a public health practitioner.

After six years at CDC, I understood the value of information. My wife and I had settled there. We owned a home. We had three kids. And, I had a good job and fully intended to stay there for my career. CDC tended to have people doing the research, and I was very interested in how that research could make a difference.

However, I realized that I was much more interested in being part of a team, working with public health practitioners and public health nurses, and the media. It just seemed to me that the best approach was to really get out there and see how this research can make things different. So when I saw an opportunity to come back to Madison and work in a health department with a variety of people—not only researchers, but also with people who are practicing public health—I jumped at it.

You're a Wisconsin native, right? So you were coming home?

I was born and raised in Madison. My father was a young professor in

† The Fox River Valley is in Northeastern Wisconsin

the law school and I was the fourth boy in a two-bedroom apartment. We had six kids in our family. Four of them followed in my father's footsteps and went into law. Another brother got his PhD in agronomy.

I was the black sheep of the family. Law did not interest me, since I was really never interested in arguing for a living. We had a very strong tradition of eating together, the eight of us sitting around a table and, invariably, we began a discussion that soon would move into an argument, to people taking sides. Of course, my mother knew better, probably the smartest one at the table, not to get involved. Maybe being the fourth kid and just watching this happen, I just saw the futility in it.

Now, I realize that in society we need people to argue and come to resolution, but it seemed to me that truth is often somewhere in between. That's why I was interested in science and medicine. When you're doing research and asking questions, you're really trying to build consensus. You're trying to get many opinions, all working together on a single solution, as opposed to going into the court room and having a prosecutor and a defender, and either winning or losing.

I knew I wanted to be a doctor in second grade when I had the textbook on human anatomy checked out all year long. Now, I don't actually remember reading it or studying it very much, but it showed my interest in human anatomy, the human body and health. Pretty much from then on, I assumed that I liked science. I liked math, in particular, and was always sure that I'd go into medicine. I did take some breaks along the way, but I eventually applied to the University of Wisconsin, here in Madison.

You're a different kind of physician. You don't see patients.

I do not see patients. It is unusual, especially coming from a clinical training program. When I started, I was in a "flexible" internship in internal medicine. The work that I do now is fairly simple. I sit at the intersection between the practice and academic community. My goal is to translate research into practice, so that the things that really smart people learn in academic settings actually make a difference. In a way, the practice community considers me to be a bit too academic for their taste and the academic community considers me to be much too practice-oriented, so it is an odd position to be in. I just try to work in both worlds.

Many of the reports we do are done by students who conduct the work during a one month elective, or during a semester course. They're very intelligent students, and work really hard, but they are students and they're just learning. These are skills that, when they get into the workforce, they can bring to public health agencies and really become productive.

But if you just look at the numbers and don't communicate them, it's like doing a clinical exam without giving the patient any prescription.

You are incredibly good at communicating complex, statistical information in an understandable manner. How did you develop that ability?

I never thought I was very good at this and maybe that's why I am good at it. I don't take a very sophisticated approach. I look at the data like it's a puzzle. My job is to solve it. It's easy to make mistakes. You've got to be careful. You have to remember not to make a mistake and lose credibility.

When I arrived back in Wisconsin, and joined the State Health Department, I decided I needed to have a way to get information out. At the time, Wisconsin had an epidemiology bulletin that was published. I asked whether I could contribute material, and they said that I could.

However, the cost of the publication was significant—mailing to all the physicians in the state. I had no budget, so I decided to go to the medical society and ask whether it would be interested in publishing a paper. The Wisconsin Medical Society has been, without a doubt, the single most important partnership that I've developed since graduating from medical school. I met a guy named Russ King, who was with the medical journal at the time. And after my meeting, he listened intently and then said, "Not only can we publish a paper, let's do it every month. Let's call it a public health column. And if you can deliver me content, I'll publish it."

Now, he happened to publish it in the socioeconomic section of the journal, so it didn't go through peer review. It was reviewed within the Wisconsin Division of Public Health, and I had colleagues who gave me advice. But it was not reviewed by the editorial board. That began a monthly column that really put us on the map for getting information out to the state—both to physicians and the media.

Over the years, obviously, we became interested in formally submitting the papers to the medical journal. They are now peer-reviewed. It really provides the single best source of information on the health of the citizens of Wisconsin.

But I've been criticized by a number of colleagues because they've viewed this as a way to artificially increase one's resume. They see it as self promotion. I can understand that. Within academics, the pure pursuit of knowledge is the gold standard—to have the papers published in a peer-reviewed journal with a national or international reputation. And although I do that occasionally with my research that's more focused on discovery, I also consider myself a practitioner of public health. And these publications—the *Wisconsin Medical Journal*—really demonstrate the practice aspect of public health.

When research is done at universities, it's often disseminated through national peer-reviewed publications, which by the way, almost never get back to the public, policy makers and to physicians. Well, we like to come back with information we have on the people in the State of Wisconsin and put it out right away. Decision makers might as well make a decision based on the best evidence available, rather than no evidence at all. In a very short time, we became a source of information about health in the state.

I remember one instance involving the Governor where your media relationships almost got you in trouble.

I got a call from a reporter who simply wanted to ask about what I would recommend in a theoretical case, where an individual had an elevated cholesterol, slightly elevated blood pressure and slightly overweight. It seemed to me to be an innocent enough question, so I answered, as all public health physicians would, that this individual should improve his diet, exercise, and if he smokes, either cut down or quit.

Well, the next day in the paper, I read the story. The reporter had gotten a hold of Governor Tommy Thompson's numbers from a recent medical exam and they quoted Pat Remington. Of course, I was working for the Thompson administration, in the Department of Health and Social Services.

Now, one might expect me to be in hot water with Tommy Thompson, but he took that and turned it around and used it very positively. He did change his lifestyle. He started exercising. He lost weight. I'm sure his blood pressure and cholesterol improved, and to this day, he really is quite a fanatic with respect to fitness and personal responsibility. I wish everybody could respond when confronted with those numbers—we now call the metabolic syndrome—so positively.

I later saw him when he came to Madison for a press event. I was going to give him one of our pedometers, which I'm wearing here today, and he said that he already had one. He had already put on 10,000 steps that morning and it was just 7:30 or eight o'clock.

Well, after working for more than 10 years at the State Health Department, I decided to move over to the University to join the faculty to teach and continue to conduct applied research. And much of my work at the University centers around how we measure the health of the community and what works to improve the community health.

Today, I think medical schools are broadening their focus, not only to teach students to diagnose and treat disease, but also to think about ways to improve health and prevent disease. And to do that, we really, as a system and as a society, need to think about approaches outside the clinic.

Physicians today are much more aware about the importance of what we call upstream determinants of disease—thinking about the importance of education, the environment, economic development, and the influence of industries, like the tobacco industry or the fast food industry, on health. All these things really shape the health of individuals and society as a whole. The traditional health care system was relatively uninvolved in examining these factors and working at strategies to improve health at the community level.

And so, one day I got a call from our press office to talk to a reporter about what makes Madison one of the healthiest cities in the nation. Well, this reporter came from *Men's Health* magazine and Madison was a finalist among 10 cities being considered for the healthiest city. When he called, I said rather than you coming to my office, just take a taxicab to the Capitol, walk down State Street, and I'll meet you at the Memorial Union terrace. It was a Friday afternoon and we met and talked for a couple of hours about Madison, about my experience, and why it's such a dynamic and vibrant city.

After our meeting, he walked over to Bascom Hall,[‡] went to a jazz bar, took a taxicab, and left town. Well, three months later the *Men's Health* magazine came out and sure enough, Madison won and was classified as the healthiest place for men that year. The reporter commented that he didn't see one overweight person in the entire city of Madison. Of course, it didn't hurt that he walked down State Street,[§] on to the campus, saw all the college kids on the Memorial Union terrace, and then went to a jazz bar.

But the other surprising thing in the article was that I didn't realize he wasn't asking me about statistics and measures of population health. He was doing a story about me and my experience in being active and involved in sports, so it had an uncomfortable, personal focus about Pat Remington. He described my appearance and my various attempts to remain active and fight off the inevitable aging process.

I do participate in amateur sports and I'm not a very competitive athlete. I did get a bit of ribbing from my friends when they read the quote that said, "Pat Remington is the epitome of the Madison man." They took great umbrage, such that the rumor got out that I was being razzed and the *Capital Times* did a front page story about the trials and tribulations of how hard it is to be called the epitome of being the Madison man. It could be viewed as my 15 minutes of fame in a magazine where the cover has guys without shirts on and six pack abdomens.

For me, it was a nice opportunity to mix my professional perspective with a humanist, public interest story. I've learned enough about the importance of diet and exercise, two fundamentally important things, and I read a lot of cutting edge information about diet and exercise. But it gets down to pretty simple stuff, so what I try to do is just eat simply and eat less. As we age, we expend fewer calories, so I try to exercise a little more. But it seems that I fail as often as I succeed. I find it very difficult, personally, to exercise every day. I don't walk as much as I should. I ate four chocolate chip cookies today just because I exercised over the weekend and felt I earned them.

‡ Bascom Hall is a prominent building high atop a hill on the University of Wisconsin campus.

§ State is the main street that goes directly from the State Capitol to the campus of the university.

If 90% of the time you do the right thing, 10% of the time you can eat anything you want and sit around and watch TV. But what I try to do, most important, is create an environment where then my decisions are easy.

Knowledge is important, and so are your attitudes and the information you might have. If I tell you ice cream is bad for you, but you have a half gallon in your freezer, every time you open it it's going to be staring you in the face. If you don't buy the ice cream, you're not tempted.

Some of my colleagues are purists. For example, they don't eat ice cream. They don't eat meat. They won't have a cigar once in a while. I tend not to be absolute in my lifestyle—I do all things in moderation. I enjoy a cappuccino ice cream at Babcock¶ just like anybody else. But I know that I can't have one of those every day, so what I try to do is surround myself with a healthy environment. I chose to live in a town where I could commute to work. I don't have a parking pass for my car so I can't drive to work. Well, now they have flex meters so I have to pay by the hour. Fundamentally I'm pretty cheap, so for years I didn't have a parking pass and I never drove to work. That forces me to use alternative transportation, usually biking or walking.

I try to make sure that in the morning I prepare a healthy lunch. I try and bring an apple and a yogurt, or something healthy so that it's there when I want it. If I leave it to later decide what I'm going to eat, I'll get a candy bar or a bag of chips, just like everybody else who eats on the run.

The most important thing is to understand how to create an environment and systems that make healthy choices easy. I try and surround myself with people who like exercise, and I find that when I don't feel like it, a friend will call me and say, "Let's get out." We know that's a predictor of lifelong exercise, having a partner or group of friends who are committed to it. This weekend, I went out with friends and went biking. I wouldn't have done it if it were up to me alone.

The next major frontier in our research on health is going to be in stress reduction, and in sleep. I'd probably get an F in both those health habits. There are relaxation techniques, and the health benefits of those are just being discovered. But we need to somehow fit that in to our lifestyle, our busy work environment. There's good evidence that good quality sleep is important. The environment in which we find ourselves isn't really conducive to relaxation.

Now, I'm hoping that the approach I take {to exercise hard} instead of relaxing is actually a reasonable compromise. But we may find in 10 or 20 years, that that didn't work. I focus on the "big three;" a good diet, alcohol in moderation, and avoiding cigarettes. Then, all the other things, like dietary supplements or green tea—I have a cup of green tea here—really are

¶ Hall on the University of Wisconsin campus, where students learn to make ice cream and other dairy products.

at the fringe. Then, good mental and spiritual health, with relaxation, may add, if not years of life, quality of life that you have.

We try not to take the work that we do too seriously. It's very hard when the research and the writing you do is about healthy living and then people I've known for 20 or 30 years, come up to me, sort of hold their head down, as if I am somehow going to preach to them, or apologize for maybe not exercising as much.

Somehow, I would really like to completely disassociate that, how to differentiate the work that you do. I go to work and I do it because it's my job. I certainly don't take it out into social settings. Some people think I'm constantly thinking about healthy living and lifestyle, so I often find it amusing when people come up to me and the first thing they do is apologize for having a cigarette. Or I actually see them put out their cigarette and then look at me like they're 14-years old. You know, busted again by Remington.

But being in the city I grew up in, when I have a reputation for being an expert on healthy lifestyles, there are people in this town who know the truth about my past and they find it ironic at best, and hypocritical, perhaps, at worst, that I'm out there actually telling people how to be healthy.

The other thing is what I do in my health promotion side. I do tend to take risks and people think it's ironic that someone who's talking about healthy choices will go out and mountain bike and bike at night in a 24-hour bike race with head lamps. Just this weekend, I was up riding on the west side of Madison in front of three of my friends, hit a rock and did a complete front summersault. I get up, and love it because of the thrill of it, but recognize that there's something that just doesn't make sense for why people take risks.

That really does get back to my main message that we need to understand the benefits and the risks. For some things in society, we acknowledge the risk because there's great benefit. I equate that with doing sports—riding a bike fast or rollerblading. I know there are risks there. But the benefits—not just health benefits—outweigh the risks. It's fun.

But when I see things like cigarette smoking, or horrible diets that lead to obesity and diabetes, individuals really haven't calculated the true cost, true risks of that fun. So what we try to do is make it fun not to smoke. Make it fun to be active. Make it be fun to eat a healthy diet, and then take risks when the risks are relatively minimal and it's enjoyable while you do it.

How much of illness actually is preventable?

Oh, a huge amount. It's astounding, really. There are lots of things we can do to help promote our health, not just exercise and the right diet, but stress reduction and, obviously, not smoking cigarettes, and access to good health care.

Now that being said, a study was done and published last year, that looked at the proportion of adults with five healthy lifestyle factors—not being overweight, eating at least five servings of fruits and vegetables, not smoking, drinking in moderation, exercising. What percent of the population had all five? It was about three percent of the population. One out of 33 people, has figured it out.

It's very hard to maintain a healthy lifestyle in today's society. Can we get some industrial engineers to reengineer society, so that it's health-promoting and not disease causing? How do you redesign this environment? We were very passive in how the environment has been designed—not just chemicals in the environment—but the physical environment, with computers and technology, automobiles, urban design. We didn't think about health. We just designed it based on convenience. But if we think about what defines a healthy environment, then we can make people's decision-making much easier.

Cigarette smoking is far and away the worst public health problem, not only at present, but throughout the 20th Century. And I predict that through the 21st Century, worldwide, there will be more death, disease and disability from cigarette smoking than any other condition. Everyone recognizes the toxins that are present, but it is an unbelievable drug that addicts kids and then makes it virtually impossible for people, once addicted, to quit. Only after repeated attempts can people quit.

What we're discovering is that we knew there were clear harms of a lifetime with smoking. The estimate is that 350 or 400 thousand people die each year. If 250 people die in an airplane crash, the federal government spends hundreds of millions of dollars finding out the reason why. That's for 250 deaths. That {smoking deaths} happens in 10 days in Wisconsin alone, and we haven't put more than a few million dollars in trying to prevent that during that same time period. It really is a disproportionate investment of resources. There's no greater imbalance between the burden of the health problem and what we spend on solutions.

The other amazing thing is we know the answers. We know how to fix this problem. It's not like Alzheimer's disease and the epidemic of obesity, where we understand the problem, but we really don't understand the solutions.

With cigarette smoking, if we raised prices significantly, as European countries have done, if we made it illegal to smoke in any indoor environment, funded an intensive mass media campaign, combined with severely limiting the tobacco industry's ability to advertise to youth and restrict kids' access to cigarettes, we would see a tremendous decline in the number of kids who start cigarette smoking. When it was done in Canada, there was a 45% decline in cigarette smoking. We could do that tomorrow.

The second thing is that we know that if we provide free or low cost smoking cessation, we can help smokers quit. With high taxation on tobacco products, mass media advertising, and smoking cessation, we could cut deaths and disease from cigarette smoking by several fold, in just a few years. Yet, we don't do it. That to me is why cigarette smoking represents the single most important public health problem. The sheer magnitude of the problem—about one in five, one out of six deaths—is caused by cigarette smoking, the single leading preventable cause of death, and yet we have the solution.

There's also an imbalance between how the public perceives risks from environmental contaminants. You go out and smell polluted air, or you maybe drink water that has a slight odor to it, or wash your vegetables, thinking there might be pesticide residual. Then, think about inhaling two to three thousand chemicals in a cigarette. One cigarette has more harmful chemicals in it than most people are exposed to in a year in the environment. One to five cigarettes has significant harmful affects on individuals, and we've so minimized those effects and so amplified the fear of health effects in the environment, that we have a really distorted view of what really is a public health problem.

Most of the research that has been done on the health effects from passive smoke is from talking to non-smoking spouses of people who smoke in the home. Again, this is a chemical that is dose response related, so yes, the whiff you might get from another person's cigarette walking out the door of a public building is not going to kill you. It's not going to harm you. But working in an environment for months or years where levels of cigarette smoking far exceed any federal standard that we have for any other chemical, it will harm you. We know it will. We can measure the effects of that.

The most logical disease that people are worried about from passive smoke is lung cancer, but actually, we only suspect about 3,000 deaths each year from passive smoking. The estimate is that 50,000 people die from heart attacks. That seems so implausible that most people don't believe it until you look at the research.

Passive smoke causes the platelets in our blood stream to be stickier, so people are predisposed to heart attacks. When you go to a smoky bar, you're at a substantially increased risk of having a heart attack—now, maybe not everybody. It's very easy to paint your own perspective when you're thinking about a health risk. For most of us, who don't work in an environment where people smoke all day, we don't go home and cough at night and wake up with a smoker's cough, having never smoked a cigarette. We don't really realize the level of exposure that other people have in the workplace.

So it makes sense to ban smoking indoors, but there's another reason to ban smoking indoors, beyond the fact that it's good for people not to be exposed to passive smoke. It is part of a national campaign to denormalize tobacco. The tobacco industry spends over $10 billion per year promoting tobacco, its image, normalizing it for youth and for young adults. The only weapon that public health has in this battle is to enact polices which can then denormalize tobacco.

With smoke-free bars, you can't have a drink and a smoke at the same time. We've uncoupled the link between the two. Some people would call that social engineering, and that's exactly what it is. It's an intentional campaign to not only protect non-smokers, which is the explicit rationale, but if we had a society where nobody could smoke indoors, we would have far fewer opportunities for young people to learn how to smoke.

These smoke-free campaigns are as much directed to those individuals who are trying to quit or who never smoked, by uncoupling the indoor environment from the ability to smoke. It's far more important when you get down to the real crux of the matter in these policy debates than protecting a few people from being exposed to cigarette smoke.

It's far more important to have University of Wisconsin students to come to Madison, engage in their lifestyle, going out to bars and having a drink without having a smoke. That's a much more important policy outcome than the reduction in passive smoking exposure for those people who work in the hospitality industry.

But that's a hard argument to make because that's really protecting people who aren't really asking to be protected. That's promoting a social agenda, a policy agenda that's directed at the tobacco industry and not at passive smoking. But it's very much part of the campaign. The primary goal may be to protect every person from environmental tobacco smoke. But the secondary goal is when people can't smoke indoors, there will be fewer people starting to smoke and more smokers quitting.

What's your take on the tobacco industry's interest in promoting weak statewide clean air laws?

I have a litmus test. If the tobacco industry is in favor of something, I'm against it—before I even ask what it's about. Because there's no way the tobacco industry would ever promote something that doesn't help its bottom line. Your board of directors would be fired immediately and your stockholders would revolt. Stockholders want to see profit in the company. If it's good for their bottom line, it's bad for public health.

Clearly, the movement that's happened in California, the City of New York, Connecticut and even in Ireland, is seen as a major threat to the tobacco industry. Smoking and drinking go together, and protecting places where people can smoke indoors is an extremely important agenda for the tobacco industry.

This is the classic, I will give an inch and take a mile. They'll give an inch and allow a statewide ban on smoking in restaurants. Most communities are moving in that direction anyways. Then, they'll go around, parade the fact that this is the best thing to happen for the health of the public.

There'll be some restaurants that will go smoke-free, and that will protect some people working in the hospitality industry.

However, the mile that they take is that they will preempt forever, the ability of local communities to enact any stricter ordinances. But this is really the intent of the local tobacco control community, to ban smoking in every indoor environment, in every place where people are employed, and in every public place.

The good news is that 15 years ago, when the tobacco industry preempted local ordinances, nobody knew what preemption meant. At least now, it's part of the lexicon. We talk about preemption and its effect on public health, but it's a bad bill and, fortunately, we have very smart people who are working on this on the public health side. Wisconsin does have a tobacco control program—$10 million a year—which is not where it needs to be, given the magnitude of the public health problem. But at least it provides enough of a community of public health advocates, that they smell a rat on this public health policy.

Some of the things I talk about, like smoking, I experimented with as a teenager, but never got addicted, so it's never been a personal struggle. But I understand how hard that can be for people who are addicted. The one thing that I try to do, and it's very hard to do, is to separate my prescription for society from what I would prescribe for individuals.

It's inappropriate to blame individuals, and it's hard for individuals to change, given the society, given the environment, so I try to focus my message on society and policy makers and not really sort of preach to patients or to individuals.

Can you tie public health progress to policy work that you've done?

Well, that's very difficult. It's like the clinician whose patient finally quit smoking or loses 50 pounds. Was it something the physician said? Often, you say no. We say the patient finally decided to go cold turkey.

Similarly, in public health, did our work in tobacco have anything to do with the progress we've seen in reducing smoking among youth? The clean indoor air policies are being disseminated across the state, tobacco use rates are down, people are cutting back and quitting.

I see it as just incremental contribution to health improvement. It's hard really to link one certain act or one certain report that we put out with one monumental public health accomplishment. I think of it more as ammunition. I'm providing information to those people who really toil in making decisions in health care and public health. If they can use the information I put out on public health problems, or on evidence-based approaches, then I'm helping them do their job.

The difference between individual approaches—educating the patient, personal responsibility, is really the focus in medical school. How to make things better? Simply provide information to people, give them information at their fingertips and they'll make the right decisions. And if they don't, frankly, then they're not taking responsibility.

However, if you think about almost every public health problem that we have today, we have created a toxic environment for kids, for young adults, even for older adults and seniors, where it is almost impossible to do what the doctor says. It's almost impossible these days to get your kids to be active, five, seven days a week and not be sitting around and watching TV, or instant messaging, or playing video games. That environment is extremely challenging for a clinician to combat—same thing for young students going to college, or off to the workplace—the environment of alcohol as a social norm, or of drinking and smoking in bars and taverns. Those two behaviors are so tied together that we now see increases in smoking rates in college, where before, most people who smoked, were smokers by the time they were high school graduates. We see continuing increases in smoking rates in colleges because of the connection between alcohol and tobacco use.

Now, clean indoor air policies may have an impact. Young adults can go out. They can socialize and have a drink or two, and yet it's not necessarily combined with cigarette smoking.

Lawyers may argue at each end of the pole that it's personal responsibility or public health policies are the answer. The better approach is the combination of the two—to have policies in place that provide as healthy an environment as we can.

We compromise individual freedom for the collective good. We agree to drive at a certain speed limit, to stop at certain intersections, to pay taxes, not to smoke in indoor environments, and compromise what many of us would consider to be individual freedoms because it's good for the collective public. And yet, that alone will clearly not solve our problems. There is an important role for individual personal responsibility that, once provided with the opportunity for good health, ultimately ends up with individuals having to make the right choices.

How has the Internet changed the work that you do?

When CDC developed its mortality data set, I could go in and answer questions about trends in any cause of death for men and for women, by race, by county, by year, over all the states for the last 25 years. So it's an extremely valuable resource offering immediate answers to my questions, and everybody can access it.

So much of my research in the past was focused on understanding mortality rates in Wisconsin. Now, the State of Wisconsin has enriched that with birth records, with hospital discharge records, with survey information. We're to the point where the information on the Internet far exceeds our ability to examine it.

It used to be that one would say we need more data. But I think we're now at the point where we're data rich. What we really lack, though, is enough people who are really thinking the right questions, the important questions, and then have the skill set to examine the data, and not make mistakes.

Just this week, the medical school has had approval to change its name to the School of Medicine and Public Health. To me, that's a really great day for public health in this state, and medicine, because the partnership is stronger than either can be alone.

But when I came to the university 10 years ago, I really changed the type of work that I was doing. I got a big grant from the NIH.** I started doing research. I started teaching a course and I really tried to reinvent myself. I was able to do it. I was able to write research papers. Jeff Davis {state epidemiologist} said to me, "How are things going?" And I said, "I'm not sure I'm cut out for this job. I'm able to do it, but it's different."

And he said, "Pat, they didn't hire you to come and do their job. They hired you to do your job."

In academics, you really do have the academic freedom to create the type of research and the type of teaching that you believe in, and so I did change at that point. I wanted to get more involved in teaching, so I started creating new courses. One year, I taught three different courses, one on physicians in public health for medical students, one on public health principles for practitioners, and one on how you measure and monitor population health.

The second thing is that I got back to working with students on the applied work of public health, looking at health information, putting it into a short, concise report and, in effect, doing what I did back at the State Health Department. I didn't do that consciously. I just sort of moved back into that. And that really has brought me full circle to going back to what I did at the State Health Department, but much more closely linked with the students and with the other faculty at the University.

Many public health problems are deeply rooted in social and economic problems—poverty and racism, and deep societal ills, and so it's very hard to solve those problems overnight. But it's a lot easier to ignore them. You can't force everybody to jog and eat right. But you certainly can provide an opportunity that makes it easier to make those choices.

Has the definition of public health expanded?

When I worked at the CDC in 1985, there was a seminar about violence as a public health issue and there was actually debate after the seminar as to whether this was an appropriate topic for a public health seminar. Well, yes, the definition of public health has broadened. We focused in on infectious diseases, things that were caused by the environment, and if you made the environment healthier, then people were healthier.

** National Institutes of Health

What we've discovered is that we've broadened the definition of public health as we've learned more and more about the causes of violence, chronic disease, and depression. The roots of those problems lie in society, lie in problems not of individual decisions, or in individual behaviors, as much as how society handles its redistribution of wealth, or in how to assure equal opportunity or equal access to health care. And those issues really deserve a population-based approach.

So yes, we thought that violence was only a criminal justice issue in the past, but then we discovered that violence has determinants and that programs can be provided. We talk about conflict resolution, the relationship between firearm ownership or gun safety locks or trigger locks—all of these determinants, which are preventable, then realize that violence has become a public health issue.

I think about it as if a doctor were sitting with a patient with a problem. This is the way I'm teaching a course. I'm giving a lecture in neoplasia, which is cancer. I used to talk about cancer epidemiology, what causes cancer? I used to have the students regurgitate the facts. What are the causes of cancer?

I'm changing how I'm teaching this course now, in that what I'm going to say is that they are confronting a patient who has colon cancer, metastatic[††] to the liver, and who is 55 years old, 40 pounds overweight, and smokes a couple of packs of cigarettes a day. What does this patient need? The obvious thing he needs is surgery, maybe radiation, certainly chemotherapy, and then all of the related medical care treatments, quality of life issues, palliative care, etc.

But then, I ask them to get outside the clinic and think outside the box, where we as a society and you in the community could have prevented this colon cancer from occurring. Or, what could we have done as a society to have prevented it from occurring so late? Could we have detected it earlier?

They need to understand what the risk factors are for colorectal cancer. Do they know that 75% of colon cancer can be prevented? Do they know evidence-based approaches to finding colon cancer early, and what the costs of those are? And what's effective and what's not?

I'm really trying to think about how we best provide care to the patient, but also how we, as a society, assure the conditions in which people can be healthy? How would we have prevented that through exercise, through better diet, through smoking cessation or smoking prevention? How could we have really accessible screening, so when you turn 50, you're reminded to come in through universal healthcare, or access to health care. You don't have to have certain people fall through the cracks and others get routinely screened.

Just having them think—they may not, when they get involved with

†† Spread from another site.

their jobs as physicians, be involved in the up-stream determinants—but I think they need to be part of the solution. If the health care system isn't going to be part of the solution, at least they need to support the other community practitioners who are trying to prevent disease and promote good health.

Because I study population health, I often look back to 100 years ago. I'm amazed at the ignorance of the physicians, at the turn of the century, about the important causes of disease, the fact that they knew very little about contagions, or the nutritional causes of disease. We didn't understand that cigarette smoking caused cancer and other diseases. And yet, at the time, I'm sure the physicians in the medical community thought they were the most enlightened people in the community and respected as such.

Well, it's no different today. We are ignorant about what we don't know. Some day, we'll look back and discover our ignorance about the important determinants of health. When I try to think about things we're doing today that we really don't appreciate—one theme is the importance of stress and its impact on cardiovascular disease, cancer risk, premature aging—that there are people out there attempting to understand mind-body connections. Sometimes they're ridiculed because of soft science and the ability to measure stress. Well, at the turn of the century, we couldn't isolate bacteria, we couldn't treat infections. I'm sure people dreamed about the day when we could treat and cure pneumonia.

I heard a story from the epidemiologist Richard Peto from England. He talked about how, as a male physician, he didn't smoke. He exercised. He ate a proper diet and he maintained his body weight. And yet, despite doing that, his risk of cardiovascular disease was still significantly higher than women, significantly higher than it would have been had he been born in a developing country, or lived a hundred years ago. It's that fact that we really don't understand how we can continue to reduce the risk.

In this country, we'd probably like a pill to reduce all the potential risks from stress and its related health impact. But it's going to be more complicated than that. It's going to involve understanding the relationship between the mind and the body and the importance of balance and relaxation.

Present in societies that have high rates of longevity is a commitment to strong family and a purpose in life. We don't measure that right now in a physical exam. We don't measure that in populations. Physicians in busy practice might do better to think about relaxation, and balance in life.

Now, you're going to hear, obviously from people who are so busy that they are willing to trade off some risk of disease because of the enjoyment, the pleasure of working long hours or working at recreating at a fast pace. But if there are ways to put balance in life and improve health outcomes, most people would be willing to listen.

We have that evidence today that the attributes of your job are extremely important. It is not just whether you have stress and it's not simply the hours worked. It's the feeling of control. Jobs which have a low level of control lead to higher rates of disease and mortality. Jobs that have high rates of latitude of control are related to longevity.

The other factor that's important is there are these studies that looked at type A personalities. Early on, they thought type A was a risk, but follow up studies found no association. When you divide type A in two parts— Type A, but hostile, in other words, really pressured and pushed, but feeling hostility and anger, those people do have high risk of disease, whereas simply being Type A and being motivated and busy and active was not associated with disease.

So again, we have very crude tools to dissect these attributes of stress and of the relationship between our emotions and our mental health and disease. We have simple screening questions for mental status. We measure resting pulse rate for a measure of stress, as opposed to really understanding how hormone levels are, or what brain wave activities are.

There are always problems that arise. Some we can address. Just as we fix a public health problem, infectious diseases or vaccine preventable diseases are significantly reduced, violence, depression, and racial and ethnic disparities now are incredibly important public health problems. So we continually have to define what's unacceptable and provide that information to people who can make a difference, to the decision-makers.

Where I think we should question personal responsibility is among those people working in agencies, organizations, industry and corporations. Understand the impact of not only what we do as individuals, but also as a society, and then take responsibility for those decisions.

Since you don't have those personal relationships with patients, how do you find job satisfaction?

I get great rewards in teaching students, and for the rest of my career, that will be the main part of my practice. When I see students develop skills and gain confidence in being a public health practitioner or researcher, it gives me a great reward. I'm also rewarded by the sense that I'm helping people in public health understand the power of information, the power that we have by defining the unacceptable.

But, as physicians become more interested in improving health in individuals and communities, information on public health becomes relevant to physicians, but it also becomes relevant to the public in general, and the media picks up on that.

We just published a paper on teen pregnancy rates. Clinicians oftentimes begin to deal with the problem when a young girl comes in pregnant, and deals with the repercussions of a teen pregnancy. When we publish a report on trends in teen pregnancy in Wisconsin, physicians are interested in it, but also the community, the media, and public health.

I got a call from Kenosha, from a reporter. She was simply trying to replicate in her community a study that we did at the state level, to make it relevant to her community practitioners and the decision-makers in Kenosha. I'm always learning something about what we do and how to do it better. I realize that when we put out a paper like that which gives a statewide perspective, we're missing an opportunity to, at the same time, include a local perspective.

Almost every issue that's of interest to statewide policy makers and the media will be of interest locally. We should have accompanied that with, here's a website to get your local teen pregnancy rates. Here are the evidence-based practices that work in schools, in families, and in communities, that help prevent unplanned pregnancies among children. We didn't have that. We got a lot of attention about the story, but we really didn't have the local information, and we didn't have what people could do with the information. We did more good than harm, but there were missed opportunities in that recent story and hopefully, next time we'll do a better job.

Chapter Eleven

Doctoring Health Policy

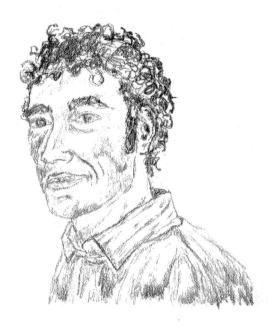

"There are a lot of problems with the health care system right now, so that's a big part of the reason I'm so interested in it."

Peter Vila, Pre med student
University of Wisconsin-Madison

Doctor Patrick Remington walks in carrying a stack of papers.

"Look at this," he says. "I've got a really sharp graduate student who wants to become a doctor and I can't keep him busy enough. I gave him this assignment last week," Remington says, incredulously.

The student is Peter Vila, who's in his mid 20s. He was working on his Master's Degree in public health when we met. What Peter finds so seductive about medicine are the extensive problems in the health care system that he says must be fixed.

Peter's convinced that physicians are the ones best suited to propose health policy changes that can make a big difference in the public's health.

I heard a good analogy by a sociologist at a conference. He said saying the U.S. health care system is the best health care system in the world is like saying the Italians have the best auto industry in the world because they make the 600 horsepower Ferrari. Who drives a Ferrari? One out of many millions of people, right? No one has access to that. Overall, the auto industry is not Ferraris. It's your every day thing; your regular '92 Toyota Camry. Our health care system is like this: If you have money, it's great. It's the best in the world. If you don't have money, you don't have access to it and it's a big problem.

I studied molecular biology and philosophy in my undergrad work and I feel that was my time to just learn and not be too serious about what I was going to do for a career. I couldn't really see myself being a lab scientist or a philosopher later on. But it was good to learn, and it helped prepare me in a lot of ways.

What I'm doing right now is getting a Master's in population health, MS, which is more research-oriented than the MPH. We're just learning about how the health care system works, a lot of epidemiology, a tool to study the distribution of disease, and biostatistics, to analyze all that data. It's basically a set of methods we learn to study the health of populations.

The more time I spend here, the more I want to get involved with policy because it's fundamental to making changes. Through politics, that's how it's done. As a physician, that's something I'd be well prepared to do. You understand how health care works. You're in the health care system. There are a lot of problems.

Some people might think that would be the reason not to go into it. Does any of it concern you as you might try to practice medicine later in life?

The number one complaint I hear from physicians now is they're losing their autonomy or that they're losing their salary. And for the anesthesiologists who were making like $400,000 a year, it probably wouldn't hurt. From my perspective, anyway, I'm not doing it for the money. Whatever I'm getting paid, that's fine. I'll make enough, I guess.

The thing for me is that I really want to get in there and fix it. No one person's going to get in there and fix everything, but there are so many problems that you learn about. And I'm just in a classroom. I'm not out there, so I may have some misconceptions.

Health disparities are a huge problem, and this is at all levels. And you don't realize it, because the people in power, the people making decisions, every day average people, have health care, have jobs, and have access to health care, basically, whereas, lower income people don't. And if you don't have health insurance, you can't go to the doctor because you can't pay for the $2,000 bill.

My dad's situation is that he had to work from a very young age, so he just did the first thing he could do so he could start making money, because his mom was in the hospital. She ended up dying when he was like 15, so he had to work to pay off the medical bills.

He's an auto parts executive. He's a very knowledgeable guy. He can talk about anything. We can really get into philosophical conversations about stuff and politics and whatever. My mom is a teacher. She teaches Spanish. I was born in Miami, Florida, a first generation American. I was the only child. When I was younger, I had an older sister that lived with us. She's from my dad's previous marriage.

I moved around a lot. We moved to Indiana when I was about six, and I was kind of raised in Ft. Wayne. I did a lot of schooling there until high school, when we moved to Detroit. I lived there for a couple years, and then I ended up in Wisconsin, where I finished high school, did my undergrad, and now my Master's.

What I'm doing now is very population-based. How do you measure health in communities? What programs would you put in at the state level or county level to try and have an effect on these things—immunizations, seatbelt laws, helmet laws, tobacco? Things like this, that you're not going to see in the doctor's office.

The doctors might recommend that you stop smoking, or that you wear your seatbelt, but those aren't effective across the population. A big reason for why I'm here, now, is to bridge this gap between public health and medicine. When you talk about traditional medicine and what medicine does, it's very individualized. It's very treatment-focused, not so much an emphasis on preventive care, not so much on the population.

I hope other schools and other academic communities embrace this whole idea of marrying public health and medicine because they do have a lot in common, but traditionally they've been two very separate disciplines.

Will having a Master's degree in public health enhance your chances of getting into medical school?

Yeah, I think so. Medical schools want to see that you're interested in the field and you're serious about what you want to do. With an understanding of public health, you have a much deeper understanding of how the health care system works and what you're actually doing as a doctor. A lot of people don't realize that as a doctor, you have a lot of power to go to your legislators and talk to them. That's the stuff I'm learning now, and I'll be using it for the rest of my life. They're very effective tools for creating social change.

You have to think about it from a career perspective and ideally, the healing aspects of it, the altruistic part of it, that's very appealing. Now, if you're going to do that for the rest of your life, you'd better be a little more prepared than that. In other words, having the added tools under your belt that epidemiology and biostatistics have to offer will make me a much better physician, in my mind.

I've always had an interest in science. In undergrad, I studied molecular biology. It's a very powerful thing to be able to go to work, and heal people. Your health is just so fundamental to everything else. We take it for granted. Without your health, you don't have anything, really. And it's kind of a strong idea to be able to help people with that. The mission of public health, similarly, is to assure people conditions in which they can be healthy.

I definitely haven't been able to do what I want to do, which is to actually provide care. If you're not a doctor, you can't do any of this stuff. But when I go to a clinic, there are things you don't have to have a medical degree to do. Give somebody a shot or take somebody's blood pressure.

I'm volunteering at Meriter Hospital in the ER, and you see really what these people do day to day. It's very dynamic. It's really kind of a seductive thing to me to be in there and to help save people's lives, one step at a time. As a volunteer, you don't do a whole lot, but you basically make sure patients are doing okay. You talk to patients. The doctors are cool. They let you in to watch the surgery. You just observe.

A lot of what I do is patient transport, so if they need to go get an x-ray, I'll take a patient to the x-ray room or for an MRI. You get to know the hospital pretty well, going around to all these different places, and you see how the hospital works.

How confident are you that you'll get into medical school? It's very competitive.

It's extremely competitive. I wouldn't say that I'm confident that I'm going to get into Harvard or Stanford, but I'll get in somewhere. I'll apply everywhere, and whoever takes me and wherever I get in, that's the best fit for me, and that's where I'll go. I won't go to the Caribbean. But I'll hopefully go to a good med school. Maybe if I don't get in to where I want to go my first year, I'll take a year off and do some research and apply again. I'm actually going to be applying this summer, so I'm taking the M-CAT in the spring of next year and all summer.

What's M-CAT preparation like? Is that something you study for?

Yeah. Maybe if you're some kind of crazy genius and you remember all this organic chemistry and physics that you learned in your undergrad, you can get by without studying for it. I am not, so I'll be taking that prep class. Yeah, it's just a lot of general science knowledge and biology and stuff like that.

Do you have any trepidation regarding the amount of training you're going to have to go through?

It's intimidating if you look at it, like wow, the next 15 years I'm going to be stuck in loopholes. It is a long process, but that's part of the journey. You need to enjoy every part of where you are. I like where I am right now. Hopefully, it will be like that every step of the way, and if it's not, then I know I'm not doing the right thing and I should look elsewhere.

I found out, early in my college career, that I was not one of those people who could look at a book and just know it. I'm smart, but I'm not that smart. I learned that the hard way. There are people who are that smart. They never go to class and get a four-oh.

I had a 4.0 last time I checked in my graduate career. My undergrad, I had a 3.3. I'm not your 4.0 from third grade kind of student. Intelligence wise, I know I'm fine with it, and if I really want to do it, I can do it. That's why I'm taking a lot more time and actually doing it in grad school.

How do you study?

What I do if I have a test coming up, I'll try to give myself a week, a little bit every day at a time. I can't handle study binges, eight hours at libraries. I don't do that. Put in a couple hours every day. That's really all you need. For me, that works. It's very adaptive. There are different types of studying, so I'd be one of the people who go to class and sit there and sometimes fall asleep in lecture and sometimes listen, but most of the time I try to stay pretty active there. It's tough trying to swallow 15 weeks of material and do well on an exam without actually being there.

So are you pretty sure public health will be your emphasis, or might that change, too?

That might change. It's really tough to know what you want to do before you actually go through the rotations in medical school and try out what you think about the specialty. It may not be what it's like to practice it, and maybe you don't like that practice, or maybe you like this other one that you never thought of before.

If I really like the preventive medicine kind of stuff, I'll stick with that and really do public health. If not, maybe I'll just go into some specialty. Maybe I'll go into cardiology and apply some of these ideas I've learned in public health to cardiology, specifically.

How are you going to pay for medical school?

It's really expensive, especially in the better schools. It's like $40,000 a year. Loans. That's the best you can do. My dad's not rich. He can't afford that. I certainly can't afford that. I'm living off a graduate student's stipend right now. But you take out loans, and, hopefully, you can pay them off before you die. I'm pretty responsible with my money, so I don't think it's going to be that big of a deal.

What about the effect on your social life? You have to put in a lot of time to become a doctor. Have you thought about that and whether you're willing to make those sacrifices?

That's funny that you ask that, because last night a bunch of the guys from the class—we all went out and we were talking about med students and you don't have a life any more after you go to medical school. But all these first year kids I know, they're going out all the time. Certainly, I hope that I'm not going to be going out all the time. There's a balance. Everything in life is a balance, and it gets to the point where what really matters is what you should be doing. And if you're going to medical school with the intention of going out and having this great social life, maybe medical school isn't what you should be doing. So yeah, you may have to sacrifice a couple nights here or there, but that's okay.

Do you think you have the right temperament for being a doctor, with the pressure and the stress?

That's definitely something I've thought about. It is a huge responsibility, especially in neurosurgery or something. You're operating on people's brains. One slip up, and the guy's dead. It's a risk I'm willing to take. That's definitely the hard part of it. I would think a lot of doctors have a hard time dealing with their professional mistakes. You are going to make some mistakes. It's going to happen. Nobody's perfect. It's inevitable. That's just something you have to deal with. It kind of develops your character. It's also the power to do good things.

What about the hours? A lot of doctors work huge hours.

I'm definitely not going to be one of those guys putting in 80 hours a week at the hospital. I want to have a family. I want to go to my kids' baseball games, so that will determine my choice of specialty because there are some specialties where you live at the hospital, and there are some, like dermatology, where you have more of a 9-5 job and go home at the end of the day.

I don't think I'd consider myself a workaholic—maybe at times. I like my time outside and enjoy the rest of life, as well. I play guitar, so I've always been really into music. I've been playing a lot of open mics and stuff. It's fun. It's challenging. That keeps me busy for a lot of my time, and I just try to stay active.

I just picked up windsurfing and kiting, which is really dangerous. I might as well do it now while I'm young and stupid. The more you immerse yourself in different things, the more you just get out of life.

Have you met any influential doctors yet?

A lot of the doctors I've met have been academics rather than clinicians, so I guess I have sort of a biased sample. These are the guys that do the practice for a couple years and then decide it's not for them. They're all about the knowledge and the research. Those guys are some of the coolest people I've met. Those guys are the ones that definitely influenced me and my career path and continue to do so.

Most of the people I work with are either MDs with an MPH or MDs with a PhD, so that's a big part of the reason why I'm doing this path, because all the people I see are in positions of leadership with an MD.

Pat's Remington's like, my everything—my boss, my advisor, and my mentor. I spend a lot of time with Pat. He's a great guy. He's another one of those people who has really been a big, influential person in my life, and I am sure he will be for the next couple years. I'm very lucky to have met him. He really just has a way of coming down to your level and being like, "Alright, let's get something done."

Your whole 10 years of becoming a doctor is a test by fire. You just get hammered by these doctors; at least that's what I've heard from my friends. You talk about leadership development, that's really what it's all about. When you're a doctor, you just have to develop a sense of what you want to do and how you're going to convey that in a practice setting or hospital.

It forces you to be a leader. If you can't be a leader, I don't think you should be going into medicine. Yeah, I'm confident enough to be where I am right now and to go in to medical school with the attitude that I need to go with taking the criticisms, the tests, and the long hours, but it's a process.

You're going to have to go before some committee to make your case before you're admitted to medical school. Have you thought about what you'll tell them about why you'd make a good doctor?

I would be a good doctor because I'm motivated to change people and society, from a public health perspective. It's applied science. You're taking all this knowledge and doing something about it. That's why I'll be good at it, because I'm not just interested in it intellectually, but health to me is something that is so fundamental to life. I really want to have a part in providing that for people, trying to find the best way to keep people healthy.

The way our system works is that people do matter, and by you going to your legislator and talking to him, that's going to potentially make a difference. That is at least going to get them to bring something up that they haven't brought up before. And that's really how you get these things done.

Here in the U.S., even here in Madison, South Madison, we've got these huge disparities. Just go down to the south side clinic and you'll see the kind of things you wouldn't see elsewhere. Even in Milwaukee, it's one of the most segregated cities in the United States. The amount of disparities you see, it's like a third world country in these low-income populations. And these people aren't taking part in the political process. The only people who are tend to be the more affluent people, who don't realize there's this problem with disparities. And there really needs to be a voice for the low-income population or the disadvantaged to go through and take part in this.

Physicians have a very large role in that because they see these people every day, really. I want to do it because you're not only exposed to the whole community—you see all of them in your offices, day to day. And not only are you there to heal them, but really to connect with them and, hopefully, encourage them to change something in their life.

Are you optimistic that any real change in the health care system will happen?

I'm very optimistic about it, and maybe it's because I'm in this setting, an academic institution. But I think that every day you see more evidence of it in politics. In Massachusetts, the Governor is proposing a statewide, universal coverage plan, and he's a Republican.

Bush really hasn't done anything about it. Hopefully, the next presidential candidate will be able to do a little more with that. Really, what it comes down to is it's not an attractive political issue because the problem is a lot of people have the misconception that if you go to universal coverage, or if you switch to a system different to what we have now, the quality of care is really going to go down. That's all propaganda propagated by the media and by interest groups that don't necessarily represent the evidence. A big part of change in health care is going to have to happen through getting rid of the misconception that quality is going to decrease.

Another of those misconceptions is that if you nationalize the system, it's gonna automatically be like this communistic, socialistic thing. No. There's ways of having a universal health care system in the way we have it set up now. There wouldn't be drastic changes. There could just be expansion of Medicare or Medicaid, or something like that, individual-mandated insurance.

The bottom line is that something needs to be done. The big part of the reason why it hasn't gone anywhere is because there are so many options, that you can't get all these different people to agree. And while they all may agree that something needs to be done, they all have different ways of doing that. We just need to pick something and do it. We need to get past this kind of writer's block we have now in Congress.

Editor's note: Four medical schools accepted Vila. He chose to attend Mount Sinai School of Medicine in New York City, beginning in fall, 2007.

Chapter Twelve

Wrench in the Killing Machine

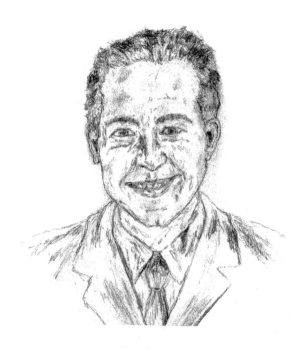

"My mother began smoking, probably in the '50s, and that's when a lot of American women began to smoke. In fact, that would be my Christmas present to her every year—a carton of Winstons."

Michael Fiore, MD, MPH
Internal Medicine & Preventive Medicine, Madison

It was one strange phone call. A woman asked for a copy of any letter the Wisconsin Medical Society received from the University of Wisconsin Center for Tobacco Research and Intervention {CTRI}. Dumbfounded, I paused before asking who she was, where she was from and again, what exactly she wanted.

She gave me her first name only, Michelle, and would not tell me who she worked for. Then she asked again for letterhead copy. "Why should I give you this? For all I know, you work for the tobacco industry," I said, jokingly.

I e-mailed Michael Fiore, MD, a veteran smoking-cessation expert who directs CTRI, to fill him in on what transpired. It turned out that this woman worked for a lobbying firm that represents Big Tobacco. At the time, Fiore was a witness for the United States Department of Justice lawsuit against the tobacco industry. What "Michelle" wanted the letterhead for remains a mystery to me, though some people suspect it had something to do with discrediting Dr. Fiore.

When I began writing health-related smoking stories as a radio reporter in the 1980s, I actually used to call the Tobacco Institute for comment. Whenever there was yet another medical report demonstrating the harmful health effects from smoking, the Institute's response was pretty much the same, no matter what the latest research found. "There is no scientific evidence conclusively linking cigarettes to…"

This mantra eventually became so ridiculous, that "Saturday Night Live" created a hilarious spoof of a defensive, tobacco industry spokesman played by Martin Short. With his hair slicked back and plumes of cigarette smoke all around him, the character would nervously look from side to side as he responded to the reporter's questions. "I didn't say that. You said that."

It became abundantly clear that the tobacco industry had few legitimate insights to share about the issue, so I eventually stopped including its "perspective" in my reporting. Michael Fiore, however, was another story. He frequently provided the authoritative quote I needed.

Despite everything that is now known about tobacco's dire consequences, it's an industry that is still very much alive, even if many of its former customers are not. Taking on tobacco is always a serious challenge because Big Tobacco has vast resources to defeat clean air proposals and promote smoking as a glamorous, independent, legal, adult choice.

Big Tobacco has this history of pigeonholing individuals, seems to be about one per year. They'll go into the individual's records. They'll question their integrity. They'll subtly influence the university's capacity to get other research dollars. This was back in the '80s and early '90s. It's not so flagrant now.

{Researcher}Joe DiFranza said four-year olds know Joe Camel as well as they know Mickey Mouse. He lost his job. It had an incredibly chilling effect on the field. Money has power. Everything about tobacco is about money. Universities make a deal with the devil, so they don't lose other potential funding sources.

At the trial at the Department of Justice just a few weeks ago, one of the witnesses, the one who was hired to dispute my testimony, reported that he had made $2 million in one year in direct fees paid to him to be an expert witness to counter claims of tobacco control. That's enough to buy Harvard researchers, if some of them choose to be sold.

But science is not perfect. It evolves over time, and we get better. If one were to examine the work of any scientist, one would find the nature of scientific discovery is that we try things. Some of them turn out. Some of them don't. Some of them are unequivocal; some of them are equivocal. This lack of scientific certainty is really the basis of much of the tobacco industry's case—that we haven't done clean, clinical trials with humans who we've exposed to tobacco in a way that proves X, Y, or Z happens. Of course, it would be unethical to do that. It's all garbage—that's the short answer.

We've learned over decades that tobacco is a classic "dose-response" risk factor. The more you get, the higher the risk of cancer, cardiovascular disease, and pulmonary disease. We also know there's no safe, lower threshold of tobacco exposure. There's a compelling case that secondhand smoke is a cause of lung cancer. Secondhand smoke is a cause of cardiovascular disease. The more you get, the greater the risk.

The more interesting data in recent years has been on the cardiovascular side. It appears that some of the damage from tobacco smoke is more acute in cardiovascular disease rather than from lung cancer. That's why Stan Glantz, the one who does the writing on this, talks about 40,000 U.S. cardiovascular secondhand deaths, but only three or four thousand lung cancer deaths. In contrast, direct smoking causes 100,000 lung cancer deaths.

How did you get so focused on smoking? Were there smokers in your family?

My mother began smoking, probably in the '50s, when many American women began to smoke. My Christmas present to her every year would be a carton of Winstons. I was a very young boy. It was just a very common Christmas gift. All of my uncles smoked, and most of the people in the family did. My father was the exception, and really disliked it.

I grew up in Boston, in a poor, ethnic Italian family. My father, although he was born in America, grew up in Italy, came over when he was about 13. My mother's parents are both from Italy. My existence was a street in Boston with four houses in a row, which were all family, with my grandparents in the middle of them. Neither of my parents finished high school. They were from the era of the depression and worked starting when they were very young.

I'm the youngest. I have an older sister and brother. I'm the only one who went into medicine.

Do you remember when you first became interested in science?

It was more medicine, actually, than science. A lot of our life was built around 30, 40 family members spending Sundays around my grandmother's table. At a very early age, I can remember being told the family needs a doctor and you're it. I can remember a couple of times coming in, maybe as young as seven or eight, saying, "What about meteorology?" Somehow, I thought weather was interesting. That's great, but being a doctor will really make a difference and it's sort of a way to become successful and help people.

Even though it came from the family early, I can imagine, in other circumstances, sort of rebelling from it. But somehow I embraced it, and it was perfect for me. I love being a doctor, the relationships I can have with people, making a difference in people's lives, one person at a time. I love preventive medicine.

I went to an inner-city high school. It was basically custodial care, so I went to college not particularly well prepared. It was an incredible transformation. I went to a small liberal arts school in New England. At that time, it was almost all men. It had just gone co-ed the year before. About half of the students were prep school kids. It was a school that had been in existence for almost 200 years. It had incredible tradition. It had a long history of producing a lot of businessmen and bankers of New England. I just showed up the day school started in September of '72.

A teacher told me, "You should apply there." So I did. They gave me almost a full scholarship to attend. It was a wonderful experience. It really taught me about the world, and I got a great liberal arts education. But I also got to understand the good, the bad, and the ugly of our society, and the power structure, relationships, and making things happen. I went from an incredibly green, naïve, urban, ethnic boy to a—sophisticated is probably too much—but I was a little more worldly when I completed that experience.

What was medical school like?

It was incredibly hard, but fine. I went to Northwestern, in Chicago. My grandmother was just petrified, because in her mind Chicago was full of gangsters. I told her most of them had been locked up, so that would be okay.

I made wonderful friends. I got a great education. It's where I first began to focus on prevention. I had a great mentor there. His name is Jeremiah Stamler. He's still alive, in his mid 90s. He's one of the nation's, sort of, fathers of cardiovascular epidemiology. He helped define the link between high blood pressure and cardiovascular disease through large epidemiological studies. He's an old lefty who was blacklisted in the '50s during the McCarthy Era. He was mixed up with this whole crowd of cardiovascular epidemiologists who, ironically, even though he was Jewish, bought land south of Naples, on the Amalfi Coast, and built villas. They also did a lot of the Mediterranean diet studies that showed that sort of thing was healthy. Through that, he taught the class. It focused on prevention, and just totally clicked for me that that's what I wanted to do.

Doctor Stamler had enough contacts there through his work that he hooked me up with some people over there, and I moved to Italy. He opened doors for me that then led to sort of a little side path. I moved to Italy for a year and a half.

My family all spoke dialect Italian. Hearing Italian was very comfortable for me, but I didn't really speak it. I went over there and went to intensive language school for two months. And because I had heard it all my life, I was able to speak proper Italian fluently within two months.

For me, it was much more of a personal, cultural experience. It wasn't a professional experience. I worked in a hospital, but that was really the excuse for being over there. The wonderful thing for me is that I knew no Americans over there. I was totally hooked in with an Italian group, and they took me in like family.

What I did, in essence, was take a fifth year of medical school. I actually went over in the middle of my senior year and stayed almost a year and a half. While over there, I even thought about not returning. But I couldn't be licensed there, so I came back and did internal medicine at Boston City Hospital.

When I went to Italy, even though I had fulfilled all of my requirements, I was putting my graduation off for a year. I asked the school to write a letter that I had fulfilled all of my requirements and was the equivalent of a medical doctor. My mother framed the letter and put it up in the hallway. She was so proud.

My father, until the day he died, would always want me to give him my business card. He was a custodian in the Boston School System, and just loved to take out the card and say, "My son is a doctor, and this is his card."

I didn't even attend my own medical school graduation, because I was overseas at the time. I don't believe I had a party. It's important for me to be understated. That's a big part of me, to be understated.

Why is that?

Culturally, I don't want to come across as arrogant or a fathead. It's particularly an issue that I'm sensitive to now, because of some prominence around the tobacco issue—how I carry myself in a way that is appropriate and respectful.

Tell me about your early training.

I did internal medicine at Boston City Hospital. It was the hospital for the poor in Boston. It has a reputation of training cowboys. You're on the front lines from the first day; you do everything. Incredibly sick people, incredible responsibility, work like a dog, incredible esprit de corps. There were many nights that I was painfully tired. I probably wasn't ready for that.

There was a giant African American population that went to that hospital. Two people come to mind. One was an old African American man who had disseminated prostate cancer and was in extraordinary bone pain. We're in an era of such high-tech medicine, where tragically, people are not allowed to die. I'm always impressed when somebody recognizes it, and will allow it to happen, and often insists that the system and the technology not unduly prolong their life. Just to see this guy die with dignity with this incredible bone pain—that taught me quite a bit about how to carry one's self.

It was at a time when people would stay in hospitals often for weeks or even months. They still had wards back then—wards where we would have 12 patients. In the TB wards, you could wheel the patients out to a screened in patio, so they would get some fresh air to help with their tuberculosis.

I also had a rather dramatic family event. When I was an intern in the family unit, my mother was admitted to the intensive care unit with a toxic cardiac arrhythmia. At that time, you were on call every other night, so you would work a 36-hour shift, be off for 12, and then work 36 again.

My mother came into the hospital and it was just so bizarre being one of the doctors on her ward. And, of course, I wasn't directly taking care of her, but she was sort of waving at me, saying "Hi!" to me, since I was on every night. She was in for about a week.

When she came in, the cardiologist said, "We don't know why you're having this arrhythmia, but we think your smoking is exacerbating it and you need to stop."

She did, and it fully resolved and she never had an arrhythmia again without any treatment. That was dramatic to me.

I did three years at Boston City; that's what it takes for internal medicine. I stayed on at Harvard and got a Master's in Public Health, and there, focused on chronic disease epidemiology again.

One day at Harvard, I was talking to some buddies and they said there was this great program at the CDC—the Epidemic Intelligence Service— sort of the disease detective thing, which is a model for TV shows. They choose a hundred, mostly physicians, every year to be on the front lines of epidemic health outbreaks in America. You go to the CDC and get trained. Then you either get assigned to a health department and work out of a state, or work out of the CDC.

I chose chronic diseases and was assigned to Wisconsin. That was back in '85, so that's how I got here for the first time. I was trained and boarded in internal medicine, because I had a Master's in Public Health and had done this Epidemic Intelligence Service training, and was eligible for preventive medicine if I did one more year. I went to Washington to work with the U.S. Office on Smoking and Health.

And at that time, Surgeon General C. Everett Koop was in charge of the Public Health Service. He was working very closely with that office. It was very small, but it's the office that produces the Surgeon General's reports. I just became totally engrossed in that, and that became my passion, my career.

At that point, first I was very junior on the totem pole. Doctor Koop is an incredible guy—he's truly one of my heroes. He was the first pediatric cardiovascular surgeon in America. I would be in meetings with him—sitting in one of the chairs around the table, rather than at the table with him. But I got close enough to him to admire him. Since then, though, we've become very close. I talk to him at least once a month, and visit with him as often as I can. He's invited me into his life in a way that I feel very privileged.

I worked in epidemiology. For example, one of my first tasks in the area was looking at trends in tobacco use at the time. I published a series of three articles in JAMA {*Journal of the American Medical Association*}, probably in '89. That put me on the map in tobacco trends in cigarette smoking in the United States by gender, race, ethnicity, and education, which really defined the dramatic differences based on vocation and economic status. I came up here on July first of '88. The articles were published and got incredible attention, so all the national news people came up to film. I started with a bit of splash here in Wisconsin around the tobacco issue.

How serious a health problem does tobacco present?

It's a dubious distinction – being first, in terms of the number of deaths. But one of the biggest communications challenges I see is to avoid crying wolf, and to convince Americans that not all risks are equal because, of course, the slippery slope argument that everybody makes is that if we control smoking, then the next thing you know, they'll say we can't eat a Big Mac. It feeds into the tobacco industry's perspective, and they promote it. But it isn't equal. It's entirely appropriate to say something that has such extraordinary, clear impact on health as smoking should be regulated, whereas there are plenty of other potential things that don't warrant such regulation.

As a society, we don't tolerate the needless exposure of innocent people to toxins. Consider this scenario – what if I were to go into a pub here in Madison and say I felt it was my right to sprinkle a little asbestos dust around me. I should be able to do that—exposing the workers and patrons because I love to sprinkle asbestos dust. The absurdity of that argument is exactly what the tavern league, but most of all, the tobacco industry, advocated. People should have the right to sprinkle a little bit of a carcinogen in our environment, that they should have the right to sprinkle a little bit of an agent that causes myocardial infarctions and strokes in our environment. It really isn't about individual rights. It's about public health and we have an obligation to protect public health.

Has there been much progress?

Sure. It's slow. The way I measure progress is in rates of smoking.

We're approaching 20%. It was 43% in 1965. That's an incredible public health achievement. To me, it ranks among modern medicine's greatest achievements. We're in a 100-year war against tobacco, and we're about at the halfway point.

It's been the initial recognition and dissemination of information about the health effects of smoking, starting in the '50s, and the early heroes of that effort who did research and published it. The first Surgeon General's report in 1964 was an incredible wake up call to our society. The relentless power of more and more scientific data that say tobacco is deadly, along with families across America bearing the health brunt of this.

It's criminal, in terms of what the U.S tobacco companies have done, in terms of imposing this deadly addiction, particularly on developing countries across the world. China—giant market, biggest cigarette factories in the world. In some Asian societies, the rate of male smoking is 50, 60, 70%. It's where we were right after World War II with men. I don't know if the distinction by education is true yet in Asian societies. My sense is that once you get to that rate of prevalence, it has to be pretty much everybody.

But education is a big factor in this country, isn't it?

Oh, it's dramatic. The rate of smoking in college grads today is about 10%. It's really been de-normalized for them. And that's a success. But what have we done is to relegate the burden of tobacco use to the least advantaged members of society. What about the poor, the least educated, those with co-morbid conditions—psychiatric illnesses, dependency on alcohol, and other dependencies, a lot of chronic diseases?

One of the things I despise most about the tobacco industry is when they say that if we raise the price of tobacco, we put an unfair burden on the poor, when just the opposite is the case. The unfair burden on the poor is to relegate the illness and death from tobacco to them, and tolerate that in our society. To condone it is criminal. The best way to help those individuals to break that addiction is to raise the cost of it.

Particularly, a large tax increase is unequaled in terms of its impact. We've included in some policy work we've done that can model very specifically, that if you raise the price by x dollars or cents, you'll get this kind of a decline in smoking. There's nothing else that will do that for you. The amazing thing about it is that it doesn't decrease state revenues because it's not a one for one decline.

One of the things the tobacco industry fears most is to denormalize tobacco use in our society. And we've seen in every state that has gone smoke-free—Massachusetts, California, New York State, and most of New England, tobacco use rates go down, people think about quitting, kids are less likely to start. It's the most important thing we can do.

Some feel that those who want to quit already have, so why bother?

People do talk about hardening the target. That's how it's described in the cessation literature. The people left who are smoking are the most addicted. But you know what? We need to recognize that the population of smokers is very dynamic. Every day, 2,000 kids become addicted smokers. Every day, a thousand people die of a disease directly caused by smoking.

Are there hard core smokers? Without question, but if you look at the pool of people who smoke, it continues to reflect a wide spectrum of people in terms of their dependence and their capacity to quit. The most powerful supporting statistic is that since the year 2000 we've made some progress. Smoking rates have gone down since that time, 15% or so, from about 25% to about 21% of all adults. There are clearly more poor people who smoke, more chronically mentally ill people who smoke, more alcoholics who smoke, more very ill people who smoke. But in total, the smoking population is still very heterogeneous.

There are some people for whom quitting smoking is extraordinarily painful, who've tried many, many times, and have just not been able to do it. With the right medicine, the right counseling, the right social support, and the right chronic care that this sort of tobacco dependence requires, everybody, ultimately, can quit.

The one thing I've gotten so sensitive to is what a burden tobacco is for most people who use it. There aren't a lot of people running around out there who say, I smoke and I love it. For the most part, they are people who are addicted. They hate it. They are embarrassed. They feel weak. They feel stupid. They feel like they are letting themselves and their families down.

I have extraordinary empathy for smokers, and it really bugs me—although I think we're doing a better job of it these days—but the last people who should be blamed for this tragedy are the people addicted to tobacco.

One core component of quitting is wanting, but that's the tobacco industry's argument—that it's all about personal responsibility. But, do I tell you that controlling your diabetes is your personal responsibility? Do I blame you for being of weak character because you don't control your hypertension on your own? Of course not. We treat these as a chronic diseases.

We work with people over time. We partner with them. That's what medicine's about. Why do we buy the tobacco industry's argument that it's all about free choice? It isn't. These people for the most part, became addicted as kids and have a physiologic dependence that warrants treatment, just as any other chronic disease warrants treatment.

The hold that tobacco has on people varies, and some people are able to put it down and walk away from it and seem to have a relatively painless path in doing so. But they're relatively uncommon today. Here's the statistic that tells me that more than anything else: 80% of U.S. smokers today have already tried to quit and have relapsed. That speaks to the fact that most people are unable to just walk away from this drug. There are all sorts of factors that come into play. Genetics, I'm sure, plays a role—not yet defined. The social environment in which we live plays a powerful role. The ubiquitous nature of the tobacco industry's $12 billion advertising and promotion plays a role.

It's a complex factor, the fact that it's incredibly cheap. Doctor Koop first said we'll make a difference in cessation when it's as easy to walk down to the corner store to get treatment for tobacco dependence as it is to buy a box of Marlboros. We make it very hard to get treatment for tobacco dependence. We make it very easy to buy a pack of Marlboros.

We've made progress in Wisconsin. About 70% of covered lives have insurance coverage for at least one of the treatments for tobacco dependence. What we don't do is make the treatments barrier-free. What we don't do is promote them. What we don't do is encourage people to use them. Why? Everybody is interested in the healthcare dollars going out today, even though they may save more dollars a year from now or two years from now. The immediate return on investment in this era of incredible health care inflation rears its head because many insurers view treating tobacco dependence as a new expense. Making a powerful business case to treat tobacco dependence is actually something we focus a lot on.

We're moving in the right direction. The things we have now, we wouldn't have even dreamed about 10 years ago, so there's progress. Science can be done at many levels, but where science is needed most is at the policy level. How do we deliver the treatments, how do we increase demand for treatments?

One thing is mindset—how we think about this—because breaking the habit de-medicalizes it. We're much more into trying to medicalize this addiction. I'll give an example.

A patient visited me at our smoking cessation clinic and was incredibly embarrassed. He continued to smoke, though he knows everything there is to know about the health risks, and is a very educated individual. He cannot conceive of himself being able to function without smoking. I got an e-mail from him on his quit day, and for the first time in his life, he has five weeks without tobacco under his belt. I put him on lots of treatments including high dose nicotine. He got hooked up to the Wisconsin Tobacco Quit Line. He's had some one on one counseling in our center. I mean, we're treating him like a severe chronic disease, working closely with him.

The tobacco withdrawal syndrome has been well-defined. One thing we've learned about tobacco dependence, it's a life-long chronic disease. For virtually all smokers, you can take it a day at a time, but you need to commit to have not even a single puff. For most people, even a single puff is the beginning of a slippery slope back to daily smoking. The relapse curve begins to flatten in about six months after quitting, but even between one and five years, one-third of the people who have been good will relapse.

By five years, it really starts to level off. Most people will relapse within the first two weeks after they try to quit—a giant amount of early relapse. What often trips them up is a powerful withdrawal syndrome—irritability, difficulty concentrating, disturbed sleep, unable to function.

What do we do with patients trying to overcome alcohol? We often put them in a 30-day residential facility. What do we do with a tobacco smoker? We say quit, then deal with your wife, your kids, your job, and all the stresses in your life, and overcome this very powerful dependence. For a lot of people, it's just too much.

Different medicines do different things. Nicotine medicines basically replace the nicotine in cigarettes. But, it's delivered in a different way, unlike the nicotine in cigarettes that is delivered through the alveolar bed, and thus these medicines are less reinforcing.

We're involved with a study with the National Institute on Drug Abuse and a small start-up company for a nicotine vaccine, with the goal of actually developing antibodies to nicotine. If it works, after taking this vaccine, when you take a drag of cigarette smoke, the absorbed nicotine will bind to the antibodies in your bloodstream and then none of it gets to your brain because it is a compound too large to cross the blood-brain barrier, so the cigarettes are no longer reinforcing. It's in the very early stages, years off, but if that pans out, I mean, what potential. Potentially vaccinate all kids, and all adults who want to quit.

What do you think of legal efforts to thwart the tobacco industry?

I refuse court work on almost a monthly basis. I have no interest in being an expert witness. I don't think that plays to my strengths and it's not something I really want to be involved in, but I was asked by the United States Justice Department and I felt I couldn't say no to the government.

Well, the government has launched the largest civil litigation* in U.S. history against the tobacco companies. It's been a tough case for the Justice Department. There's been controversy about both sides influencing witnesses, as well as changing their science-based remedies to penalize the tobacco industry.

Understanding and treating tobacco dependence has always been what I do best. It takes an enormous amount of time, and really keeps me focused. It may sound egotistical, but I'm now one of the nation's leaders in cessation. But, cessation is only part of the battle—tobacco control is broad. There are other basic policy, science and clinical issues. Even with that—where can you have more impact on American health? I would sug-

---

* On August 17, 2006, U.S. District Judge Gladys Kessler found that the tobacco companies violated civil racketeering laws and defrauded the American people by lying for decades about the health risks of smoking and their marketing to children.

—Source: Campaign for Tobacco Free Kids

gest there is no area with greater potential for positive impact than helping smokers to quit.

The Department of Justice asked me to come up with a cessation remedy for America, which I estimated to cost $130 billion over 25 years. At the 11th hour, they changed that $130 billion to $10 billion—a small price to pay for the tobacco industry. That's really a tragedy. What an injustice. What an opportunity lost.

CHAPTER THIRTEEN

PRETTY SMART

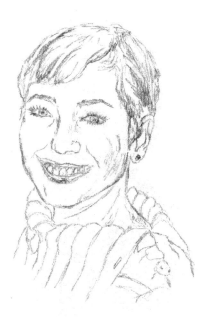

"The personality of someone who competes in the Miss America pageant is similar to every single student in medical school. We're all very competitive. Nothing stands in our way."

Tina Marie Sauerhammer, MD
Surgery Resident, Madison

There can't be too many surgeons who operate in stiletto heels. For Dr. Tina Marie Sauerhammer, shoes symbolize that other part of her life. She's a surgeon in training, but she's also a former beauty queen who made it to the finals of the Miss America pageant. Being a heartbeat away from that title made perfect sense in the context of Dr. Sauerhammer's life.

She's a petite woman in her mid 20s with big, brown eyes. On the evening I dropped by her home for the interview, she was wearing a sweater, red lipstick and rouge, with her dark hair tied back.

Doctor Sauerhammer had just returned from a 12-hour shift, but her face didn't betray the long hours or the stress of such training. It's a good thing doctors are trained when they're young, because they need all the stamina they can muster to get through residency.

Speaking of youth, Sauerhammer was 18 when she graduated from the University of Wisconsin-Green Bay, as valedictorian, no less. Ever watch that TV show, Doogie Howser, MD? Doctor Sauerhammer is the real deal.

The first time I competed for Miss Wisconsin, my parents were at the pageant cheering me on. There was a message for my dad on the answering machine, from the University of Wisconsin Transplant Center, saying, "We have a kidney donor for you. Call us right away."

Unfortunately, my dad did not receive that message in time. He never told me. I never knew about that whole story until several months after the fact. The organ only has a certain lifetime, so they go down a list of potential patients who will be recipients of that organ transplant. If somebody is not calling back, obviously, they have to move down the list and call somebody else.

My dad was diagnosed with Wegner's Disease—an autoimmune disease that basically affects your sinuses, your lungs, and also your kidneys. My dad has always been sick, in and out of the hospital a lot.

It was during medical school when his health really started to decline. He was first diagnosed with kidney failure. That's when he was put on a waiting list for a kidney transplant. He was dialyzed, secondary to his kidney failure.

That was really difficult for me because I was here at school. Meanwhile, my mom and my dad are at home. When I was a third year medical student, I was home for the holidays, and that was when my dad ended up passing away at age 45, on his birthday.

I was visiting my best friend in Chicago, and I was going to come back home later that night, but early in the morning my grandma called me. She said, "Tina, you need to come to Green Bay. Your dad is in the hospital."

It was just the oddest thing, because my dad had been in and out of the hospital constantly. I can't remember a holiday, like Christmas, when he wasn't in the hospital. It was this common occurrence, but I knew something was different.

I ended up driving from Chicago to Green Bay that night and my dad was in the intensive care unit. It turns out he'd actually coded a couple times during the day, and I had no idea. My grandmother and my mom didn't want me to know how serious it was. He was septic. He had a widespread infection, and basically, they just couldn't keep his pressures up and he just succumbed to his disease. It was probably just a few hours after I had seen him in the hospital, when he passed away.

He was on the waiting list for a kidney for four years. I think it would have prolonged his life. It would have given him a better quality of life, as well. Every other day, he needed to be dialyzed and even on his off days he barely had enough energy to carry on a normal conversation. He barely had enough energy to walk from this side of the room to that side of the room. He really had no quality of life, and I could tell. I could see it in his eyes.

Had he had a kidney transplant, he would have just had a happier life. Even if it prolonged his life for two years, he would have seen me graduate from medical school, or he would have been with us that much longer.

When my dad passed away, I took a second look at what I wanted to do. Even though I knew I would graduate medical school, I wasn't ready to continue moving forward, because I didn't have a fair shot at accepting what had happened to my dad.

Luckily, I was on rotation near Green Bay, and close to home. That helped a lot, but it was definitely a challenge for me to make the decision to continue on with medical school. I was right then and there ready to just say, stop. I just can't do this anymore. This is the point where I just need to put things on hold. But one thing that my mom and my grandmother told me really helped me to keep going and complete medical school: "Your dad would really want you to continue on."

My dad's dream was to become a doctor. His family never had the means to send him to college and get the appropriate schooling, so it was really important for me to live out my dad's dream.

I ended up competing for Miss Wisconsin, my reasoning being that I wanted to be Miss America, so I could be a spokesperson for organ and tissue donation. I can help save the lives of people who otherwise would die without organ transplants. I just wanted to give back to my dad.

Was your dad like you? A big brain?

I would describe him as a scholar. He was definitely where I got my brains from. I'm the first person in my family to be a doctor and the first one to even graduate from college. All I know is that I wanted to help people. I wanted to be a baby doctor. As long as I can remember, that's just what I wanted to do.

I was born and raised in Green Bay, Wisconsin. My dad was born and raised in Green Bay, as well. He initially was a meteorologist in the Air Force, stationed in Korea, where he met my mom. My mom was an artist in Seoul. They met, and came back to Green Bay. Growing up, my mom and I always watched Miss America on TV. We always watched, as long as I can remember.

My dad worked at Ft. James, which is a paper mill, and my mom opened her own sewing business. She's a seamstress. Just with the Korean culture, first generation from Korea, she wanted to give me everything that she never had. Education was really important for both of my parents.

What was school like for you growing up?

There's a school called Montessori Children's World in Green Bay. This school, in particular, emphasized learning by the senses, so I started there when I was two. I went there from preschool all the way through eighth grade. With Montessori training, it was learn at your own pace. By the time I was done with Kindergarten, I tested out into third grade. By the time I was done with seventh grade, I actually already completed my high school curriculum. I had already completed chemistry, calculus—all these different subjects during my middle school years.

I wanted to graduate with the rest of my class. After that year was completed, I had the opportunity of either going to high school or the option of going to a prep school somewhere on the East Coast. Then, the third option was going into college.

My decision was not to do another four years of high school when I'd already completed all the classes, but, to go forward. That's when I made the decision to go to college after eighth grade. I was 14-years old when I started.

You must have felt a little out of place.

Being an only child really helped me. As I was growing up, I always interacted with people several years older than myself, with my parents, with adults. I was a lot more mature than other people my age. I really didn't feel any different at all.

What about socially?

I don't think they even knew I was young unless I told them. Once I told one person, of course, word spread around very quickly. I had a ton of friends when I was in college and, looking back, they were some of the best days of my life. I still keep in touch with my friends from college. And even to this day, my friends in med school are several years older than myself and I don't think it's odd in any way.

How was it for you, academically?

Ever since I was two years old, I knew that I wanted to be a doctor. Of course, when you have that mindset, every single step you take leading up to medical school and residency is to get to the point of becoming a doctor, and it's very competitive to get into medical school.

I worked really hard during college. It's hard to say whether it was difficult for me, but all I know is I worked the hardest I've ever worked in my entire life. In the end, it didn't seem that difficult for me, but I think it was more because I put that much more effort into it. I needed to do well in order to get into medical school.

At first, you can be 14 and go to college, and there wasn't too much hype about that, because you don't know how well a 14-year-old is going to do. You could either fly or flail.

For the most part, it was really towards the end, when I graduated from college that there was a lot of press around me, because I graduated as Valedictorian of my class. I was the class speaker.

I hear about 14-year-olds and younger going into college and a lot of them don't do well because the social aspect is really important. You have to have an outgoing personality, or want to do well, in order to thrive in that kind of environment. Fortunately, I was able to do that. In the end, I think that's why people were interested.

I was 18 when I graduated, as the youngest person to graduate from UW-Green Bay. We had a reception after the ceremony and all my professors from my college years came. Everyone from my calculus professor to my premed advisor came. It was wonderful. That was another thing that really helped me a lot. The staff at UW-Green Bay were so helpful in incorporating me into that environment. My success has everything to do with what wonderful teachers they were.

Was there a downside at all, going to college at such a young age?

I don't think there was a downside to it. If I had to do it all over again, I might have taken time off between college and medical school. Medical school is a completely different world. I really wasn't anticipating the change, the transition. For me, it was even more difficult because I was not only starting medical school, but I was moving away from home for the first time. When I was in college, I lived at home with my parents, so the college transition wasn't that great for me.

Medical school, you really have to be very focused. I can't tell you how many times I second-guessed my decision to go to medical school, whether this was really something that I wanted. The most difficult part is when you're younger. You see your friends or people who are your own age, doing other things. When I was in medical school, my friends my age were in college and they were having the best years of their life. It was really difficult for me to focus, at times. But that would be the only thing—the one downside.

Did you have any trouble getting into medical school? Was your age a factor?

It definitely was a factor. It's a factor even now. People wonder, "Well, she's young. Medical school is a lot different than college. Is she going to be able to do it?"

The thing is, every place I go, just like at UW-Green Bay, there always has to be one person who really believes in me and really thinks that I'm able to succeed. It just takes that one person to have faith in you and you'll be fine.

I was looking all over the country. UW-Madison Medical School was the first acceptance letter that I received and I said, "That's it. I'm staying here." I'm really glad that I decided to stay home and be close with my family.

You said you had an interest in medicine since you were a little girl. How do you know that didn't stem from this saga with your dad?

When I was younger, I saw my dad really sick. It gave me some exposure to medicine in that way. But if anything, looking back, it would have driven me away from medicine.

The night he passed away, I was thinking, *I'm in medical school and there's nothing any doctor can do to save my dad.* At that point, I realized it's not necessarily what doctors do that save people lives, it's actually what other people can do for each other, like organ donation. If there was one person who made the decision to be an organ donor, he'd be living right now.

The role of the physician is not just to heal people and make them better—a lot of it is to be a teacher and to advocate different things, be it organ donation or something for patients.

Is that why you returned to the Miss Wisconsin competition?

Well, the Miss Green Bay pageant got wind of one of the articles printed about me and they ended up contacting me and asking, "Oh, would you be interested in competing for Miss Green Bay?"

After I graduated from college, there were all these people who were interested. "There's this 14-year old who went to college. Now she's 18. She's graduated."

What a lot of people don't realize is the Miss America organization is the world's largest scholarship program for young women. They see someone who's very interested in academics, scholarship, so they see that as something that I might be interested in. They were right. But they contacted me right before I was supposed to start medical school. At that point, I said, "No way. I really need to buckle down. I don't have time for this."

But between my second and third year of medical school, I was ready. I said, "You know what? This would be a wonderful opportunity for scholarship, a wonderful opportunity to meet people, just to do something different." At that point, I really needed to take a year off.

I thought that if I won Miss Wisconsin, I'd be forced to take a year off, and that would be a perfect excuse. That's what I ended up doing. I won Miss Green Bay, and went on to Miss Wisconsin, and was third runner up. I had no intention of doing it ever again, until my dad passed away.

The second time I competed, my whole goal was to become Miss America so that I could be a voice for organ donation. You have to compete for a city title first and then a state title and then, go on to Miss America. I competed for Miss Madison and won, competed for Miss Wisconsin, and won, and went on to the Miss America competition.

You don't really think of smart people being in beauty pageants. Tell me what that experience was like.

The personality of someone who competes in the Miss America pageant, for example, you'd be surprised. It's similar to every student in medical school. We're all very competitive. We see something we want and go for it, and nothing stands in our way. But it's completely different, in completely different ways.

We compete in swim suits, which is the stereotype; what Miss America actually started as, an evening gown competition, and then talent competition, which has the most weight in our score.

What most people don't see is the interview portion. That's really important. As part of our interview, we each have to have a platform which, if we win a title, we would promote throughout the year. Of course, mine was organ and tissue donation.

My talent was the cello. In preparation for it, I don't think I worked as hard for anything my entire life. I really wanted it.

You had to take a full year off. What did the medical school say about this?

In medical school, I was doing Miss America. Everybody was so supportive. Everybody was so excited for me. Throughout the year, as Miss Wisconsin, it was so wonderful. Everybody just completely embraced it.

Did that disrupt anything, being out of the medical mode for a year?

I don't think it caused any problems for me. I didn't have to disrupt anything, other than starting residency a year later. Personally, I wasn't ready to start residency right after medical school. The year as Miss Wisconsin allowed me to really open up and learn so much more about myself. First, it gave me an opportunity to meet a lot of people in the medical field, which is amazing. To this day, I've done so much work with people all over the country in medicine, in surgery.

Every opportunity I have to speak and to teach people, it was almost being a doctor in a different sort of way as Miss Wisconsin. It mentally prepared me for the years to come. It gave me the opportunity to do something completely outside of medicine for a year before I really buckled down and started my training.

I remember my year at Miss America. It was kind of the bookworm year. There were two Harvard graduates, there were two law students, there was me, and there were a couple premed students, as well. It was really interesting to see our diverse backgrounds, and for the Miss America organization, it was wonderful. For the first time, I think they did away with that stereotype that this is just a beauty pageant. This is an organization where women can have the opportunity to have scholarships for whatever education or career that they choose.

When I competed at Miss Wisconsin, a lot of the girls were very competitive in sort of a negative way. Going to Miss America, I was a little concerned that it would be the same way. But it is not at the national level. Every one of those women were just wonderful. They each have stories to tell, and they're just so much fun. They're just amazing, and I'm glad I had the opportunity to meet them and spend time with them. I ended up winning $50,000 in scholarships.

As Miss Wisconsin for that year, I advocated organ and tissue donation. What better way for people to listen to you than when you say, "I'm actually a physician. I went through four years of medical school and I'm not only talking to you about this from my personal experience with my father, but also as a doctor." It really gave me that extra touch when I spoke with people. On top of that, of course, everybody has the stereotype, oh, she's just a beauty queen. But when they learn about what I did with my career and with my education, that changes their mind.

What was your main message?

For me, my message was to share my personal story. You can preach about whatever topic you want until you're blue in the face, but people don't listen to you unless you have a voice. For me, my crown was my voice. It was kind of my megaphone to talk to people.

The other thing that touches people is that you have a personal connection to it. Anyone who's involved in organ donation, most of them, will have a story to tell. There's a reason why they're so passionate about organ donation. You ask them, and your heart will just melt.

There are so many myths about organ donation. To teach them about the facts of organ donation, that helps a lot. Any person who comes in and says, "I don't want to be an organ donor because I'm scared my body is going to be disfigured, or they're not going to try to save my life. They're going to take my organs instead." Also, people are not aware of what it takes to become an organ donor.

Did you get a sense as to whether you were making some progress in changing minds?

I did. A lot of times, it would touch me after I had a speaking engagement. People would come up to me afterwards and say, "You know, I was really skeptical, but I think I'm going to make the decision to become an organ donor." But I didn't just change the mind of that one person, because that person will tell their friends and their family.

Organ donation and how it's progressing through this society, is due, in part, to Wisconsin contributions. Doctor {Hans} Solinger is the chairman of transplant surgery at UW, and he was somebody who took me under his wing and had a huge role in what I did with organ donation throughout my year as Miss Wisconsin.

He was also close with Governor Tommy Thompson. I think they were at an event one day and Dr. Solinger was just not himself. He seemed kind of sad. Tommy Thompson asked, "What's wrong, Hans?"

"I just lost a patient today who was waiting for a kidney transplant."

Tommy Thompson was just so surprised. "You mean people actually die waiting for a transplant?"

Doctor Solinger said, "Absolutely. Not enough people are donating."

That was the turning point. That was when Tommy Thompson started to make all these legislative acts. When he became secretary of HSS, it became nationwide.

How much of this is the physician's responsibility? I hear that physicians are reluctant to ask that question, especially after they just lost a patient. The family's grieving and the last thing they want to say is, "By the way…"

It's very difficult. In the last year, during trauma surgery, I've dealt with that personally on several occasions. When an organ donation is pending, we'll have special people from the organ procurement organization who are trained in approaching family members. It's a group effort. It's an important conversation, because we have to decide whether we need to prolong this in order to preserve those organs, or do we just stop care now and that's the end of it. It does impact how we care for patients.

Recently, we had a patient who committed suicide. He had a gunshot wound to his head—a non-survivable head injury. There was nothing that could be done to save this person's life. His brain wasn't damaged to the point that he lost all his reflexes. We were still maintaining him on the ventilator. At that point, we had to have a conversation with the family, saying, "There's nothing that we can do to save his life. Eventually, he is going to succumb to the trauma."

I had to ask them. "First of all, if you're interested, organ donation is an option for you. Your son is young and he could save a lot of lives by donating."

His mother said, "No, absolutely not. He would have never wanted that. He doesn't want his organs ripped out like that."

I explained to them that this was not going to disfigure their son's body. It's difficult because at that time, they're grieving. They're not really thinking straight. His brother said, "I think we should donate." She said, "No, I don't think we should." It went back and forth.

That happens a lot with family members. In the end, they chose not to donate, which is unfortunate because he was a young guy. One person can save up to 50 lives.

Have you considered becoming a transplant surgeon?

It's in the back of my mind, always. One of the most fascinating operations is a kidney transplant. I remember the first time I saw a kidney transplant. You have the white, pale kidney, and once you have all of the arteries, veins and everything hooked up, right before your eyes you can see the blood flowing into the kidney and it transforms from white to pink to red. It's a beautiful thing.

However, I also love to see my family. I want to have kids. I want to be there for my children. I have a strong interest in transplant surgery, but in the end it's something that I'm not going to choose to do because of the difficult lifestyle. People do it and I completely admire them. Yolanda Becker, who is one of the transplant surgeons, is amazing. She has two kids and she's able to do all these things. And I said, if she can do it, and all these other people can do it, so can I.

But for me, I can still advocate organ donation, and be a part of it by speaking to people and doing what I'm doing currently, as opposed to being an actual transplant surgeon.

When I went to medical school, I thought that I was going to be a pediatrician. That was my plan through medical school, and I ended doing my surgery rotation. It was my very last rotation of my third year and I completely loved it. I was on call and we were so busy. We were in the operating room and I remember this one case we were doing. We were taking out someone's small intestine. I was sitting there because as a medical student, you don't do very much. You just help retract and expose things. I wanted to get in there and start sewing and cutting and doing everything that they were doing. At that point, I really made the decision that this is something that I want to do.

I struggled with that, because family is so important to me. I think surgery is the right field to go into. When I told people I was going to do surgery, nobody was surprised. My mom said, "Oh, yeah, I already knew that you were going to be a surgeon."

"Why didn't you tell me?"

She was like, "You just have to figure it out for yourself."

But I love working with my hands. I play the cello and the piano. I look back and it's obvious to me now. Of course, I want to be a surgeon. Someone has a problem, and we surgeons go in and fix it.

Internal medicine doctors have a problem, and they like to think about what the possible causes of this problem could be. You're either kind of one or the other. I want to see results right away, too. I love every single thing about surgery. I want it to be technically challenging, whatever I end up doing. I want to work with kids. I want to operate on children.

I'm in my second year. General surgery is a five-year program, so I still have three and a half years left. After I'm done with general surgery, I can either go out and practice privately or I could continue on with a fellowship and specialize.

I'd like to stay in Wisconsin, because my family is here. I love Wisconsin, but as long as my mom is willing to move with me, if I end up moving elsewhere, there's nothing holding me back.

My second year, you don't get to the operating room as much as you would like. But right now, trauma surgery has started. It's fun. Winter months are a little slower, but I love the operating room. It's an intense learning experience, for sure. It's trying at times. I get tired a lot. But in the end, it's like medical school. You just have to stay focused. You have to look at the end goal that I want to be a surgeon.

What's a typical day like in a surgical residency?

They have rules about that now. Back in the day, it was completely different. We can't work more than 80 hours per week. There are rules that say you have to be out of the hospital for at least 10 hours. Things have changed for the better, definitely. Right now, I work on the day team, so I'll be there at six in the morning and I'll come home lots of times at seven o'clock—a 13 or 14 hour day.

That's a big improvement?

A lot of people are shocked by that. "I couldn't imagine working 80 hours a week."

We have to take call every other weekend, which is in-house. We have to stay in the hospital. But every other weekend I have off, so the time that you do have, you make the most of it. I've traveled the most that I've ever traveled before. I get on a plane and go to New York or Vegas, just to get away. That's what I like to do with my free time—just get away completely and do something different.

Today you started at 6 a.m.?

I was in at six and I got back here around 6:30. {It's about 7:30 p.m. now}

How do you feel?

I'm tired. The first thing I want to do is eat, and then sleep. I love to sleep. The thing is, we have to study on top of that. A residency is different than any other type of job that you do. You take things home with you. It's not just doing things at work or the hospital. You go home and have to study, to prepare for the next day. It's a continuous process.

Where do you get the energy? How do you manage to do it?

Well, the weekends off are wonderful. They're very good for rejuvenation. I'm doing this because I want to help people, because I love operating, because this is what I wanted to do, for as long as I can remember. We always talk about this in residency and ask ourselves, why put ourselves through this? We make our decision. We're in residency because we want to be. If we didn't like it, we could quit and not even think twice about it.

There are tough days, but we love it. There are bad days, and today was what I would consider a bad day. It's definitely kind of a roller coaster. You just never know what you're going to get.

What was bad about today?

I wasn't as prepared as I should have been. Sometimes, I get in the operating room and I'm working with someone and I didn't know the anatomy as well as I should have, or trying to get patients out of the hospital can be a chore, sometimes.

Then, on the other hand, we had a kid who came in who was in a car accident who had this huge cut. His whole arm was deformed. We took him to the operating room and it was me and the staff, and we fixed it. That was like the greatest thing I've done, probably all month. I was so excited about that.

Even with the day, you have this low point and then you go to the operating room and have this really cool case and you have this high point. At the end of the day, you go home and things are okay, and the next morning, you wake up and do those things over again.

What about stress? Doesn't it freak you out that a patient could die if you do something wrong?

It does, and more so each year, with more responsibility. As you progress in the program, the more responsibility you are given. One good thing about residency, you have this responsibility, but there's always someone you can turn to for help. It scares me to think that some day I'm going to be on my own. At that point, I'm the top of the pole and there's nobody else to go to after that.

But you really need to have faith in your training program. This is such a strong training program that it's going to give me the best training that I could get. At the end, after the five years, I'm going to be comfortable dealing with all sorts of situations I wouldn't be right now.

What do you like to do in your spare time?

I love to eat. I love going to the movies. I love shopping! It's an addiction of mine. I recently got engaged, so we're planning a wedding, as well. Ever since I met Alec, I'm just really excited about having a family and everything that goes with it.

One downside of residency is that I hardly call my friends or my mom as much as I'd like to. It's kind of difficult.

I've dated a few people during residency and medical school. A lot of men, a lot of people, are not understanding of what we do. It's more difficult for women, because we're supposed to be at home cooking dinner and all these things. But it's difficult for them to understand that our jobs are just as important and demanding as the next person's.

Alec, for example, he is absolutely amazing. He's just so understanding. I've never met anyone like that before. It takes a special person, because they go through it with us. When we're on call, they're almost on call, as well.

Alec's friends have asked what it's like to be dating a doctor and he said, "Oh, it's so great. Hearing the stories is like the best part." That's one of the wonderful things about being a physician. We're so privileged to get these glimpses, to be so intimately involved with our patients. Nobody else gets that opportunity.

For example, we ask patients if they are taking drugs and people will tell you. People trust doctors and they will tell them anything. What we ask, they answer.

Do you get razzed by your medical colleagues about the beauty queen stuff?

I still do, to this very day. There are some physicians in the hospital who kind of tease me. I'm wearing scrubs and I have these high heels. I wear some of the craziest shoes with high, stiletto heels. It's the whole Miss Wisconsin/doctor thing. I have this thing for shoes. I'm addicted to shoes.

In this last month, I've been in trauma and we had clinics once a week. That's kind of our time to dress up. Every single time we have clinic days and I'm wearing these high heels, I get traumas that come in.

My chief right now is a female, as well, and all the med students are female, too. My chief likes to wear high heels, so it's just the two of us walking in our stilettos. We have lead on.* We have trauma patients coming in, bleeding all over the place. I'm like, please don't get blood on my shoes.

At least two times in a month, there will be patients who recognize me. It's fun. They won't say anything at first and then they'll be like, "Oh yeah, you used to be Miss Wisconsin." I always blush because it was such a long time ago. It's fun to think back, but I'm also happy to be where I am today.

In the same way that beauty queens have this negative stereotype, doctors have a stereotype, as well. Their stereotype is more, we don't have personality and we're cold people. We don't have many interests; we're just kind of focused on the books. That's totally not true. It was nice for them to have a spokesperson on the opposite sort of the spectrum. We're physicians, but we also have other interests.

So are you completely done with the beauty pageant part of your life?

I am. I'm aged out. I'm glad I did it. Looking back, I don't think I would ever do it again. A lot of times, I'll look back because I was runner up and I was this close to being Miss America. Had I been Miss America, it almost scares me. Where would I be right now? I probably would not be in a residency. I probably would have chosen a different direction; more public relations type of position.

---

* When trauma patients arrive, the doctors wear lead aprons to protect themselves during x-rays.

IV

Performing Artists

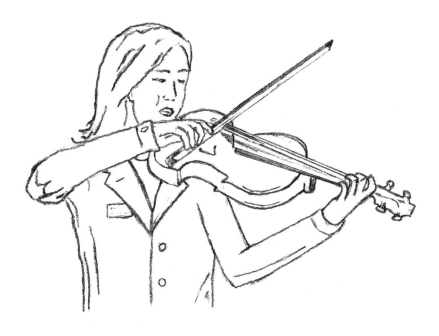

"Fine art is that in which the hand, the head, and the heart of man go together."

—John Ruskin

CHAPTER FOURTEEN

PHYSICIAN MUSICIAN

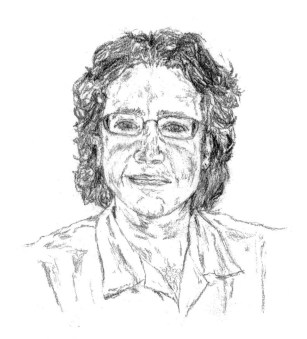

"Surgery is like playing the piano. It requires the touch. Without the touch, it sounds like a mess. Without the touch in surgery, you can really do some damage."

Adam Dachman, DO
General Surgeon, Dodgeville

A surgeon and a musician, Adam Dachman frequently discovers new connections between his medical life and his musical one. They lead to revelations that continually inspire him to better perform in each venue. I've talked with Dr. Dachman over the years about the healing power of music, as he's a pianist and composer who's recorded multiple CDs.

In his early 40s, Dr. Dachman practices in a small, farming community with one hospital, about an hour west of Madison. The hospital tour he gives me triggers memories of what Dr. Dachman has experienced there over the years.

My very first surgery in Dodgeville turned out to be a chest case. I ended up doing a thoracic surgery on a man with lung disease, and I did it with a scope. Nobody had even heard of thoracoscopy *at the time, let alone see it done. The whole operating room was filled with doctors from around here.

I'll never forget my very first incision—a small incision in his chest. I must have hit some subcutaneous vessel and there was just this Old Faithful gusher under the skin. I remember putting my finger in the hole and my heart rate went up just a little bit and I stayed calm. I'm thinking, *Oh, I can just see it now—The first front page of the* Dodgeville Chronicle— *"Dachman's First Patient Bleeds to Death on Opening Incision."*

Wasn't it a bit nerve-wracking to have all your colleagues there?

Yeah, but fortunately, I had this background of performance around people. At the time, I didn't really realize it was going to suit me and keep me composed, keep me poised, but it did. I just kept my cool and completed the procedure and everything went fine.

From that day forward, it's just been a real success. People have been in ORs to watch me do things and have come from other cities to watch me and help me, and I've had examiners come out and board-certify me.

When did your interest in surgery begin?

I was between 10 and 13 when I started doing dissections. I had just a real fascination and my mother recognized it, and brought home a microscope and dissection kit, and frogs, and pigs, and rats. I did my own science experiments. I opened them up and looked at them. After that, what I wanted to do with my free time was look inside things—absolutely fascinating. Just seeing how things were wired and put together—the heart, the lungs.

My mother would take me to the library in Niles, Illinois, where I took out my very first atlas of anatomy when I was seven years old. I wandered the shelves of the library all by myself. It was my little universe. I would go into the music room to listen to music. The anatomy books just flipped me out. I couldn't believe that we were that complicated inside.

I took out Grant's Atlas of Anatomy and I took it home with me. I still have it. That's one heck of a late fee. It was due back in, something like, 1969!

Tell me about your family.

My grandparents were immigrants. All their families died in the Holocaust. They came through Ellis Island. They were all escaping, basically Europe, trying to keep themselves alive and escape the Nazis.

I was an accident. I was the third and final child. I have two older sis-

* The insertion of a narrow tube with a mirror or camera attachment, through a very small incision.

ters. They call me Doctor Brat. They're very sarcastic about me. I guess they think I was my parents' favorite child because…because I was!

I was born in '62 to a relatively poor family. We lived in apartments. My father was a salesman who never finished college. He pretty much had a high school diploma and half of a two-year college education. Then he got married and had my sister and had to work to raise her.

I grew up in an all-American suburb of Chicago, a good place, going to school, taking piano lessons. I was five when I started lessons. I took lessons all through college, so I was a musician long before I was ever a doctor. I was really ordinary.

Life was good. I grew up not knowing bigotry—not too much anyway. I grew up in a really diverse neighborhood—lots of townhouses very close together, lots of kids, lots of free space to run around and play in parks. We left our doors unlocked, and the worst thing that ever happened to me was that my bike got stolen in my back yard when I was 10.

The thing about growing up in suburbia in the 1980s is that individuality is one of the tougher things to have when you're in high school. Really showing your colors, and standing out and just being yourself, is not easy. It wasn't for me. We couldn't afford to take fancy vacations, and we couldn't afford to eat out a lot. We couldn't afford to have the coolest pair of jeans that all the other kids wore. I had to take what my parents could afford.

My parents shopped on Roosevelt Road in Chicago. They had friends that were jobbers. They sold everything out of these rented spaces. They wholesaled their clothes and their shoes. They all had deals. I never had clothes that looked like anybody else's.

I went to Glenbrook North High School—which has produced some interesting people. It produced John Hughes, the director, who put out "Sixteen Candles" and "The Breakfast Club." "Ferris Bueller's Day Off" was filmed at my high school. It also produced that awful story about hazing, and some fraternity or club where they threw pig intestines.

It was a difficult period. I had a lot of trouble feeling confident about my talent and my individual background. I was from a relatively poor background and I went to an affluent high school. I had talents that wouldn't be known to the high school until I was a senior.

Teachers came to me because I played the piano. I played at home, but I never had the confidence to play in school. Teachers would say, "You made it through high school and we didn't know you had this talent." I missed the boat in high school.

My uncle, who was a very successful businessman in Chicago, said to me, "So Adam, what are you going to do after high school? What are you going to do with your life?"

I said, "Well, I think I'm going to be either a rock 'n roll musician or I'm going to be a doctor. I'm thinking about surgery."

He said, "Wow. It sounds like you're going to have to make a choice because those are different life styles."

I said, "What do you mean?"

He said, "Well, a doctor is going to be standing in one place and a musician is going to be on tour all the time, moving all around. That's kind of a crazy world, too—the whole music scene. You sure that's really what you want?"

I said, "You know, uncle, the world of music is really strange and whenever I see it on television, it really rubs me the wrong way. It almost frightens me, and I'm a home guy. I like having a family. You're making a really great point."

That was a turning point in my life. I was really lucky to have that kind of conversation with an adult, and it really helped define the rest of my life up to this point, seeking out that stability and that one location kind of life-style, as opposed to having to go around on a bus or a plane. That's when I really decided, I am going to be a doctor.

I wanted to be three things in life. I wanted to be a doctor, a musician and a farmer. As a young man, my parents hooked us up with a farm family in Hartford, Wisconsin, that had a program that was like a bed and breakfast on the farm. You could come up and experience the farm life. And this for me, at age 10, was an amazingly magical thing. That's how I really got interested in Wisconsin.

By the time I was a teenager, we finally started to fall into some affluence. My father started to do some work that brought in some reasonable revenue, and all of a sudden, I could afford, fortunately, to go to college. I was finishing high school and my parents insisted that I would be the one who would have a college education. I was the first kid in my family to actually complete college.

It was a pretty important moment. They were very proud. I applied to Carroll College. I chose Carroll because it was close to Hartford. It was close to the people that I knew and the area I had come to love. They really helped me become a musician there and I still have close ties with a professor in the music department. I studied piano and biology.

My training in music continued through college. I kept both things going, and it was a real struggle. My music professors would see me struggling and I would constantly say, "I think I'm going to have to give up my music. I've got to get straight As. I've got to get a grade point to get into med school and I can't do anything besides study."

They're like, "No, no, no. You can't give up this talent. It'll be an asset to you. You might not see it now, but it will be." They kept encouraging me.

My premed advisor said, "I don't know. I don't think it's ever been done before here. If you don't have this tip top grade point average, I don't know if you're going to get into med school. Maybe you should be thinking about whether you really want to be a doctor. Maybe you should think about just being a musician."

But I was so determined about being a surgeon that nobody was going to tell me to do something else. My premed advisor played the devil's advocate, which probably was a good thing. He was a son of a gun and was not a guy that built you up. He was a guy who tried to break you down. But that kind of personality in my life was so unusual. I had so many people who tried to build me up and tried to build my character. To meet a guy who was my nemesis—that was my premed advisor. I had to prove him wrong. And so there was a real strong push that kept me motivated to get the grades and still do the music, and I did it all through college. He would say things like, "You're not a good technician. You're not a good student." I had to prove him wrong.

Do you think that's what he had in mind when he was telling you that stuff?

Sometimes I wonder. We were a whole band of wannabe doctors at Carroll College. Whenever I speak to anybody who went on to become a physician, they all had the same exact experience, and not one of them feels any fond thoughts of him.

I finished college, moved to Chicago for two years where I did medical research and started a music composition company called Adameus—a spin off of Amadeus. I started playing the piano for big events. Had my picture taken with a lot of cool people—Oprah Winfrey, Michael Jordan, and ultimately got into medical school in Iowa.

I had finished med school and residency and I had moved back to Wisconsin. I went back to Carroll College for homecoming, in 1995. I found {the advisor} at the homecoming football game at halftime and I introduced myself.

He said, "Oh sure, I remember you."

I said, "I just wanted you to know I became a surgeon and I'm a musician, as well. I just wanted to say thanks for your guidance and let you know that I did it."

I remember all the years of feeling anger and bitterness and dislike for him. But I never shared one ounce of bitter water with him. He seemed like he had mellowed. He appreciated that I stopped to speak with him and was glad that I achieved my goal. It was warm, but it was lukewarm. I felt lucky that I had the chance to go to him and let the past be the past. It was a great experience. I ran into another student minutes after I met him and said, "Did you see our counselor?"

She said, "Are you kidding? I've seen him and I wouldn't go near him. He's the biggest A-hole I ever met in my life. There's no way I am going to talk to him."

I said, "What are you doing now?"

She said, "Well, I'm the chief of gynecology at Northwestern Memorial, in Chicago."

Maybe there's some method to this guy's madness.

Yeah, I thought that too. Maybe that was part of his program, to harp on you psychologically, so that it would motivate you. That's an interesting person to meet on the yellow brick road on the way to the Emerald City.

When I went to med school there were some characters, but they never got to me. I graduated from med school in 1990. When I came to the reception area after I left the graduation hall, I had 180 grads from med school with me, I had my cap and gown on and a fake diploma in hand. I had just taken the oath and walked into the reception area and my mother was just beaming with joy and pride. She put her hands on my arm and looked me in the eye and said, "I am so proud of you." She gave me a big hug and a kiss.

I said, "Thank you, mom. But I have just one question. Now, can I be a musician?" It was just meant to be a light hearted thing because she said to me when I was growing up, "You can be whatever you want to be as long as you're a doctor."

Pretty much walking that walk of wanting to be a musician and a doctor. The farmer thing was still kind of background. I always say the happiest moment of my life was the day that I got into medical school. I worked so hard to get into medical school and it's so competitive. It took me three applications to finally break through the wall and get in. I guess that is just the way the stars had it for me and I'll never forget I actually heard by telephone.

I had interviewed at some med schools. I was going away on a trip in February, 1984, and called the med school secretary, and said, "Look, I'm going away and waiting. I'm holding my breath, waiting to see if I got in. I am going to be away from the mail, and I was wondering if you had any information?"

She said, "Hold on a minute." Barbara Fox. I'll never forget her name— the med school secretary. She took about five minutes and she said, "Well, you know what? Fortunately, I can tell you. I want to congratulate you. You've been accepted to the class of 1990."

I was in the kitchen. I was all by myself. I jumped so high, I swear I must have hit the ceiling. I screamed. I just started crying. I told Barb Fox I loved her. I started making phone calls all over the planet, telling people I had been accepted. I was absolutely frantic.

Then, from Iowa, we moved to Detroit, and I did my surgical residency there for five years, through Michigan State University. They say, go where you want to train; not where you want to live.

But when I got to residency, the culture of the residency was for the most part, "Young doctor, you are licensed to kill. You are dangerous. You know nothing and you lie. Residents lie. You'll tell me you think you know something when you're not sure, which is another way of lying. You'll tell me you know something just to make yourself look good in rounds when you really don't know what the hell you're talking about and somebody could get hurt."

I always respected that immediately because the interesting thing is it's true. The average human being, when you talk to them, will stretch the truth. They'll tell you something based on an assumption, based on a few facts, rather than based on the actual truth, which in public can work sometimes to make you look good.

But in medicine, if you don't know, the best thing to say is, "I don't know, but I'll find out." Either you know or you don't know. In between can hurt somebody.

Some residents continue down the path of assumption, and continue down the path of not really respecting that intellectual integrity, the law or rule. Those residents do tend to get more abuse than others. I've seen it. Some residents really react rebelliously against that authority, even though it's in the best interest of the patient.

There are elements to residency that some residents don't adapt to well, and they should. They need to. There are other elements of residency, however, which truly are abusive. You can also argue, hey, the longer you're around seeing what happens, the more experience you get, and it makes a greater depth of knowledge and confidence and intuition. It makes you more of a Jedi† around the hospital. And I'll tell you, I was the last of the old school. I did those long two-day things, with no sleep. I also had the advantage of senior residents dropping out of my program due to its rigors, so much so, by the time I was a sophomore resident, there was only one other resident ahead of me, so I got to do chief resident cases in my second year.

By the time I was a chief resident, I probably didn't even need to do my chief resident year because I was already an attending, in terms of my skill, because I had so much experience. By the time I got out of residency, I was well poised to come to a place like Dodgeville, where the community really needed a surgeon who could do virtually anything that needed to be done.

Yeah, abuse in residency, it's still there. It sort of passed from one generation to another. The abuse mostly is, "I don't want to hear you whine about how tired you are. I don't want to hear you whine about how far it is to check that x-ray again because you missed what you shouldn't have missed."

People sometimes talk about abuse, when in fact, that's just safety. I never talk about my residency as being abusive. I did have some abusive attendings. I did have some degrading attendings. To this day, when I see them at meetings, when I say hello to them, I really try to open myself up

† Star Wars reference that refers to characters that gain their power from doing good in their communities.

intuitively to who they are and where they are, energetically speaking, in the world. Some of them haven't changed a bit, which I feel sad for them because they're missing so much. Their particular personality type robs them of much of life's joy. I look back at them and forgive them for the abuse they handed out to me. I don't hold on to it.

Vascular surgeons were notorious for having you assist them in the OR and you were trying so hard to technically help them to the best of your ability and look for guidance and suggestion on how you can do the best job possible, and all they can offer was, "You're doing a bad job," or "Doctor, I need you to suction that blood. I need you to suck, suck, suck!"

"I'm sucking the best I can."

Their line would be, "That is very scary."

And that's all you get from them is that kind of sarcastic attitude. Well, it's like, if you think you can do it better, show me how. Of course, you never say that, otherwise you'll end up with some discipline. Any kind of attitude was perceived as being insubordination.

When I went to med school, I had such a gift of two years growing between college and med school and doing my own thing and having my own level of success. I carried an air of confidence with me that people just didn't mess with. I had my music. I was a damn good musician and composer, and had had success. I always had something that no one could take away from me, which is why I've become such a staunch advocate for music education. It's something you can do as a youth. You can't become a doctor as a youth. You can't become a lawyer. You can't become an engineer. You can become a musician as a child, and it gives kids such a personal sense of accomplishment.

Fortunately, most of my attendings knew that I had talent when I came in; knew that I had a brain. I also had kids. They viewed me as being a real person, where some of the residents who came in were younger than me and less advanced in life, so they got abused more because they didn't have maturity. They didn't have compassion, or intelligence, or the experience level to not be abused, which I felt bad for.

It wasn't until I was a surgical resident, believe it or not, that the chief of surgery at my program, who really took me under his wing, a colonel in the Reserves, six-foot-five, white hair, mustache, brilliant surgeon, great hands, just a great guy. It was my first year of surgery residency. He says, "You know, a surgeon needs to be nuts about anatomy." It was the first time anybody in the profession said that to me, and it was like, boom! It struck back to the days of my childhood. Somebody who was on the other side, a surgeon, finally, was brilliant enough to say what needed to be said long ago.

I'd been through med school, gross anatomy. I excelled in gross anatomy. I was a TA[‡] in gross anatomy. Subsequently, after my first year, I

‡ Teaching assistant

taught all the incoming students and PA§ students, and the podiatry students, and made a few extra bucks doing it. I was always straight As in anatomy in college, and in med school. But you have to be nuts about anatomy. That's what surgery is. Taking the anatomy and knowing it like the back of your hand and being able to reroute it, manipulate it, work with it, touch it, feel it, instrument it.

It's like playing the piano. It requires the touch. You gotta have the touch. Without the touch, it sounds like a mess. Without the touch in surgery, you can really do some damage.

It's like gardening. I had a girlfriend in high school who was into horticulture. She taught me how to handle roots and transplant things and graft things. I created amazing gardens in multiple houses, and it's that same kind of thing—working with the hands, and working with the tissue in a way that respects it and treats it within the limits of what it can handle.

In 1995, I was in Detroit, doing my residency. At the end of the residency, we were searching around for opportunities. A couple of weeks later, I got a phone call from our administrator here {Dodgeville} who invited me out. It was the last hospital that I'd looked at. I came out in the middle of February of 1995 and the snow was everywhere. It was ice cold. I just immediately liked it.

It was close to Madison. The people were great. The hospital was growing and modern. It had Lands' End,¶ it had more of a diversified flair. The long and the short of it was that I established roots here and started my practice at this location and my name has been on that window ever since.

There are two operating rooms here—very large, very modern, and well-equipped. It's all we really need at the moment, due to the population. When I got here, it was pretty much a boundless sense of possibility. They'd never heard of some of the things I was capable of doing when I got here, surgically speaking. When I came here, it was really very much, Dr. Dachman, the highly-trained modern surgeon that's going to bring the hospital into the 21st Century, because they had older doctors who didn't have all of the modern technologies that I had when I trained.

I was worried that this was going to be a country hospital that didn't have facilities and wasn't modern. But when I came here, it reminded me of where I had come from in Michigan. It was attractive. It was comfortable. It was new. Everything was just shiny, spic 'n span and modern. I was very impressed. They really needed a surgeon badly, so I felt a really strong sense of need out here and decided to fulfill it.

Even though we're in the country, we still have an obligation to bring the community forward, medically, and provide them with the best that

§ Physicians Assistants

¶ Catalogue company that employs 4,500

they can get anywhere. It's always been my mission to make sure that nobody does a better job than we do.

Right now, we're running about 28 beds. We're a critical access hospital, which basically means we're really important out here. But it also means that we're supposed to stay fewer than 28 beds. If we go above that, then we're no longer critical access. It's kind of this balancing act, so we need to know what we do well and we need to know what we don't do well. We're not doing heart, lungs, transplants or brains. But we're doing a lot of the bread and butter, nuts and bolts community medicine, trying to do it as well, if not better, than anyone else.

At what point would you need to send somebody to Madison?

What we can do here is help stabilize the patient for transfer. If they end up here, then it's our job to make their chances of getting to Madison better, so that in the transit, they're not bleeding to death or having an airway problem. It's our job to secure their airway, establish vascular support so their blood supply is adequately protected, their fluid supply is protected. And then, get them there, because it's not our role to handle multi system traumas. It's more our role to focus in on single or double kinds of issues. Once we start getting into multiple systems that are really threatened, we need to bump up to a facility where there's more manpower and more facility. There's one more trauma surgeon here. He's been here for 30 years.

I've never been overwhelmed. I can only think of one night during a blizzard, in the middle of January one year, I got called in, total white-out. I risked my life to get here, literally. There was a fella who was in a bad accident. He had a ruptured spleen and he was bleeding pretty badly. He was going into shock, so we took him to surgery and opened his abdomen and ultimately stopped as much of the bleeding as we could. But I knew that he was going to need some services that we didn't have. He was going to need some fancy x-ray services with angiograms, angiography and a technique called embolization, where they use angiograms to find blood vessels and squirt them with foam that stops them from bleeding from the inside. I stayed in the operating room with him until he could fly. They put him on the helicopter and flew him to UW, took him right to radiology and embolized the vessel.

He made it. He went home about 10 days later. It was an example of how we can work as a team, even though we're at two different locations.

Somehow, I got here, in spite of the fact that I didn't have chains on my vehicle. It's arguable as to whether he would ever have made it to Madison by ambulance. There was no other option than me.

The most absolutely life threatening emergency that I have ever been called to was at a different hospital altogether. I was here in Dodgeville eating lunch at my desk at noon one day when one of my colleagues in a nearby town was in the operating room. She was doing a case and had inadvertently injured the patient's vena cava—the largest vein in the abdomen. The patient was bleeding to death. Two holes in a garden hose-size vein way back in the abdomen—two feet in, literally, in this very obese patient.

The doctor said, "I need you here. This lady is going to bleed to death. I don't know what to do." I got into my rocket. We call it my red Mach 8—without a radar detector. I flew to Darlington, which normally takes 20, 25 minutes. I got there in about 12 minutes through the back roads.

I got there and these guys were just covered in blood. The hospital is really rural. It's bare-bones medicine. I got into scrubs. Got into the operating room and these guys were literally holding their hands over these holes because every time they lifted their hands up—and the hole—you could only see maybe two inches around in a circle through this ten inch incision. The lady was so big that by the time you got down to that big vein, everything was kind of caved in. So I spent the first five minutes just getting everybody calm and the next five minutes packing everything off. There was no transfer opportunity. There was no way to get her anywhere else. It was either me or it was heaven.

We got exposure of the holes. I sewed them both shut and we let the clamps off the veins that we had to control them. To take care of the vena cava, we had these sponges on the clamps that were pushing down on the veins, just stopping the blood flow. And once we let them up, the vein immediately filled up with blood again and then the suture lines held. There were no leaks. Everybody took a big sigh and then … I remember walking away from the operating table and taking my gown off. I was literally soaked from head to toe with sweat. I had never sweated like that in my life. That was the most extreme experience I've had in this area. We normally don't go there.

In Detroit, it was an every-day thing to have somebody die on an operating table from bullet wounds, or a ruptured aorta, or something terrible. I took care of a girl in Michigan. She came in one day shot up with bullets one night. One of the attendings and me—I was the chief resident at the time, took this kid to surgery and opened her belly, and had a couple of holes in her vena cava and it was the same thing. This was before I came to Dodgeville. We got control of the veins and we sewed up the vein holes at that time. Same story. We took the sponges off, the vein filled out, didn't leak and she went home seven days later.

I'm thinking, my God, it was that kind of experience that saved the Dodgeville patient's life. Created the mettle for me to be able to do it, to stay calm. It created the skill and experience for me to be able to fix the problem, so I was glad that I'd spent those five years in the war zone to come out here to paradise to be able to save, you know, if it was even just one life, from that one case.

But out here, we don't usually get those cases. I've not seen one single gunshot wound in 10 years out here. The only ballistic penetrating trauma

I've ever seen here was a man who accidentally shot himself with a nail gun right in the pubic bone. The only thing that saved him, really, was the Levi's jeans heavy denim over the zipper area—caught the head of the nail so it didn't go in any deeper. Poor guy. All he needed was a good pliers and some anesthesia. I put my foot up on the table and pulled the nail out. He went home the next day and did fine.

When we take someone to surgery electively, which is what we do most of the time out here in this environment, where they plan their operation, it's extremely unlikely that they're going to bleed to death. Nobody's ever died on one of my operating tables.

I don't want to jinx anything, but death post-operatively here in Dodgeville is almost never seen. I don't think I've seen anybody die after an operation in two or three years. I talk to other general surgeons, and it's one or two a month. It's because the community that uses this hospital is an active community—farmers; hard working people. They take care of themselves. They're in reasonably good physical condition, so it's a good thing.

I have to be ready for anything. As the years go, by we've learned how to triage our patients. We know what to send and what to keep. We don't want anybody to die because of something we don't have, technologically or personnel-wise. We only have so many people working here because we're a small community. It's a balance which I think is a good thing from a quality of life perspective.

As we walk through the halls of the hospital, some of these memories come out. A fellow came along, a mythic character, a legend, a traveling guy, kind of a vagabond from Texas—bushy mustache, sideburns, thick gray hair, tall, southern accent, cowboy boots, cigarette smoker, so many smokes that his finger nails were stained from the cigarettes. He always had a butt in his hands.

I set him up for some elective surgery, but before he ever got to the elective surgery, he landed in the emergency room with a life threatening bowel obstruction. He had hernias. He went home only to come back with emergency bowel obstruction a few days later.

He was in the hospital for about 10 days, and I saw him at the clinic. In those 10 days, I got to know him more. It turned out that he likes to paint country artists, primarily music people, the giants, and I was so impressed by his story. His southern accent—it was like talking to this authentic cowboy. He just totally touched me. He had this free spirit.

He was a total failure with women, in terms of having any long-term relationship, but he was a lady's man, nonetheless. This guy had so many girlfriends in his lifetime. But he couldn't hold one down and told me about his love for Elvis. I never had an appreciation for Elvis. Ever. I wasn't into Elvis. The whole thing was kind of a tacky joke. But I eventually went to Graceland. We did the Elvis Presley tour and when I left, I was literally just completely elevated to a different place. I had an appreciation for the musician for the first time. I didn't realize the depths of his musical abilities and the magnitude of what he did, musically. He redefined music. His accomplishments were truly amazing. I had no idea.

When I came back, I really got into Elvis Presley. That was what, almost 25 years after he passed away, that I, the first time, really paid any attention. I shared all this with this fellow, the Southern man from Texas, and he said, "I saw Elvis when he was just a kid down in Brownsville when he was just comin' out and the loudspeaker system was crude, people were so loud and people were screaming, you couldn't hear a word he sang."

We realized, we both love Elvis and I said, "You're such an interesting guy. I don't meet people like you. You've inspired me. I was really hoping that you would…"—he was hurting financially—"I'd like to pay you to paint me an Elvis portrait for my studio because every studio needs a portrait of the King."

So he was like, really honored. And I said, "I'll pay you whatever you ask me for." So after he was discharged, he spent the next few weeks painting an Elvis portrait. And while he was painting, I got this inspiration and I sat down and wrote this song called the *"Southern Man"* about him. The lyric goes:

> *Cigarette fingers stained moustache, too*
> *A southern accent, a toothless fool.*
> *He loves to paint pictures in shades of reds and blue*
> *Livin' colors, he loves Elvis, too.*

And then the chorus goes:

> *He's a Southern man from Texas*
> *A Brownsville station dude,*
> *I met him one day when things were bad*
> *And he showed me the way to you.*

So it turns out to be this love song. And the Southern man is talking in the song, says: {singing}

> *Now paintin' is like lovin,' said my southern friend*
> *Gentle brush strokes flowin, repeatin' till the end.*
> *There's no rushin' a woman when her heart's on the line*
> *It's like paintin' a portrait one color at a time.*

So then it goes back to this flashback.

> *Let's go back to that summer night when we were very young*
> *I could not keep my hands to myself and I made you turn and run*

I was talkin' about this girl that I had moved too fast with. Then, it goes back to this paintin' is like lovin' thing. You have to hear the song.

> *Paintin' is like loving, said my Southern friend*

Gentle brush strokes flowing, repeating till the end
There's no rushing a woman when her heart is on the line
It's like painting a portrait, just one color at a time.

So I went back to our spot, along Route 62.
It was a foggy night, but it was crystal clear that I was after you.
When our eyes made contact, my heart began to pound
I slowly moved closer, what I heard was the sound
Of the Southern man's voice as I gently touched her hand.

It's this real funky, jazzy swing number. It's never been released, but I've been working on this tune for years, so I recorded it for him in proto-type form and on the day that he brought me the Elvis portrait, I gave him a copy, a couple copies of the "Southern Man" CD. He just said, "Doc, you've got soul." That's all he said. That's all he needed to say. That's probably the best compliment I could have gotten from somebody about my music.

I gave him a wad of cash and was just so happy that I had known this guy and he left me with this lasting piece of like, legend. I hope that one of these days that the *"Southern Man"* gets heard by the world.

How did he do on the painting of Elvis?

It's cool. It's a young Elvis, sort of before he really makes it. Just on the edge of his real fame. There's this edge in his eyes, of almost like a foreshad-owing of what's to come after, the years of all the success. It's brilliant. He did it in oil, and it hangs in my studio.

It is, to this day, the most vivid recollection. This wasn't so much his medical story as it was this guy rubbed off on me in a way that was about sort of about life and the pain, the break ups with women, and like learning how to love, making it a metaphor for lovin' is like painting. You've got to go one brush stroke at a time. It's just one color, one brush stroke. There's no hurrying it.

Surgery's just like that. You can't rush. It can only happen so fast. If you rush it or hurry it, you're going to tear something, damage something and make an irreversible mistake. Through this man, he gave me another angle through which I was able to understand my own life.

At times, I wonder who gets more out of the relationship. If anybody's really paying attention with their patients, really in attendance with them, it's school. They're teaching us about life in a way that we can only learn by having that experience with them. It becomes a really gratifying, fulfilling experience.

After about a year of being out here, and really establishing myself as kind of the wizard of surgery who can do all these high-tech things, and get in there and fearlessly save lives like that, the day to day wasn't so intense. I've got 99.9% control of what I'm doing. I'm not taking in stab wounds and really sick alcoholics, drug addicts. I'm mostly taking care of hard working people who need care, and schedule it.

That led to me picking up golf, which I dabbled with a little bit as a resident in surgery, because some of my attendings invited me. I wasn't a golfer prior to my surgical residency, but my attending surgeons—a couple of them were golfers. One in particular, who's my greatest mentor, frequently took me to his country club in the Detroit area. I decided that it would be a nice icebreaker for me and the docs, so I started inviting docs and started to golf. I became a pretty good golfer. I was golfing two or three times per week.

In 1996, I was golfing so much that I scratched my head one day in wonderment about all the time I was spending on the golf course. My whole life has been controlled by others. Now, suddenly I'm realizing that I can actually have some control of my destiny, so golf was a way to create space for myself. No sooner did I get that awareness, I put my golf clubs away and bought a grand piano. I revitalized the musical Adam that had been put to sleep years prior, when I started medical school.

I always played and I always had a piano—an electronic keyboard that kept my fingers going. During residency, I played for parties and a few events. I kept writing some songs, as well, but I left my really passionate years of music behind.

The time that I was spending on golf, I spent on writing music and recording. I strung together enough sessions to get the first album recorded, and produce the CD with the jacket and everything else, and developed a little bit of a marketing plan of sorts and started a little corporation. All of a sudden, I ended up on the front page of the *State Journal*** as a headliner, one morning in May of 1996, when I played with Garrison Keillor. The headline was, "Surgeon Plays his Way into Famed Humorist's Act," May 18, 1996. It's in my office, hermetically sealed on a wood plaque.

All of a sudden, I started really getting serious about my music, so I started doing some performances. I started committing to a second album. It wouldn't be for four years that my second album, "Center of My Heart," would be released, which was a more genuine attempt to take where I was in time, and place it into my music.

I've managed my own affairs completely, which has been very difficult. I'm primarily a surgeon and a father, and music has just been my passion. I've never done it for the sake of making money at it. I've always done art for the sake of art. Whatever has happened is because somebody heard it and then somebody else heard it and somebody else heard it and then it comes to some attention. "Hey, we liked what you did. Can we talk to you about something?"

That's led to my latest project, an international project with 23,000 discs distributed so far, which is my biggest distribution ever. That is

** The Wisconsin State Journal is Madison's daily.

called, "Music for Life," and is produced by a company in Ohio called GSW Worldwide. They market for Genentech—the world's second largest biotech company. They produced a CD featuring my music, and commissioned me to write a theme for their company called, *"Keys of Hope."*

Well, *"Center of my Heart,"* that features stories and songs about people I've taken care of. I created imagery in my mind which is the summation of many patients wrapped up into one song. I wrote a song called *"Spirit of This Woman."* That was based on many of the patients that I've had who had breast cancer. It's a song that begins with an introduction of a young woman in her 30s, going on 21. She's an adult, but she still has this young spirit inside of her who likes to travel and likes to live and really soars, and how people are inspired by her presence and how she offers something to the world around her.

Then one day comes where she's delivered this news that things are not the same. She's facing a life-threatening problem and all in all, it ultimately leads to the doctors working sleeplessly to save her life and her spirit, and ultimately, she passes and dies. Her spirit soars to the sun.

For me, it's a very sad song. It's not a song that puts any fluff behind the diagnosis of breast cancer. This particular song is really a way of my dealing with some of the women who've passed away from breast cancer who I've seen, which, fortunately, is not the majority of women. And the song was my way of really paying tribute to the women who didn't have the happy ending, but had the sad ending. It's a way of immortalizing their spirits in a musical form, and also I got some comfort out of writing it.

I performed it on Capitol Hill, right in front of the Capitol on a huge sound stage a couple years ago—thousands of people.

I had written another story about a young woman who passed away. I went to her funeral. She left a beautiful family behind—four kids. Her funeral was absolutely devastating. It was so sad. And I stood way in the back—there were just no seats in the church. I was with some nurses. We were all crying. There was a song playing, "When I'm looking down to you from heaven, my tears will be raining down on you." I'd never heard that song before. It was like she was singing to her children who were left behind. I could cry right now just remembering it. We were all soaking wet in tears. When I play that song, I really try to inspire people to let go, to let them cry. This is the time for tears.

I wrote a song called *"You were with me from the Start."* I've performed it all over.

> *Why does it take loss to bring us all together?*
> *You were here and now you're gone*
> *Like wind blowing on a feather*
> *Is it all just random or is there some command?*
> *God above, I know there is*

And I know it's in His hands

His eyes so bright and filled with life
All the way to the end
When the Angels shut them for all times
And brought you to their land
Is there hope that we'll survive
And keep your soul alive?
I know there is
And then realize we all stand side by side

Then the chorus goes:

The tears come fallin' down
My eyes are filled with sorrow
The years keep spinning round and round
And I know that tomorrow.
You'll live inside my mind
And fill my aching heart
That's the way it's always been
You've been with me from the start.

Then the next line goes:

When did we grow so cold that we forgot to cry?
Does it always have to be that someone has to die?
Is there a life without some tears?
I know it would be a lie.
So let them run on down my cheek
And trickle from my eyes.

It became a funeral song. I have a song that people play at recitals. I've got a song that people play at relays for life, and people sing at funerals and it's a really befitting funeral song. It was written at a funeral, literally. That's where it was inspired. I never knew that I would write a funeral song. I have a rock 'n roll background as a teenager.

I have not written a song that was inspired by going through a death with a patient. I don't have that many people die, thank God. And the few people that have died, I went down with the ship with them. Part of me died.

How do you break bad news, rare as it is in your practice?

We will do everything possible that modern medicine has to offer, knowing that there are no guarantees. We'll explain everything about risks and complications and leave it up to you whether you want the treatment. We will tell you how successful or not a particular treatment is, and we will work with you as a team, so you're part of the decision-making process.

But remember, once you make decisions about taking treatments or not—even if we do everything that we have the power to do, medically, we're still left coming to the great interface. While you're hoping that your pain won't reoccur and your cancer will go away, I have to tell you that not only is that my hope for you as well, I want you to be open to all possibilities for healing because they don't always come in that particular form.

Sometimes they come when the cancer isn't responding to the treatment. We've done everything we can, medically, and there's nothing else we can do. The possibilities for healing still exist. They're not solely dependent on me or anyone else in medicine telling you you're cured. Because remember, in the end, we are all, already dying.

When a patient says, "I am praying for a miracle."

I say, "What is it you are praying for?"

"I'm praying that the doctor makes my ovarian cancer completely go away and I'm cured."

And I say to them, "Then, you have an expectation. From a place of expectation, all other possibilities are eliminated and until you realize that you must let go of all expectation."

We can break down these old barriers where we have separated science from spirit. Let's just realize that this separation is nothing but an illusion that keeps us from moving at light speed. The minute that we can all walk into that place of endless possibility, that's where miracles come from. Miracles happen when we have no expectation and where we are completely open to any and all possibilities.

You can empathize, but you can't sympathize with patients until you yourself have been on the receiving end to a magnitude level equal to theirs or greater. In 1995, when I came to Dodgeville, I had the flu. I thought I did. But I also had severe abdominal and pelvic pain. I could barely walk that day.

But it turned out, I landed in the hospital with acute diverticulitis.[††] Then, it all kind of made sense. I was hospitalized here for two days on antibiotics. A CAT scan showed some fairly severe diverticulitis. I had had multiple episodes that I had pretty much always figured was diverticulitis, but really didn't want to do anything about it. But I kept getting pain episodes, pain attacks, feeling bad.

I never knew why people came to the emergency room. I never knew what signal triggers them to cross a particular threshold that something is really not okay and not just that something that is going to go away. It's something that was scaring me.

I had about 36 hours of pain that kept getting worse and it just kept building. And it got to the point that I was kind of paralyzed and I didn't know what to do. I was trying to talk myself out of it. I was trying to talk myself through it and coach myself that it was going to get better. Of course, that's why we have wives. My wife looked at me and said, "You're

†† Condition where small pouches in the colon become inflamed or infected.

going to the hospital today to make rounds. Why don't you just stop at the emergency room?"

That was a nice little gentle way of getting me there. I got to the hospital and I didn't make rounds that day. I went right to the ER. I called ahead and told the ER doc I was coming, and she made all the arrangements. Within an hour or two, we had our diagnosis and I was hospitalized.

I visited a surgeon in Madison, who could do surgery that I normally do on people, and set it up for seven weeks into the future when I felt I could take a month off. During that seven weeks of waiting, I really experienced a lot of stuff—anxiety, a lot of mental gymnastics, literally trying to talk myself into a cure without having the surgery. It was an elective surgery—it was not one of these surgeries to save my life. I could have recurrent episodes and history would suggest that in my case, if I didn't do this, I was going to have more trouble. I'd had multiple episodes.

The surgeon and I talked and he said, "You need the surgery." I said, "I know. I don't want to have it. But it seems to be unavoidable. It's spoken loudly many times."

And so, we set it up and I went through it. I kept a journal about my experience and the one element was that the fear and anxiety that I had created for myself was so powerful that it just drained me. Fortunately, I had some personal coaching and some spiritual coaching, and really built myself up to a level of fearlessness and surrender. It was a real place that I had never been to.

The surgery was the most authentic thing that I had ever done, even more authentic than getting married, more authentic than going to medical school. Those things had an out. This didn't. Once I was going to be put to sleep, there was no turning back. I was going to wake up different—large incision, staples, my insides rearranged with all the potential risks associated with that. And so for me, it became a real elevating experience of transformation. It transformed me into an intellectual being who could take on anything with my mind. It transformed me into somebody that was a spiritual being who had intellect as a tool, but that tool would only fit into so many different places in life. And that ultimately, faith would be the only thing that would carry me through. And that was an experience they can't teach you in medical school. And you can't learn that by being on the delivery side of medicine.

My surgical experience was just an absolutely amazingly healing experience. It was transformational. It was so much more than an operation on my body. It strengthened my spirit, immensely. I spent a week in the hospital, came home. This was right around Christmas. I had a nice holiday and it was very warm and family oriented. It was a perfect time to do it.

I felt that in my personal surgery, there was something lacking, that my surgeon did not really share himself with me. Yes, he gave me his time and his competent technical skills, but I did not feel that my surgeon gave me the opportunity to fully express myself with him after the surgery. I felt it was kept to the bare bones minimum, check the vitals, check the incision and walk out.

Isn't that pretty much how it goes with surgeons?

Well, not this one. I really make it a point to give my patients an opportunity to express themselves to me. Old people—they have so much to tell you after the operation. So much inside about what they've gone through. Not everybody has that need, mind you. I felt I did. I didn't get the opportunity. I'm just glad everything went okay.

I would have discussed my personal gratitude. It wouldn't have taken long. No matter how hard I tried to think myself through this, I ultimately had to lie down on the table and let everybody treat my body and have an element of letting go. I would have liked to share the insight with the surgeon, so he could have felt like at least he heard me, so he could have been grateful for sharing that with me, just some kind of a moment, creating the space.

When I say that, I mean creating the time and the opportunity, where somebody can safely express themselves about whatever is on their mind at the moment, and be heard. It's so important for a patient to have that opportunity. It adds to the healing and gives them the sense of being complete and whole; not just a body that was operated upon, but a whole complete individual.

When we're treating a patient, we're treating the entire world. That's my particular belief—that we're all connected to each other. There is no separation. Any separation that we concoct, is purely an illusion, is purely just some way that we artistically create walls between us, separations between us that don't really exist. We're all each part of each other's lifetime.

If we all elevate our consciousness to the level of, when I sit with Steve Busalacchi, I sit with the entire world. When I stand, I can't stand for myself unless I stand for you. I can't stand for myself unless I stand for the patient. I'm not fully myself, unless I'm fully for everybody else, because without everybody else I'm no one. That kind of approach is my approach. That's the way I walk into the room.

My colleagues say that surgeons are the hardest ones to do surgery on. It's hardest to go through an operation that you yourself have performed many times each year because you know what can go wrong. You know all the possible complications. You know all the subtle millimeter nuances of the best result. Millimeters can define an excellent result from a good result from a poor result from a bad result. Ultimately, it was a question of letting go, then elevate it to a whole new level.

I produced this whole new album called *"Keys of Hope."* And the whole notion of *"Keys of Hope,"* for me personally, it's been a way for me to share another element with my patients. Here, have this. It's an expression from me. It's just another part of me that I want you to have. It's nothing other than that. There's no ulterior motive here. I just want you to have this. I think that it will help you to understand your surgeon a little bit better. I really think surgeons need to share themselves with their patients.

Surgeons will take pictures. A lot of them love golf, sports, cooking. Some of them just love their kids and love their dogs. Some of them are just nuts about cars. Share that with your patients. They love to see that you're a person. It gives them such a warm contentment to know that not only are you highly regarded in the community as being an excellent technician and great surgeon, but it's nice to know that when I'm with you, you make me feel like I'm a person, and not just a piece of meat.

When I hear stories about orthopedic surgeons who see 20 patients an hour, my heart feels terrible. Now, these guys are mavericks as business-men, and the hospitals love them because they generate revenues that are astronomical. But ask any patient who has really been through one of the more painful specialties, which orthopedics is, and ask them just how much their doctor participated, and their ultimate healing experience, and they'll agree: "He gave me 30 seconds to look at my staples and got his nurse to take them out."

"Yeah, I thought he was great."

"Well, why did you think he was great?"

"Well, he did a great job."

"How do you know he did a great job?"

"Well, 'cause it got better."

"Oh, good. Did you know there's a difference between orthopedic sur-geons that not only do a great job, but that actually let you know that they care about you and let you care about them for a few minutes, too? And that you could also feel not only like an orthopedic patient, but like a hu-man being with them? They're out there and they're just as good."

These guys that do a thousand cases a year, I can't say they're any bet-ter technically as the guy who does 250 cases a year. Once you do a cer-tain number, you're just as good at the job as somebody else. Now, what distinguishes you, now what really makes you a healer? Medical schools and residency programs really do have an amazing opportunity to use what would be considered to be the greatest body of work that has ever existed in mankind's history as it relates to development of the spirit and the devel-opment of human interaction.

Medical training really needs to include a spiritual element that is to-tally lacking. Medicine could move so much faster if it could just get out of its own way.

How can spirituality be integrated into a science program, essentially?

There are experts that can be woven into medical school training. People who have expertise in spiritual transformation, who are working in healing realms that don't utilize needles and knives, who do not use x-rays and sound waves.

We have great tools. The mind is only capable of going so far in any given time. I think we should have more trainers in medical institutions who have personal experiences that have a mission and a charter from the medical schools to teach it. I think once the medical schools decide to include this in their training throughout the whole four years of the medical experience, to have that "what does the patient experience?" side of it, to have the weekly or monthly update on the human factor.

I trademarked something called The Human Factor. I'm working on it right now. It's a DVD. It's a video that talks about my musical presentations and how they transform, help to teach the powerful human relationship we have with our patients. It's called "Transforming the doctor patient relationship, one note at a time."

The human factor celebrates the interaction we have with patients. The human factor should be taught in every medical school and in every residency. The human factor, basically, is that non-technical aspect—that one-on-one, treating the whole person, aspect, where it's not just a logo or a slogan. It's actually something that's experienced at the bedside or in the exam room. It's that, "Let me find out who you are." Who is this person who's got this disease, and is there anything about me that you want to know, and allowing for that to happen?

Tell me about another patient so I get a better feel for what you're talking about?

I had a patient who walked in one morning to do a consultation for him. He was a cute old guy who had these funny looking fingers and when I walked in he had this old man face, "Hey, dere doc. How ya doin?"

"Good morning. My name is Dr. Dachman."

"I know who you are. They told me you were comin' to see me. You know what's wrong with these hands?"

I said, "I have no idea."

"Oh, when I was a boy. I got caught out in the snow and I got frost bit and this is the way my hands have been ever since."

These kind of stubbly fingers with half finger nails. I said, "Wow. That's really sad."

He said, "Yeah, but I never let it get in my way. I hear you're a musician."

I said, "Yeah."

He says, "You have to take care of those hands."

I said, "My mother's been telling me that for a long time, but I've never listen to her. Really, I still use table saws and..."

"You can't be doing that."

He told me about his musical interest. He had cancer and was really at the end of his life.

When I walked out of the room, this was one of those mythic people I met that just, boom, hit me. I went right to my office and closed my door, right in the middle of my day and I sat down and wrote the lyrics to a song called "*Hearts and Hands.*"

It probably took me at least a year to come up with the final version. There are fiddles. There are sliding guitars and vocals with harmonies, drums and bass. It was a real production, and he got to hear it before he passed away.

He liked it. He approved. And, he was really a complete experience for me—to be able to have that, along with the medical part of my experience with that patient. It's not just about being a surgeon. It's not about doing these amazing technological things. In 10 years, it's become completely about the human factor of medicine.

CHAPTER FIFTEEN

PLAYING DOCTOR

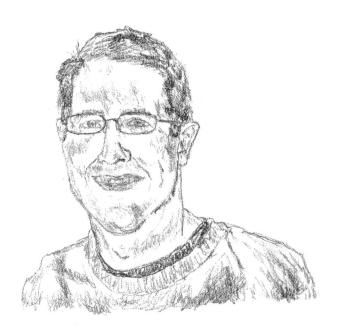

"I'm seeing a new patient every 15 or 20 minutes, solving a problem. I have no idea what I'm stepping into when I walk in that door. It's like improv theatre every 15 minutes. I totally dig it."

Mark Timmerman, MD
Family Medicine and Sports/Performing Arts Medicine, Madison

One of Dr. Mark Timmerman's diabetic patients wants to run a marathon. But regulating blood sugar during such a strenuous event can be tricky, so Timmerman runs along with him for a little insurance. Timmerman is a sports and fitness enthusiast anyway, so he's happy to do it.

Mark Timmerman is that kind of doctor. He's a popular physician, not only because he literally goes the extra mile, but because he has a gift for developing rapport with patients. In his younger years, he was so well liked that a wealthy classmate paid his entire medical school tuition for him. He never told me this, but the amateur psychiatrist in me says Timmerman's annual medical mission trips to poor countries are his way of repaying that extraordinary gift.

"I'm heading to Pakistan for a relief effort," he mentions, during the interview we had in my family room one evening.

If his generous friend had hoped to make a good philanthropic invest-ment in Mark Timmerman, she bet on the right horse. He's one of the lucki-est people in the world, not because he avoided an enormous debt load, but because he's managed to funnel his passion for sports and the arts into a pro-fession he loves.

My daughter loves Shakespeare. We go to plays all the time. One night we were watching an actor in a duel who gets a sword banged against his elbow really hard. He was wincing and obviously, injured. It looked like maybe it was part of the play, but I was thinking, *uh, uh, no, that wasn't planned.* Well, the next day, he walks into my clinic. He sits down and says, I'm so and so.

I said, "How's your elbow?"

He says, "How did you know that?"

I said, "I saw it last night."

He thought it was very cool that I had witnessed his injury. It was just such an amazing coincidence that I'd been there watching. That very mo-ment, I developed legitimacy in his eyes because I had an understanding of what he does for a living. The injury was basically, just a bruised elbow.

I'm particularly interested in the artistic athlete, and am a member of the Performing Arts Medical Association, too, so I've taken care of a lot of dancers and musicians and actors.

I serve as an on-call doctor for the repertory theatre in town. I like per-forming arts medicine, which is a different branch of sports medicine that people don't normally think of. But these people are athletes, too. They have the same needs, concerns, and problems of overuse injury, and the need to continue in spite of injury. It's their job, for many of them. I enjoy taking care of the different kind of athlete, rather than just a high school football player.

There's a play that involves a bunch of stairs, and this gal fell down and twisted her ankle so badly, she couldn't go on stage. They called me and I saw her. Before the performance, I injected her with Novocain, so she couldn't feel anything. I taped her ankle and braced the ankle, just like a football player, you kind of strap them up, shoot 'em up with Novocain and put them out there. She did great.

Had another time in a play, when there was an episode where this guy slams his glass down. He shoves his hand right through the glass and it smashes, so he's got a handful of glass and he's got to go on stage that night. He comes in and I spend most of the afternoon pulling glass out of his hand. Then, he sucks it up, we put him back together, taped him up so the audience couldn't see much of his injury, and he went back out there.

I deal a lot with string musicians because there are a lot of repetitive motion injuries among them. Backaches are really common among musicians, especially cellists. Shoulder and wrist problems for flute players and violinists are really common; TMJ or Temporomandibular Joint * issues, for trumpeters and other mouth-oriented musicians. You have to work on rehab and continue to have them do their activity, which is the same challenge as taking care of an athlete.

The first real musician I saw is a professional trombone player. She had a funny tendonitis in the hand because of repetitive motion. You have a tennis player and you kind of know the motion and you can figure out what muscles are involved and you know how to get it better. But I couldn't quite see what her problem was, so I had her bring in the instrument to the clinic and had her play for me.

I watched her use her hand and hold her hand in this awkward position and that helped me realize why she had this repetitive injury. Then I was able to splint her and give her exercises to strengthen those tendons, so they wouldn't be overused. Eventually, she got better.

They can usually rehab out of these problems without quitting?

Absolutely. When they come to the office, we treat them like an athlete. It's very reassuring to them because they realize you can always rest and you'll get better. But that doesn't help them, nor does it help an athlete, or someone who is really committed to their sport. We will prescribe rehab, bracing, and injections if needed. If you apply the basic medical principles for musicians and dancers that you do for other athletes, it pays off.

If you do tell an athlete or musician, a dancer in particular, to just rest, the game's over. You've lost your validity. You're not going to be able to convince them to be compliant because they're going to shut down and turn you off. The key is bargaining with them, letting them know that you understand that they need to do something. You have to give them something that they can do, and produce a plan for them to gradually increase it.

Give them a goal, because they're goal-oriented. Give them teaching, because in my experience, if people are really serious about a sport, or an instrument, or dance, they're focused not only on their sport, but on their bodies. They're very self-aware. They really want to learn about their bod-

---

* The abbreviation "TMJ" refers to the joint but is often used to refer to any disorders or symptoms of this region, including popping sounds in the jaw, inability to fully open the mouth, jaw pain, etc.

ies, and I spend a lot of time teaching them about what is injured, and how it will get better. I show them pictures and even anatomy texts.

If you give them that information, because they're really focused that way, you tell them that this is how we strengthen it, and this is what we'll produce as a result. This is how you'll get better. Give them a plan and a goal, they're extremely compliant because you've gained their trust and they understand you're not going to stop them unnecessarily.

Sometimes, I'll say, "Look, I won't stop you unless I have to. You're going to ruin something and not be able to do this long term. You've got to believe me. I know what you're going through." I kind of meet them half way and say, "All right, you can't run, but you can bike." Dancers in particular, "You can't leap, but you can go work on the bar for a few weeks, and then we'll work up to it slowly." They'll buy that.

This sounds like the art side of medicine. There's a psychology part to this.

Absolutely. The key to being a successful physician is being able to sell your program to the patient. You can make a diagnosis and have a plan, but unless the patient believes it and understands it, and unless it's a true relationship between you that allows for a partnership, it isn't going to work.

Do you have a ton of credibility walking in the door just because you're a doctor? How much does that buy you, alone?

Not so much, anymore. The population is pretty savvy, at least in a town like Madison—intellectual population, pretty discerning. It can be a tough crowd. You don't necessarily buy yourself a level of respect just because of your title. You really have to earn your respect in a place like this.

Right off the bat, it's really helpful to be dead honest and to say, "Look, this is not going to get better in two weeks." I had a girl who had a problem that will take her a year to get better. She's 16. She sees tomorrow, or maybe the next day, as a long-term plan.

I said, "Here's the deal. On one hand, you're not going to ruin anything, so I'm going to let you keep playing through this. But, on the other hand, this is not going to get better for months, and you're going to have to work on this every day for months for it to get better."

At first they go, "You've got to be kidding me!" It helps to be an athlete, because you really have to understand what's going on, what the motions are, what the mechanics are, to help them get better.

You're an athlete?

I played club hockey, football, and was on the swimming team. Did well in school, and didn't break any rules. I grew up in Hibbing, Minnesota—Bob Dylan's hometown. It was pretty much a classic 1960s upbringing, family of four in a little colonial home.

Hibbing's a mining town, so it's sort of backwards, rough and tumble, but a straightforward thinking, honest speaking, sort of town; immigrant town, really. It's about an hour north of Duluth. My dad worked in a construction company, and mom was a social worker. I have one sibling, Julie.

At what point did you think about medicine?

I was quite young. I was definitely oriented more toward math and science than toward English and History. Yet, I still had this service awareness that I developed from my mom, the social worker, and my grandpa, who was an Episcopal Bishop. I knew that I wanted to be in service and my interest in math, science, and service really led me to think that I would be interested in medicine, enough so that I was involved in a group called the Explorers Scouts. It's a branch of scouting that developed just to explore professions. When I was doing the Explorer Scouts, you wonder about your ability to handle the blood and guts. You don't know until you see it.

I remember the first surgery I watched. I was scrubbed in. I was bound in a gown, so I couldn't get my hands stuck anywhere. It was abdominal surgery—and there was blood and guts, literally everywhere. I remember watching it, thinking, *Hey, this is cool. I'm a natural. This doesn't bother me at all. Here I am, looking at blood and guts for my first time, and this does not bother me. This is no problem. Boy, is it warm in here!*

I mentioned that to the doctors. The operating rooms are about 62 degrees, you know, so the nurses all looked at each other and then one of them put a chair underneath me and then, boom, I hit the chair. They guided me down. I had to question my natural ability. That was the only time I had been queasy about something, and since then I've been more fascinated by it than grossed out by it.

Even in high school, I was a part of this group that hung out with doctors and watched surgeries. I looked at that as a potential profession. Then I went to college. I was a good student, but I was also pretty independent and stubborn, and didn't like the stereotypical nerd student. But I went to a very nerdy college, a competitive college, Carleton College, in Minnesota—a small liberal arts school with a lot of really good students. I was a bit put off by the narrow-mindedness of some of the premeds.

I ended up as a geology major, because I loved math and science, but I also loved being outdoors and people that were interesting. Geology majors were the most interesting in the group I could find on campus, so I spent my years at Carleton playing sports and not doing premed.

I finished, with medicine still in the back of my mind. But then, after graduating, I got a job teaching high school. I left Minnesota and I moved to Massachusetts. I ended up teaching at Deerfield Academy—this prestigious prep school in Massachusetts. I was hired as a mathematics teacher. I taught Algebra II, computer science, and pre-calculus, and was the assistant football coach and head wrestling coach. They hired me at the last minute. They needed a math teacher, a wrestling coach, and a dorm parent.

They thought I'd be perfect, so ended up doing that for three years. It was great.

I was really not prepared for medical school when I left Carleton. I was still having too much fun and was fairly serious, but not really serious about studies or myself or my profession. Teaching at Deerfield allowed me some time as a responsible adult, taking care of kids and teaching a lot of classes and working hard.

That maturation allowed me to get more serious about long-term goals. It was there that I was inspired by the on-campus doctor. It was a big enough school and prestigious enough that they had their own physician on staff. I thought, *That's cool.* That's a way that I could work with kids, work with athletes, still do teaching and coaching in a way, but about health. I was much more interested in health than mathematics, long term.

With that in mind, thinking I might even go back to prep school some day, I started talking to Peggy about going to medical school. We were married a year after college, so she was there with me.

Initially, she was a bit afraid of the hard work it would entail. Being the spouse of a medical student, and then a resident, isn't always a lot of fun, so she was nervous about that. But she also saw that I liked to work hard, and that it didn't matter where I was, I was going to work hard, that I was passionate about life, about work, and about play, and I kind of ran at a certain speed, no matter what the demands were. I would probably work hard in any environment. That's when she realized the commitment wouldn't change, just the venue.

You hear these stories about how hard it is to get into medical school, and I'd been out for a few years. I started to wonder if it would be feasible. I hadn't taken the right courses. I thought, actually, I can't even get in.

I met with this doctor at Deerfield, who inspired me. He was friends with the admissions director at the University of Vermont Medical School. He said, "Let's set up a meeting between the two of you."

I drove up to Burlington, Vermont, sat down and she said, basically, "You don't have a chance of getting in to medical school—not even possible. Your grade average isn't even that good. You've been out a few years. Nope. Ain't gonna happen."

I left there a little bit dejected, at first. Then, being the stubborn, independent guy that I am, I thought, *Okay, desperation. You want to bet?* You don't tell an Iron Ranger, a northern Minnesotan, that he can't do something because then he'll do it. That ignited me.

We decided to quit Deerfield, and moved to Minneapolis because I could still claim residency if I could go there and work for a year, take school for a year, and then I could apply for Minnesota schools as a resident, which was a great financial advantage.

I went to the University of Minnesota, and I was just an adult extra student. I took some sort of tune-up premed classes, did very well on the

M-CAT, did well in my classes because I knew I really had to hammer it. I was mature. I was determined. We decided that if I were to apply and get in, great. I would do my best for a year and apply. If I didn't get in, all right, I had a great career in boarding schools. I'd go back.

I didn't get rejected by any medical schools. I couldn't help but write a letter to the Director of Admissions at UVM, just letting her know that I had gotten in to some very prestigious medical schools, far more prestigious than UVM. I had to do that. I sort of thanked her for her inspiration. {Laughs}

We went to Minnesota. Mayo was the smallest and best medical school that I applied to. It was my first choice, and we went there. My family didn't have resources, so I hadn't saved anything. A friend of mine had married a very wealthy person from Minneapolis. They were at a party with us one time after I had been accepted to Mayo and they said, "Gosh, how are you going to pay for this? You know, it's not cheap."

I said, "I don't know. I'm not really interested in the armed services, but I may have to do that, because I don't know how else I'll afford this."

About two weeks later, I got a letter from them, and they said that they would like me to consider letting them pay for my tuition for four years, as their gift to science. I remember us opening up the letter together and both kind of being just silently stunned. It took a while to process it, because it came out of the blue. This kind of thing you just never expect or anticipate, or even dream of, so it took us a while to even talk to each other.

I had gone to college with this woman. She married well, really well. They spent their time giving away money. They decided this was one of the things they wanted to sponsor. They wanted to sponsor me. It was a flabbergasting experience. Then, of course, you think, maybe I shouldn't. You know, money's a weird thing, and it can change and strain relationships. I wasn't positive it was the right thing to do, but it wasn't that hard a decision to allow them to pay for my tuition. I went to medical school tuition-free.

This is incredible, especially because we had Kate, our first child, just two weeks before medical school started. We were financially strapped. It was a huge deal not to have to take out these gigantic loans.

We've kept in contact, though not close contact. But when I've gotten awards or notoriety for something that I've done medically, I'm careful to send them it. When I get an "attaboy," I send it to them and thank them for their sponsorship, sort of letting them know that they didn't waste all their money. It was about $100,000.

Medical school was a blast. I ran two marathons a year and sang in a black tie choir. I really got involved in the community, partly because I was older, and more mature. We had a family. I really felt more like a professional than like a student, so we sort of lived that way.

But also, compared to being a boarding school teacher with seven days' responsibility, classes, full-time sports coaching, and living in a dormitory,

I thought medical school was a lot easier than I expected. It was easier than my job at Deerfield. I did not find it an onerous experience. I loved it.

It also helped that I had more than an adequate amount of self assurance. If you're self-confident, that really makes a big difference in medical school, because it's such a humbling experience. You can get just crushed on some of these services with your performance, because everybody's a good student and you put yourself up against some very bright people, in a very intimidating medical environment like Mayo.

Maybe you were just a natural for this.

I think that's reasonable. I was never the top of my class, as far as pure horsepower goes. But I've always had good emotional intelligence and have been able to communicate well with people. It really made it kind of easy for me.

I've gained an appreciation for the human body, and it's always been fascinating to me. But that mind and body connection is what, after being in practice for 13 years, I think is the most interesting thing. On the other hand, you develop a distance from it, too, because I think you have to. You view a lot of it as ho-hum. Otherwise, it would bother you more. Some of the stuff you do is a little bit degrading for you and/or the patient, which, I'll often treat with some humor, and that helps. It's not always pretty.

You tend to become a little bit distanced from it—not calloused to it. But it's never like working on a car, for instance. It does become a little mechanical at times, when it otherwise becomes just too gross to think about.

When I was in medical school, we were learning how to do rectal exams. It's not a very pleasant experience. They do hundreds of scopes a day there and they have their buns up on the table ready for the scope and you just go do the rectal exam first. They leave me with this guy who's bent upside down.

"Hi. I'm Mark."

"Uh, hi." His ass is sticking up in the air.

"I have to do a rectal exam."

"Yeah, I know."

I look around and there aren't any gloves anywhere. I look in the drawers in the cupboards. There's KY, but there are no gloves. I'm nervous and he's waiting. He's naked and I'm starting to sweat. I walk out of the room and go to the preceptor, who's the GI doc. He says there's only one way to get the feel of the prostate and you gotta feel the prostate without a glove, in order to get the real feel.

I go back in the room—no way. Then, I start hearing them giggling in the back room.

What did you do?

I went out and got a glove! I walked back and they had a glove waiting for me.

Another one. I was doing a rectal exam on this guy, and I'm apologizing because it's kind of an embarrassing thing. He goes, "It's okay doc, as long as I only feel one hand on my shoulder, no problem."

I'm cracking up so hard I could barely pull my finger out.

Some people have a hard time touching. They have touch workshops in medical school. You pretty quickly don't think about it much. Mayo does an interesting thing with their training, and they still do this. Mayo is made up of only 40 medical students—20 male, 20 female. They have a decided split. You pair off and you examine each other—opposite genders. It's a really a humbling experience to have a classmate examine you. But it's intentional, to sort of help defuse some of that angst about that process.

You quickly become pretty immune to it. At first it seems unnerving, but they spend a lot of time in medical school working on that, on the psychological aspects of that, working on touch, getting used to touching others. The reality of it is we have a lot of hang-ups in our American culture about the human body. But the human body, a lot of times, is not all that attractive. You tend not to think about it in very attractive ways—certainly, not in the doctors' office. In different settings, it's completely different. I could be attracted to a woman on the street and unattracted to her in the office. My friends have said, "Oh, that's bull crap."

But you know what? It really isn't. I don't know what the dynamic is, but there's something about that setting. It's sterile and uninteresting. It's asexual. It doesn't work. But at the same time, it doesn't seem to carry over outside of the clinic.

My first pelvic exam in residency, I remember because it was a really attractive young woman and I was nervous. It was at a time when I didn't fully understand how the clinic situation would play with an attractive woman. I found it to be uninteresting, from a sexual standpoint, and that was a learning process I went through. But because I was so nervous, I did her testing, and did her exam, and finished everything up. Then, I went to take my gloves off and I realized I wasn't wearing gloves! I didn't even know! I was just mortified and I went to my clinic partner and I said, "God, Ben. I can't believe what I just did. I just did a pelvic exam without any gloves!"

Tell me more about residency.

When you're a resident in the hospital and you hear the code blue, especially at night when there are only residents around, you run to the scene. I'm energetic, and I can run. It's an emergency. You hear a code blue and you're supposed to go, so I'm proud to be the first guy there. I'm in the hallway—Ta dah! Here I am.

Then you realize, crap, the first guy there runs the code. The first doctor at a code blue[†] is in charge of the entire team from that point on—all the decision-making, all the orders for all the drugs. It's part of the advanced life support protocol that you're supposed to have learned and done. But still, it's a daunting experience when you have a real, live body there, and his life is your responsibility.

I froze. It was my first time running the code. I knew what to do, but I couldn't say anything. I was just standing there and there was a bunch of nurses and techs ready to do stuff and I'm like, uh, uh, uh. My partner Ben comes up behind me and he whispers, "It's okay. You can't hurt this patient. He's already dead."

"You're right. I can hurt a lot of patients, but not this one. There is no decision I can make that will make his life worse." Then, I was fine from that point on, and actually, we revived him.

Was that your first life you saved then?

Well yeah. I was more impressed by my paranoia than actually bringing him back. I guess it was a heady experience. I just remember being petrified.

How did you end up selecting your specialty?

I tended to have a very broad aptitude. I was good with my hands. I was good talking to people. Maybe not particularly good in any one area and so that broad interest led me to specialty after specialty, until I ended up with the most general of specialties, family practice. I'm kind of one of those who loves what he's doing no matter where he is. I loved pediatrics, but also I really loved delivering babies. Family medicine is the only specialty where you can do both. I really couldn't decide.

I had always come back a little bit to this athletic thing. It hadn't left me that I wouldn't go back to boarding school and work with teenagers. When you work with teenagers, a lot of that is athletics, a lot of it is psychiatry, a lot of it is adolescent medicine, sexuality and growth, and development stuff.

Delivering a baby is a really cool thing. But, what I like more about obstetrics is all the time you spend with the family beforehand and afterwards, and even during labor, because I tend to spend as much time as I can. I like to labor as much as I can with the family. It's one of the rare times when you're not busy. They're busy. You get a chance to talk to the father for a change. That's why I like being a family doctor and taking care of them ahead of time, so when you care for the baby and the mother afterwards, it's really a gratifying experience.

I ended up finishing at Mayo and then applying to family practice. I loved the Mayo Clinic. It's the finest medical institution I've ever seen. My medical education was superb.

---

† There is no pulse.

We decided that we would apply to a good residency program, but, more important, a great city. I did my family practice residency here in Madison. Great program, and near the end of it I had remained involved in taking care of some athletes. Athletes have always been important to me, and I've always been interested in adolescents and connected well with them. I did a lot of sports medicine education as a resident.

Then, Dean Clinic was starting a sports medicine clinic and wanted a sports medicine program, right when I was coming out of residency. They said if you go into a fellowship, we would like to hire you to do some sports medicine, in addition to family practice. I did a fellowship in sports medicine in Minneapolis, and then came back to Madison.

I started out doing a mix of half sports medicine and half family practice. It's stayed that equal mix since then. Sports medicine has taken on sort of a different focus, since primary care was involved more over the past decade. It used to be orthopedic surgeons taking care of teens. Then, with the boom in female athletes after Title IX ‡ and also with the development of fellowships that were oriented towards primary care, a lot of family doctors, and some internists and pediatricians, have gotten involved in sports medicine training to be a little broader in the treating of athletes.

For instance, sure we treat the knee sprains and shoulder tendinitis that athletes all get, but sports medicine now encompasses some special needs of the female athlete—disordered eating, stress fractures, or menstrual problems, or non-orthopedic issues, like irregular heartbeat, or exercise-induced asthma. It really fits well in a primary care bailiwick, taking care of a broad range of problems related to sports, but not necessarily bumps and bruises.

Because we also do so much musculoskeletal medicine, we tend to take care of active adults—people who aren't necessarily on teams, but people like you and me who are active and continuing to do sports into their 40s and 50s and 60s, weekend warrior issues.

With so many of us in our 40s who are quite active, there's a huge population of us who are exercising a lot, women in particular. Before this generation, a lot of women didn't exercise routinely. We have a large, growing population of both men and women who have been pretty rough on their bodies.

We will have pretty many active, elderly people which will be a good thing. But from a musculoskeletal standpoint, you're concerned about a lot of hips and knees that are giving out, developing arthritis. New replacements are better and better, but it's still hard to be active after getting them.

You might as well be as active and fit as you can. Obviously, I'm very active, and I'm not very concerned about arthritis, because I assume that

‡ 1972 federal law which prohibited sex discrimination in school programs that receive any federal financial assistance.

I'll get it at some point. But if I can be active through my 50s and 60s, and then end up struggling in my 70s, maybe that's worth it.

But as a physician taking care of a bunch of aging athletes, it will be a particular challenge to help to keep them active as their joints start wearing out. Biking and swimming are less stressful on the body. Helping people realize the importance of resistance training because strength and resistance training can lead to stability of the joints.

Strength training can be most important for the elderly because it's really the strength loss in the elderly that leads to rapid decline and inability to live on their own. You can make good strength gains doing resistance training as an elderly adult—70s and 80s. You will have declining strength, of course, but you can maintain a surprising amount of that with light weights and resistance training. High reps, low weight, two or three times a week. It will become more and more important for our population to focus on that. There have been studies that have shown improved kidney function and improved cholesterol, benefits from resistance training that you wouldn't necessarily expect.

Exercise wise, my daughter feels I go way overboard. I've done distance exercise for a long time. I ran several marathons in medical school. I've been doing the Wisconsin Ironman Triathlon§ every year for the past four years. I exercise at least an hour every day. I get up at five and am exercising from 6 until 7 every day.

On weekends, I'll do a long bike ride. I like maintaining a high level of fitness. It just makes me sleep better. Feel better. I'm a high energy person and it calms me and sort of is my relief and a release from a busy work day.

When I think about what the Ironman requires, I wonder why pushing your body to those extremes is a good thing.

There's something about a personal challenge about doing things like the Ironman that you're not completely sure you can do, even if you train for it, even if you've done it before. That morning, you don't really know if you can finish it.

To me, it's also good to have a long term goal, because it keeps me focused on something all year long. Once you get used to a high level of fitness, it's hard to put up with less. The goal is trying to find the balance between being really fit and breaking down or causing injury, so moderation is important. It's a tough balance.

After I did the Ironman three years ago, a number of patients became inspired enough to change their lifestyle. One of the toughest things in medicine is to get somebody to change their lifestyle. But I've had people

§ The Wisconsin Ironman consists of a 2.4 mile open-water swim, a 112-mile bike ride and a 26.2 mile run.

come in and say that they've lost 20 pounds, or they've gotten on a program, or they've quit smoking.

And I'll say, "I've been talking to you about quitting smoking for six years. What finally did it?"

"I figured, gol darn it, if my doctor can do an Ironman, the least I can do is quit smoking."

An amazing number of people have said something like that and I didn't even know that they knew that I did this. It's hard to convince people to change their lifestyle. That just doesn't work very well. You can tell people anything, but unless they're ready to listen to it, it doesn't matter.

People can be inspired, and I've been pleased and surprised by how many people have learned that I have done some of these things for fitness, and am carrying that torch. They want to get on that wagon and follow me without my asking them to.

Even if I'm fit and I'm asking people to lose weight, they're not going to listen to me. If I'm overweight and telling people, good luck! No way.

One of my patients once told me, "Doctor T, what I like most about you is that you're so unprofessional." {Laughs}

I said, "Thanks, I think."

"No. No. No. I mean that in a good way."

When you look at doctors and how they treat the same problem, the variation is too broad. Some of them don't treat it the right way, or in a too expensive way, or in an inefficient way, and we really should work to develop more consistent, economical, effective treatment plans for particular problems.

But the art is eliciting enough from the patient to know what the problem is. Part of my training, is a very patient-based interview process—really letting the patient tell his or her story first, without questions. Shut up and take notes. I don't care how much time it takes. Some of them take too much time and you start sweating....

The patients are piling up...

Yeah. It's really hard when you're doing a patient-based interview and they're going on forever. Some people have no sense for how long they're taking. It does two things. Number one, it allows the patient the opportunity to get their whole story out and that is very relieving to them. It also allows you to hear the important parts that you may not ask questions about.

To facilitate that, I recently went from a 15-minute appointment, which is often the industry standard in family practice and sports medicine, and stretched that to a 20-minute time slot, because I just find that I can get better information from patients and can teach better about the problem. I can focus on the art of medicine more if I have a little more time.

Now, it extends my day a little bit because I did that keeping the same number of patients on a given day, but I try to get as much done on the chart as I can while the patient's in the room, so it's a wash.

You can say, here's the traditional medical approach, and we can try that. Or, if you want, in this case, I feel that this certain thing might be more effective. If we're not going to hurt you by trying it, maybe you'd be interested in giving that a try. Sort of spelling it out for them and having them participate in the decision-making. There are times when it's important to deviate from where the traditional approach will take you.

The coolest thing about this job is that medical issues cut across a lot of boundaries. I love change. I love people. I love problem solving. Every morning I walk into the office and I've got 25 problems to solve. Not all of them are final exams. A lot of them are just quizzes.

Basically, I'm seeing a new patient every 15 or 20 minutes, solving a problem. I totally dig it. I have no idea what I'm stepping into when I walk in that door. It's like improv theatre every 15 minutes.

I know people from all walks of life, all socioeconomic backgrounds. It is such a cool thing to have such a broad exposure to our population. And not only that, but you're involved with them in such an intimate way.

For example, there was this teenage girl who was sexually active at a relatively early age, and dressed provocatively. She came in one day, and complained about some STD¶ concerns and possibly about missing a period.

"When was the last time you had intercourse?"

She said, "Well, this morning."

I said, "It's nine o'clock on a school day. What do you mean?"

She goes, "Well, in the parking lot." {Laughs}

She came to my office one day in a black dress with a plunging neckline, and looked like a million bucks and grabbed a lot of attention from everybody. She stormed in and she said, "Oh Doc, this is so gross. This old guy was looking at me in the waiting room."

I said, "Well, look at what you're wearing? What do you expect?"

She said, "No, but this guy was old."

"Being an old man doesn't make him immune to your attractions."

She says, "I mean old, like he must have been 40."

I said, "I'm older than 40."

She goes, "Oh, my God. I'm sorry." {Laughs}

How many patients do you see?

About twelve hundred. Obviously, I don't see some of them except for every six years or something. But they're all people I am responsible for, and that look to me for help, and that I become intimately related to them in some way or other. It's a really heady experience. It's such a privilege. I've grown a lot by being that close to that many different kinds of people.

¶ Sexually transmitted disease

At this point, I haven't had new patients for quite a while. Every once in a while, someone will come in who I haven't seen for six, seven, eight years and I just can't place them, but not very often.

Are you ever stumped by their problems?

Oh, all the time. I had a patient today. I said, "I don't know what's wrong. But I'll help you find out. We've got some work to do."

And the patient said, "God, that's the best thing I've ever heard from a doctor."

I said, "What do you mean?"

He goes, "You didn't make up some BS. You said you didn't know."

That's the key to being a northern Minnesotan. You just say it as it is. If I don't know, I tell them I don't know. But I'm also very persistent, and I tell the patient that. The communication part of medicine is so important and I'll tell a patient, "Look, I'm not going to give up. I'm going to help you with this problem."

I see a lot of people with back problems—problems that have gone on for a long time, and for many of these people it relates to their livelihood. It's really important for them to get this better. I'll be creative. I'll be persistent. I'll make them come back and see me. "We're going to get to the bottom of this," I'll tell them. "I don't care how long it takes. You may be tired of me by the time we get to this, but I will help you figure this out."

That fixes half the problem right there, because half the problem is their frustration over feeling like they're not being heard, or something's not working for them, or they're not moving towards something. As long as they feel as though they're moving in a positive direction, it relieves half their anxiety about their problem. That's the suffering part. There's pain and there's suffering. Even if I can't help their pain, if I can help their suffering by giving them the confidence that I'm on their side and will work with them, that's key.

How do you deal with patients who have conditions where you just can't do much? They have end stage disease, etc.

That's tough. Those of us in primary care all have patients we know and love that we've got to give some really bad news. You do it frankly and honestly. If I'm doing some testing, and it's for a possible cancer or something terrible and I think that they'll figure that out too, I'll tell 'em, "Look, one of the reasons we're getting this head CT is that I'm concerned that there may be a brain tumor. I don't think that there is, because you don't have many signs of it. And if I were really concerned, I would let you know. But I want to do this as a double check."

I really trust my exam. I spent a lot of time working on my exam. A lot of people, too often, will do a knee jerk reaction and order an MRI instead of doing a really careful exam. There's a problem with technology, too. I'm a little bit of a contrarian. The problem is that technologies are so publicized that patients will ask for it and sometimes it's not appropriate. Sometimes it's not necessary. Sometimes it will lead you astray.

Here's a good example. A football player came to me because he blew out his knee.

I examined him and said, "You tore your ACL."**

He says, "Shouldn't we get an MRI?"

I said, "Well, we can, but you tore your ACL. I can tell." I trust my exam.

But he kept asking for it. You don't want to tell a patient no.

I said, "Sure, let's get an MRI."

All right, we got an MRI, which proved me wrong. He didn't tear his ACL. Of course, MRIs are only 85% accurate. But I gave him the news and said, "I must have been wrong. I can't explain it…I'm never wrong {laughs}, but in this case, maybe I am."

He goes, "Well, great. I can go out and play."

I said, "Maybe we should spend some time rehabbing, instead."

But he got the confidence that his knee was intact. He went out, and then he really chewed it up and tore a bunch of cartilage because he did have an ACL tear and an unstable knee. The MRI was wrong.

We rely on technology. Because you can look at it, you tend to trust it. The radiologist read the picture as an intact ACL. Now, it depends on the skill of the radiologist. It depends on the quality of the film. The film also can show angles and funny pictures and shadows. It's not perfect. You don't really know until you go in there and look.

When he did end up having his knee operated on, yep, he had torn his ACL, not recently, but probably when I had seen him initially, and also had a bunch of cartilage damage. It was a little bit of an over reliance on the technology, whereas the old-fashioned exam suggested otherwise.

But is technology helping you do your job?

We've recently migrated into computer-based charts, and no dictation. This new system we have is phenomenal. I can sit in the room with a patient, and with the touch of a few buttons, I can show him his cholesterol results from yesterday, and I can graph it from the last two years. I can look at his weight and say, "Let's see what your weight has done over the last five years."

I can access a new medication I'm thinking about for him. Show him the pills. Can you swallow something that large? How much do they cost? This is all at my fingertips with the patient in the room. It's just amazing. I find it a true revolution.

The patient will say, "I need a letter for my employer." I push the letter button and it half writes it for me and then I fill in the blanks. He's got a typed letter that tells his employer what's going on.

** The Anterior Cruciate Ligament connects the tibia to the femur at the center of the knee.

It will only become more popular as the patient gains access to some of his information on the web and is able to e-mail physicians instead of calling them. As it is now, I don't do much phone conferences with patients. I usually do that through e-mail. It's just so much more efficient. The telephone takes too much time. They can't reach me. I can't reach them.

Once a patient can look at a result in his chart and e-mail a question to his physician, the nurses will be able to screen it and answer most of the questions, and give some of it to the doctor. It's all documented in the chart. It's truly the way to go.

My patients have not abused the communication. I have not found e-mail communication with patients to be overwhelming. In fact, I find it liberating because I'm not spending time talking on the phone. Between patients, I can just bang out a few e-mails.

How do you manage your busy professional life with your family time?

I was struggling to find time with my daughters. I had a hard time getting to know them. They were young, five and two, at the time. About 15 years ago, I decided I would spend Wednesday with my daughters. I wouldn't work on Wednesday. I wouldn't play golf on Wednesdays. I decided we would call them special Wednesdays and I would spend them with a daughter—and I would alternate Wednesdays.

We'll go ice-skating. We'll go climbing at the climbing gym. We'll go to the book store. When the kids were younger, I kept real close tabs on the music and theatre scene in town. There are free concerts, just a lot going on. I would just scour the papers. We'd go to some pottery studio. I've done that literally every Wednesday for 15 years, to the point where we dropped off our oldest daughter at college three years ago and she said, "So, will I see you next Wednesday?"

She's three hours away. It's not a long drive, but I said, "Absolutely."

She wasn't kidding?

She was not kidding. I go to Cedar Rapids every other Wednesday and we'll do an activity together. We've always based it on some athletic activity or something interesting, and then dinner. Then I drive home.

That's been the most important thing in my life, actually, is doing this on Wednesdays. Some patients have followed suit and have taken at least a few hours a week as a dedicated plan.

But more important, it's the scheduling. I've gotten a lot of patients to follow a schedule, like go out on Tuesday nights, no matter what. It becomes a dedicated time.

The magic of that is you're not wondering when you're going to spend time with that important person. It doesn't always have to be kids. It could be spouses, sometimes parents.

Sounds like you've got it all figured out. So do you plan to practice as long as possible?

I don't think I'll be one of those physicians who works until he's 70 or 80. I view myself as doing this job for a while longer, and at some point maybe backing down in order to focus on some interesting ways to provide medical help for people, but maybe not in the clinic every day, maybe some volunteer work. I like the outdoors so much that maybe doing more expedition doctor work would be interesting.

CHAPTER 16

FACING PLASTIC SURGERY

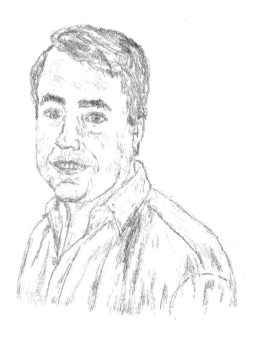

"If my patients are happy with the A, I want the A+. I'm always thinking, a tweak here, a tweak there, and seldom do they want it."

Andrew Campbell, MD
Facial Plastic Surgery, Sheboygan

Medicine's long been called an art and a science. But Dr. Andrew Campbell's connection to the "art" of medicine is much more literal. His artwork is walking all over Sheboygan—a blue collar city about an hour south of Green Bay.

A painter may express himself on canvas, a vocalist through her voice, a sculptor through his medium. Campbell, however, practices his art on people's faces. In his late 30s, he eliminates wrinkles, straightens noses, corrects horrific deformities, etc.

At his home, Dr. Campbell's interest in art is apparent. Colorful paintings are prominently displayed, while other framed pieces are piled on the floor, awaiting transfer to his new office. Doctor Campbell tells me about the art of facial plastic surgery.

~~~~~~

When I was in my training in Cincinnati, there was a lady who was driving down the road and a cow got out of pasture, and she hit it. It went right through her windshield and basically crushed her face. Every single bone in her face was broken. It hit her at eye level and below. We almost had nothing to start with. You have to start with something, and then rebuild it, so we were literally starting with her skull to put the bones back together. It took two days.

What amazes me is there really wasn't a lot of tissue that was injured. You can start with what you would consider a train wreck and nobody would ever know that anything was ever done.

Bones are, literally, like pieces of a puzzle. When it's that extreme, it's very difficult to get them back exactly the way that they used to be, and often they end up with a little flatter, wider face than you would want. You err on the side of giving them a narrower, longer face because your mistake is going to be the opposite. I don't think it's ever exactly the way it was, but you try to get it so close that they still look like the person that they were before the injury.

I had a gentleman here who was riding his motorcycle, lost control, and went face first into gravel. When he saw his face in a mirror, before we put everything back together again, ughh, it was just like hamburger. He had so many deep cuts on his face, and on the inside of his mouth. The total length of his cuts was probably 30 inches, maybe 40 inches. I had to put many pieces of tissue back together again. The lip split wide open all across on the inside, tons of cuts across his face and cheeks—some very deep. He went home the next day. I saw him two weeks later and you could hardly tell that he'd been in a wreck. One cut was a little bit swollen and probably wasn't going to look as good as I'd like to see. Everything else was almost invisible. It was uncanny. He was just ecstatic.

Somebody like this gentleman, I wanted to see back a couple weeks later. He's looking good. He doesn't want to take the time to come see me, so I'll probably never see him again. I'll never get a post-op picture.

Sometimes with cosmetic procedures, I just forget. They're happy. I'm happy. But almost all patients, I'll take that post-op photo. I'll drag out their old photo and put 'em next to each other. I'll just print them out on a glossy paper and we'll send it to them.

Why do that?

Lots of reasons to do it—one would be legal issues. If there was a lawsuit or something, you could show before and after what they looked like. More important, though, it's a learning tool, especially in rhinoplasty {nose jobs}. That's probably one of the most difficult surgeries on the face to master.

When did you first become interested in this form of surgery?

My interest in facial plastic surgery probably goes back to when I was three years old. I was able to draw and copy cartoons out of a book and make them scary close to the actual cartoon, and I wasn't tracing. I just kind of had an artistic gift that I continued to use all through school. I never really did a lot of formal training, but when I did take art in high school I won some awards for some of my paintings.

When I was somewhere around 10 years old, I was inside my house, drawing the house as it looks from the outside by memory. I had to go out and check how many windows we had, but everything else, I pretty much drew from memory. It was scary how close it looked to the real house.

I did murals in college, like a beer label for a friend. I kept that artistic side of me, and always thought I was going to be a doctor. My dad was a doctor. He's an anesthesiologist, retired. My brother's an anesthesiologist. My sisters are pediatric dentists, so we're all so kind of going in that medical direction. I always assumed that that's what I was going to be. It was never a deep, heartfelt, thought-provoking process.

I can remember saying something to my mom about wanting to be an artist, and she made that classic comment about a starving artist. Growing up in a nice house, you realize maybe that's not such a good direction to go. Physicians make a nice living and most physicians have a decent lifestyle. As I got older, it started to sink in that maybe art isn't the best way to make a living.

Where did you grow up?

In Bloomington, Indiana; born in 1967. I was the last of five children. When I was about two, my second oldest sister got brain cancer and passed away. I was too young to remember her, but it was a rough time for our family. My parents split, and my mom moved to Pittsburgh with four kids, back to where she grew up. We spent about a year there before my parents got back together. We moved back to Bloomington, Indiana, and I was raised there my whole life. They got divorced again when I was in second grade, so then I lived with my mom. I didn't really get exposed to medicine, per se, at all growing up. When my parents divorced, my dad disappeared from my life for a very long time, probably five or six years where I maybe saw him around Christmas and that was pretty much it, even though they lived in the same town.

I was basically raised by my mom, so I have to give her full credit for this. She was a school teacher. She knew that to be what most people consider successful, you need to excel in your education. She always stressed that as an important part of my life, and that's why I was valedictorian of my high school. I took my grades seriously.

I was playing football until dark and then had to do my homework. Sports makes you a driven person, because you have to keep going. You have to finish that game. You have to practice to get better. I lettered in football and hockey. If you're doing those activities, life in general is driven. That stays with you—probably for the rest of your life.

I ended up going to Indiana University, in Bloomington. Then I went to Indiana University Medical School, but that's in Indianapolis. I finally moved out of my hometown, an hour north to the big city. Between my first and second year in medical school, I married Heidi.

After I went into medical school, I was planning on being a plastic surgeon because of, again, the artistic side, and during medical school I absolutely loved facial anatomy because of its complexities.

The first years in medical school, I met the plastic surgeon over at Children's Hospital, because my sister had a friendship with him. They have common patients with cleft lip and palate, and teeth problems. After I was introduced to him, we ended up writing a couple of articles together, which is the thing to do if you want to get into that specialty. You start doing research for them.

My first rotation of my third year in medical school was general surgery. You have to do at least three years of general surgery before you can go into your plastic surgery residency.

I met an intern rotating through general surgery who was an ENT resident. He asked me why I wanted to go into plastic surgery. I told him about my love of the facial anatomy and my artistic side. He goes, "Well, then you want to go into ENT."

I said, "What's ENT?"

"Otolaryngology."

"What's otolaryngology?"

He says, "Well, we're the people who do all the surgery in the head and neck. That's all we do. It's ears, nose, and throat, and we're always working on the face. Plastic surgeons, they do boobs and butts, bellies and burns, and hands and all these flaps. We just do the head."

Well, that's all I really thought plastic surgery was, honestly. I didn't know they did burns and the hand surgery.

He said, "Go into otolaryngology." Of course, I scrambled to get a rotation in otolaryngology, because that was my elective rotation, right after general surgery. I got in and was absolutely enthralled with it. Just the people, the specialty, and what we do. I thought it was interesting to be a clinician, as far as the medicine, seeing people in the office and treating them medically, as well as the surgeon, performing operations. Other surgical specialties seldom treat people in the office with medication. They're surgeons and they treat with surgery.

You could break otolaryngology probably into seven specialties—the ear, nose, sinus, laryngology, which would be the voice box, head and neck cancer, facial plastic surgery, pediatric otolaryngology. There are a lot of sub-specialties of otolaryngology. Facial plastic surgery has its own board certification and our own Society, the American Academy of Facial Plastic & Reconstructive Surgery.

We have a board certification process that's essentially identical to what the otolaryngology {certification} is—only all it is, is facial plastic surgery. You have to have two years of experience doing facial plastic and reconstructive surgery, sit for a written examination and an oral exam. It's an arduous task, but I ended up doing that and I'm one of nine board certified facial plastic surgeons in the whole state. I was asked to be an examiner for the Board, so I've done that as well.

There aren't a lot of facial plastic surgeons. It's a relatively small specialty. We're kind of ultra-specialized.

When I talked to several fellow med students who also were interested in ENT, they said, "You need to go do a month in Cincinnati," because all of them put Cincinnati as their number one choice for residency, but they didn't get in. I did.

I had done a month of rotation there when I was in medical school and got to know all of them pretty well. I must have impressed the Chairman, Jack Luckman, because he wanted to write a letter of recommendation for me. Then, of course, you have to go through all the interviews to get a residency. You don't just apply to one program, especially in something as competitive as otolaryngology. I put Cincinnati first, and ended up getting it. That was one of three spots, and I think they had 400 applications.

When I was going through the program, where you start to get close with some of the attendings, you almost become part of that process of interviewing these medical students for residency, especially when you're chief resident. We had 450 for three spots when I was leaving Cincinnati, so it's absolutely insane, as far as competitiveness for a specialty.

I was just enthralled that I ended up at Cincinnati, and had a great experience. I did a lot of facial plastic surgery, both at the university and in private practice. I got to do a lot of reconstructive work, and then, a lot of cosmetic surgery. I felt very comfortable going in and doing full facial plastic surgery without doing a fellowship.

How did you manage to beat out all those other doctors?

On a piece of paper, yes, I got good grades, and I did some research, probably not as much as others. What would have set me apart? Really, it would have been very difficult to go to Cincinnati, having never been there before and make an impression on them, enough that they would rank me high enough to get into a residency program. But they knew me. You spend time, especially with the chairman, and he sees your interest.

He sees how you interact with people. It's really your personality trait that they're almost more interested in that than your raw intelligence. It's your work ethic. It's the way you interact with patients, the way you interact with other residents. It's the fact that you're willing to put the time and effort into researching something, if they ask you a question. They'll ask you about it the next day, and you better know everything there is to know about it.

When you do things like that, and it's in your personality, they like that. They know you're going to be a good resident. You're going to be a resident they're going to feel comfortable allowing to help take care of their patients. And, they're not going to worry when you're the guy on call. It's going to be easy to have conversations with you and you're going to be easier to teach. I think that's what set me apart.

Wasn't it nerve-wracking to work on people's faces? It's the face!
They've been teaching medical students and residents for a long time, so it's not like you're walking out of a classroom and suddenly thrown in front of a patient and expected to do a procedure.

In medical school, you start with pigs' feet. You cut a pig's foot on the skin because pig skin is very similar in thickness and density to human tissue, and just overall, all the characteristics are very similar. You sit there and sew on a pig's foot. And then, as you're a medical student rotating through surgical specialties, they may let you sew up a little bit of the wound, or they might let you do just a tiny little bit, obviously not the important stuff.

As you get into medical school or into a residency, we have to do a year of general surgery. When you're doing a year of general surgery, you get to do some hernias. You get to do some appendectomies. You get to do some trauma. They're always kind of taking you through it. By the time you get into ENT, they may show you one, and then you're doing one, and then you're teaching one.

Certainly, in Cincinnati, the great benefit I had over a lot of other programs, even big name programs, is that you operate very early in your residency. You're doing pretty complicated cases by your second year of ENT training, and by the time you're chief resident,* you're doing those weird cases that don't come across the schedule very often.

Otherwise, you're teaching the first and second year students. It's very different to do a procedure, as opposed to teaching a procedure. If you think you know how to do something well, wait until you try to teach somebody how to do it. Then, you're really going to find out how well you know it.

It's just another level of education that you get by going to a program like that, where you're teaching those other residents, who are younger than you, who are coming up. It's just a cycle. They taught me when they

---

* In your final residency year, one becomes chief and supervises less experienced residents.

were chiefs, and now I'm a chief and I'm teaching the next generation coming through.

I was so absolutely comfortable walking into virtually any circumstance in life in a hospital with my specialty. It's a good feeling to have. You can go in there with such confidence because you were able to do it as a resident.

Everybody else is going to be a little apprehensive about the face because it's the face. It's what we are. If you have a scar on your abdomen, say from an appendectomy, well, it's not that big a deal for most people. When you have a scar on your knee, because you twisted your ligaments, most people don't make a big deal about it. If you have a scar on your face, that's a big deal. That's a huge deal.

You'd better be confident. And, on the other extreme of that, you'd better not be cocky, because that's how you begin to get in trouble. Don't be overconfident and think you can do something, or maybe get around doing something that you should be doing. Don't cut corners. Do it the way it's supposed to be done. Do it well. Do it right.

Have you always been a confident person?

I was pretty confident, even as a child in high school and college. That's in my nature. I don't know if it was the art, or just my gifts I have. Even when I was in medical school, doing some of the small things, just helping to close a wound, they'd make a comment that I was gifted in that respect. And certainly in my residency program, some of the attendings would request me to help them with a case because they knew that I was technically, good. I got the Alter Peerless Memorial Scholarship, which is an award given to the most outstanding chief resident every year. Technically, that is my gift. I'm very good with my hands.

Surgeons use that phrase a lot—good with their hands. What does it mean?

There's fluidity to our motions when we operate. When you're a really good surgeon, it's almost a dance. You're not out there making jerky motions and moving and shoving something here, and pushing something there. It's all a dance with your assistant, with the suture and your instruments, and even your cutting technique. When it flows like that, your expertise is going to shine.

It's very meticulous, and it certainly can be technically demanding. Physically, there are just some people—and I've had to try and teach them—that just don't have what I would call good hands. They're a little clumsy, in a way. And yet, while you can teach them to be good surgeons, they're never going to be someone you would call gifted. I have that gift.

To be excellent, it can come with practice. Just like anything in life, certain people have gifts. No matter how much golf I practice, I'll never be a Tiger Woods, and the same goes for any other sport. That's not where I'm gifted.

But with surgery, it takes the combination of having innate gifts and abilities and intelligence, and then, obviously, an excellent education and a great experience, and high volumes of patients so you can practice—not a very nice word to say when you're talking about patient care—but you get a lot of experience. With that experience and your innate abilities, excellence emerges.

With as much education, we had a tremendous volume of patients; a tremendous number of cases that I was able to do. You become very comfortable with it, which is, obviously, the goal of a residency program.

It's great to be able to say that I truly feel I'm doing exactly what I should be doing. An acquaintance has a goal to retire within about five years. He's my age. Now, he's got other interests. I cannot imagine not doing what I'm doing, especially when I feel that I have these gifts. It would be such a waste not to use them. When God gives you a gift, you'd like to take advantage of it, which I feel I have. Sharing that gift is a wonderful thing. I did a program called Face to Face {sponsored by the American Academy of Facial Plastic Surgery} in China, where we did reconstructive surgery on patients. We do free surgery because some of the people, literally, just can't afford to have it done, even though it costs very little. They're destitute, so we provide the surgical procedure, but it is available there.

What surgeries do you tend to do there?

We can do to a decent volume of cleft noses. You do a rhinoplasty on patients who've had a cleft lip because their nose is distorted. It developed abnormally because they had a cleft lip. They already may have had their cleft lip repaired, but their nose is still distorted, so we go and fix the nose. And then, there's all the multitude of other things.

For a cleft palate, that's a hole between their mouth and their nose, so they're going to have problems eating, and they're not going to be able to speak correctly. They're almost always fixed at some point, but if they're getting to the age where they're trying to speak, they're not going to be able to, appropriately, when they have a cleft palate. You're taking somebody who has a swallowing disorder and a speech disorder and you're essentially turning them into a normal person—at least with normal speech and normal swallowing.

Cleft lip, aesthetically, is such a displeasing thing to have, and you think the kid who has big ears gets teased. I can only imagine what a child with an unreconstructed cleft lip would go through. It depends on their society, but they can literally be outcasts. Once their parents stop taking care of them, they would probably be living outside of the village. It's sad, but true.

What's nice for our specialty is that the equipment that we need is small enough that we can take it with us. We're not doing big orthopedic work, so we don't need these big instruments. I took all my rhinoplasty instruments with me.

I brought a couple of packs of scalpel blades the first year I went, and

I'd catch the nurses taking three or four scalpel blades when I asked for one. They kind of pocket the other two or three because they just don't get brand new scalpel blades on every single case.

They're cleaning and sterilizing gloves for reuse. I'm sure the blades they use, they probably use them as long as they possibly can, until they just won't cut anymore. They don't have the luxury of just grabbing another one like we do in America. The second time I went I brought a whole case of scalpels.

We tend to go in and not only operate on patients that need our help; we also educate the local physicians. We have two days of conferences before we operate. We did three days of operating while we were there, and we had about a hundred people at these conferences, so we're teaching them improvements in their techniques.

In your practice here, do you do more cosmetic than functional surgeries?

There are months where the majority is cosmetic, but there are more months where the majority is functional. It waxes and wanes. Most of what I do is still functional.

As time goes on for facial plastic surgery, you end up doing more and more cosmetic because that's really a word of mouth phenomenon. You get happy patients, and they tell their friends. But it's usually a few years later, because not everybody's ready to get a face lift at one time. It's a few years later when their friend finally decides maybe it's time to talk to the friend who's had one, and they end up seeing me.

I do market, especially now that we're building our center. We just started marketing because I want to increase the volume of cosmetic patients. We have a group of patients that have had surgery done. If a patient is apprehensive, we'll say, "Do you want to talk to somebody who's had this?" That is worth 10,000 times more than a photo album. Being able to hear from the patient who had the procedure, as opposed to just looking at a before and after picture. Anybody can show you before and after pictures, and they can cherry pick their best results. I've seen before and after that I wouldn't want to show anybody because I think it's a mediocre result. Obviously, that must be one of their good ones because they're putting it in that ad.

Marketing, there's a definite gray zone where it becomes almost unethical, but you can't really put your finger on it. I don't ever want to be put in that circumstance where I'm thinking that about my own ads. It's an unfortunate circumstance that we almost have to market to be successful. What tends to happen, as you become busier doing cosmetic work, you tend not to do as much reconstructive work. In my personal practice, as I get busier doing cosmetic work, I'll probably not do any other work other than cosmetic work.

I still do a fair amount of skin cancer reconstruction. Dermatologists may remove a large cancer somewhere on the face and it's a big enough hole that they're not able to put it back together again, they'll send it to me. That's a lot of fun because you're trying to take them back to where they were before they had tissue removed, which is almost impossible. But you can come really close, and that's a really gratifying and satisfying surgery, as well.

Putting the nose back together again to where they can go out and nobody's ever going to know they had anything done. I can show you a picture where they're missing half of their nose. You can put it together in such a way that it's almost unnoticeable.

It depends on how much of the nose is gone and where on the nose the tissue's missing. But, on an extreme, you can replace virtually all of the skin and soft tissue of the nose with a forehead flap, which is based on an artery and vein that is just along the inner aspect of your eyebrow. That artery and vein comes out from the bone there, and it courses up toward your hair.

You can base a very thin pedicle,[†] which is what it's based on, and then you can, literally, make a tracing of the area that's going to need to be reconstructed. Take that tracing, put it on their forehead, mark that out and then cut that tissue and leave it attached down by the eyebrows. You then rotate it and lay it down on top of the nose exactly where you need it. Because you traced it out, you can get an exact fit for that tissue, and then you suture it in, leaving it attached to the eyebrow.

You leave it for about three weeks, and by then all the new blood vessels have grown in from where you sutured it and now you can take down that little pedicle, that little tube that is its life blood. It survives perfectly fine on the nose.

When you take that tube away, you can also do some thinning and some sculpting of the tissue to try and make it look better. Sometimes, you have to do a third surgery where you're just going in to sculpt it, just to thin it here, maybe bulk it up somewhere else, to give it that final appearance. Now, a lot of patients are so happy with the fact that you gave their nose back that they don't let you do the third surgery because they're happy with it.

I may look at it and say if I just took a little bit here and a little bit there, it would look even better. They're happy and they walk out the door. I'm always going for perfect. Certainly, every surgery that I do that's cosmetic, I'm always looking at and trying to see what I can do the next time to make that just a little bit better. It's almost ridiculous because if you got a 95% on a test, you'd think you'd be pretty happy with that. But I'm always looking for that hundred, every single time. It's an unattainable goal. If my patients are happy with the A, I want the A+. I'm always thinking a tweak here, a tweak there, and seldom do they want it. I need to learn to keep my mouth shut, because I'm much more critical of my own work than they are.

† The pedicle is thin tissue that contains blood vessels used for the flap.

Do you catch yourself analyzing people in public?

I certainly catch myself doing that on some of the extreme cases. Sometimes those cases are beautiful people with one flaw. I'm out at the restaurant, and the waitress is absolutely gorgeous and has an interesting nose, but an unattractive nose. Those are the people who jump out.

You're always looking back at what you did, what results you got, is there anything you would have done differently? I essentially go through a rhinoplasty four times. When I first see the patient, I'll mentally go through what I'd recommend. I then change them on the computer. The third time is the actual operation. The fourth time is I look back on my results and do that rhinoplasty again. It's a learning process, continuously, even if you've done 10,000 of them.

There was a gentleman from England—a doctor at a meeting—and he'd done over 10,000 rhinoplasties and was being interviewed. The interviewer said out of all those 10,000 rhinoplasties, how many would you have liked to do over again? He thinks about it, and says, "All but one." That's just the nature of surgeons like me and him. We're always striving for that perfection that's unattainable.

But you want to make sure that the patient has realistic expectation before you go to the operating room, because if they don't, then you'll end up with an unhappy patient, and they're difficult to deal with. My job is to find out if they have realistic expectations, which typically, is relatively easy to do.

I don't walk into an operating room having never seen this patient before, and then perform cosmetic surgery on them. They, obviously, have to see me in my office. I have to talk to them. We have a relationship. I ask a lot of questions. There's a lot of body language that I observe. That's not necessarily conscious, but you just sort of pick up on certain things after a while doing this.

I'll do computer generated imaging, so I'll take digital photography, put it in the computer and alter their image, especially for rhinoplasty, so that they can see the nose I want to create on their own face. I have a 23-inch screen, and we look at these pictures together. I'll modify the result if they think it needs to be, but most of them don't. They'll say, "That's exactly what I want," and I'll tell them I can get there within about a millimeter. It's obviously not going to be perfect, exactly the way that I show them, because it can't be. But I can come pretty darn close. I know that they have realistic expectations if I show them something that I can, realistically, give them surgically.

I've not gotten in a circumstance of somebody who had unrealistic expectations, and I ended up operating on them anyway. That has not happened. I have had patients that I guess are unhappy after surgery, even though in my opinion, when I look at them, the result is perfectly fine. That, in and of itself, would have been my fault, because I probably should have picked up on that. I thought they had realistic expectations. They probably didn't, so it happens. That's a very difficult situation to be in because there's nothing I can improve on. They look great, but they're complaining about this or this or this.

Thankfully, there's only one patient who comes to mind who had an absolutely perfect result. When they're unhappy in that circumstance, you simply have to continue to see them, talk to them, make sure that they know you hear what they're complaining about, and that's pretty much all you can do. There is no final happy place that we meet. They're not happy. They're never going to be happy, and my job is just to make sure that they have somebody to talk to about it.

There's just a certain psychological profile for that person, and that person is somebody that I should not have operated on, in retrospect. I've never had anyone else like that, other than that one patient. It's interesting, because if you do enough of this you're gonna have those patients, every so often. You go to national meetings and you talk to these plastic surgeons that have been doing this for 30 or 40 years, and they'll tell you about their unhappy patients and it's an identical circumstance. It's really the patients, not the surgery or the surgeon, that is the problem. It's unfortunate that they sneak through every once in a while.

Certainly, after that one unhappy patient, I'm much more critical and I would be much quicker to deny surgery to somebody. I've done that on several occasions, where I realized that this person is not going to be happy with anything.

I had a young gentleman come in for rhinoplasty. I did computer generated imaging, and he wanted a certain area of the nose to be taken down further. I told him that it's impossible. It was up between his eyes, and he wanted that taken down quite a bit. When he was so adamant about it, I immediately realized there was no way, no matter how good of a rhinoplasty I did, that he was going to be satisfied. I asked him to find another surgeon.

It'll be interesting if, five years later, he comes in wanting a revision from the surgery he had by another surgeon, because if he does get operated on, I'm sure he'll be unhappy. It's a frustrating place to be and frustrating to have to deny somebody surgery, when that's what I do. But it's best for everybody in the long run.

Are there any cases you're particularly proud of?

Oh, a patient came in with a history of basal cell carcinoma,[‡]s and was left with a hole larger than a silver dollar. I mean, it's two to three inches. It's a good portion of their face, and I rotated a flap from another part of their face next to it. The incision for that kind of surgery goes all the way down around the ear and all the way, sometimes, down into the neck. You lift this whole big huge skin flap up, and you rotate it up to fill this hole. It's

---

‡ Basal cell carcinoma is an especially treatable form of skin cancer.

underneath their eye or to the side of their eye and when you're done and everything is healed, you can walk into that room and you can hardly tell. I walk in and I'm looking at it and thinking, *I can't even tell I touched you.* The tissue is a perfect match because it's the same area of the face. It just disappears. That gives me a tremendous amount of satisfaction, because some surgeons would just put a skin graft on. You can see that across a room. With a skin graft, I could see it across a stadium. When you use the local tissue, you get this wonderful texture and color match. If you put it together well, the scars become almost unperceivable.

A lot of it has to do with the design of the reconstruction. Certainly with cosmetics, wherever you're going to do incisions on the face, you want to hide them. You hide them in areas like around the ear, so when I do a facelift, I go back behind the piece of cartilage. I'm actually in their ear canal. You're not going to see a scar in somebody's ear canal. The rest of them are in the hair.

When I need to make an incision, say on an eyelid, I put it in the crease so that when their eyes are open they cannot see that scar. When you have again, that fluid motion of surgery, a very important part of what we do as specialists of cosmetics, facial plastic surgeons, is you don't want to damage anything that doesn't need to be damaged. We're very, very delicate with the tissue that is going to reduce the healing, essentially because if it's not damaged, it doesn't need to heal. The more it needs to heal, the more inflammation that occurs and the more scar tissue that gets laid down. So by being very meticulous, by being gentle with the tissue, you can put these cuts back together again to the point where they're literally just a fine line.

You can almost always find a scar if you made it. But on the eyelid, there are places where I literally can't find it because the eyelid is so thin and it heals so well. I'm trying to find the scar and I can't see it. I'm not going to take full credit for that. It's the human body, and the way it heals.

But for reconstruction, we try to line up these scars with what are called relaxed skin tension lines. They're where people would get a wrinkle. We don't get wrinkles that go diagonally from the top of our ear towards our mouth. That's not the direction of a natural wrinkle. That would be extraordinarily obvious, because it's not supposed to be there.

We try to hide these in wrinkles in the fold between the nose and mouth. You can hide these things in locations where you'd expect to see a wrinkle. The human mind is bombarded with billions upon billions of images every day, and we gloss over everything that we expect to see. When you see something that you don't expect to see, that's what draws your attention.

Are some patients easier to have a good result with?

Certainly. It depends on what kind of problem you're dealing with. Skin type has a tremendous influence on the results of anything that's truly going to injure the skin. If I'm going to do any sort of a laser therapy, if I'm going to do any sort of a chemical peel on skin, the skin type is extraordinarily important, and you really can't treat patients with darker skin in those ways. You just can't because you're going to end up with a lot of pigment problems.

Certain skin types are more common to form keloids, or abnormal scars, so you have to be very careful in selecting those patients with darker skin. Interestingly, the darker skin patients tend to age more gracefully or more slowly. The darker the skin, the more likely you're going to have a problem. You're going to see scarring. You're not going to be able to treat their skin with wrinkle reduction therapies that we would do on a lighter skinned person.

How often do you see patients who want cosmetic work, when they look just fine?

I've had a couple patients come in wanting things that I don't feel are necessary. Fortunately for me, those people weren't as educated about the procedure as they should have been. They thought they wanted something, when, in fact, once I kind of analyzed everything and came up with a plan, they fully agreed with my plan. It's usually implant things that they tend to want, but maybe aren't necessary to give them the image that they desire.

I was interviewed a few years back when the *"Extreme Makeover"* was occurring. There was a young lady who was on the show, and they wanted my opinion as to what was done and the results, gave me some pre-op photos of her and then of course, they gave me a picture of her on stage in her evening gown. They told me what was done and what she had—she was 37 years old. She had a brow lift, and upper and lower blepharoplasty, cheek and chin implants, and a rhinoplasty.

The only thing that I would probably have done was the rhinoplasty. I might have touched her eyelids, but everything else was a little unnecessary, but I think they wouldn't have allowed her to be on the show had all they done was a rhinoplasty, because that wouldn't be called extreme makeover.

People are having five, six, seven different things done. And that's where you can get into the unethical part, because if you're seeing patients for cosmetic reasons, you're essentially going to charge them for every procedure that you do, and adding on these extra procedures, that may not be necessary from a cosmetic standpoint, certainly is going to add to your pocketbook. It never enters my mind to do something like that, because it's not in my nature. It is unethical.

How much does the quality of cosmetic surgery vary from doctor to doctor?

I certainly do know of plastic surgeons who do mediocre work. There are certainly a lot of people out there doing tremendous volume on almost anybody who walks in the door, and they're charging a lot of money. Now, maybe that's as good as they can do. Maybe that's as good a result as they can obtain, and from that standpoint, that would be fine.

I always try to individualize a person's treatment. If I need to do a deep plane face lift to give them the results, then that's what I'm going to recommend, and I'm going to charge them more. I don't know of any cosmetic surgery mills around here. I'm sure there are.

It gets a little scary in Arizona and Texas, where people are going to Mexico to have plastic surgery. There are plastic surgeons there whose entire practice is revision surgery from people who have gone to Mexico. That's a hot topic in our industry, traveling for plastic surgery. Some people even go to Brazil, because it's cheaper. They'll go to the Caribbean, or somewhere outside the United States and get it for a much lower cost, but probably at a much higher cost to them in the big picture, because of poor results and the risk of complications. That gets into another whole scary subject. I truly believe you end up getting what you pay for.

It really depends on what procedure was done. Rhinoplasty certainly becomes much more complicated when you're dealing with revision surgery. Those are the patients I follow for years to make sure everything's okay, because the second time you go in on a nose, it's going to heal totally differently. It's going to take a lot longer. It's got a much higher chance of having scar contracture, where the tissue literally kind of shrink-wraps over the cartilage that you leave behind, so you have to make sure that you give them a very strong infrastructure on their nose. The cartilage has to be put together very precisely, and in a very solid manner, to prevent those changes from distorting the nose down the road. That's a trick. And, certainly, I do a lot of revision rhinoplasties. I really enjoy it, because it's technically difficult and there are not very many people who can do it.

If it's an eyelid problem, that can be extraordinarily difficult to fix, if too much tissue was taken out, because now you're looking at skin grafts. You're looking at some issues with the fact that if too much muscle was removed, they're not going to have tone in the eyelid. They're not going to have the muscular movement they should to close their eyes. That's a devastating problem to have. It's a difficult problem to fix, and everybody is unhappy with that one.

Facelift surgery, typically, you're going to be able to revise and fix, unless, of course, it's a nerve injury. If that nerve's been injured and they're out, say more than six months, you're just not gonna see much of an improvement and there's nothin' you can do. Prevention is the key. You don't want to injure it. If it was injured, hopefully it was just stretched and it's going to come back. Facelift scars, skin loss, things like that, you can, almost always, either greatly improve or fix the problem. That's the surgeon's job.

I don't think it's the patient's job to realize all the risks. The surgeon has to tell the patient all the risks, so they understand that they're going in to have surgery that could potentially create these problems. I'm certainly very detailed in my consent for the surgery with my patients. I go into every single detail, including risk to the facial nerve, the movement of the face, bleeding, loss of skin, scarring—all those bad things that can occur. Of course, I end by saying that these are all extraordinarily unlikely to happen, but you need to know that they could.

Usually, I can then say, to almost all of them, "I've not had these occur in my hands. Obviously, I think scarring is going to be one that everybody has because you have scars any time you cut the skin.

This is intricate surgery. It doesn't come cheap, does it?
We're talking about something that could be $25,000, when they're doing full restoration. So yes, it's a significant amount of money. They're putting a tremendous amount of trust in me to give them what they want and they're paying me before I ever do it.

It's not like they're buying a car at the dealership that was manufactured by a machine. They're buying my talent. So yeah, they're placing a tremendous amount of trust in me, as their surgeon, to do what they want me to. And yet, they do it.

From a practice standpoint, we don't have to negotiate with third party payers on how much they're going to pay me. We pretty much set whatever fee we want. Now, you obviously have to understand economics to a certain degree, because you just can't set your fees so high that nobody will walk in the door to see you. There's no Medicare or Medicaid. It's cash. They pay you before the surgery's done, so it's very easy bookkeeping.

What my patients get is a tremendous emotional boost. They feel more confident. They're less self-conscious about a flaw they have. And, certainly, I've seen a lot of young patients with oversized noses come in, who are a little timid, and they kind of hide themselves a little bit, just emotionally, and you see them when they come back and they're standing up straighter, they're looking you in the eye, they seem like they have so much more confidence. I certainly see that even from parents of younger kids who end up with a rhinoplasty. That's a truly changing surgery.

Certainly, functional patients, when they have a problem with their eyelids or their nose, and they come to me with this problem and I fix it, they're very, very happy, grateful, satisfied patients. Some of them come up and hug you.

It doesn't happen instantaneously. They have a recovery period. I usually follow people for, sometimes, years, making sure that everything's okay. You'll see subtle changes, and I want to make sure those changes are for the better and not for the worse.

I'm making somebody look younger with the other cosmetic procedures. I restore their appearance with cosmetics. The cosmetic patients for face lifting and things like that, they also again, they classically will come in and essentially, tell me that they feel better than they look. If they felt the way they look, why are they getting cosmetic surgery? They're typically healthy people who lead a healthy lifestyle. They're active. They look in the mirror and think, "I shouldn't be looking like that. That's not the way I feel on the inside." They want to match their external appearance with their internal emotions, and that's what the cosmetic surgery does. Now, they look great—the same way that they feel.

The nation's attitude toward facial plastic surgery has completely changed over 20 years when it was something that was almost looked down upon. Only East and West coast people were having it done.

And now in Midwestern America, even in small towns, it's becoming extraordinarily acceptable and people aren't pointing fingers. It's partly just time. The more people who have it done, have good results, are happy, the more word of mouth, and it becomes more acceptable.

But also, obviously, the media have gobbled this up. It's unbelievable how much press occurs around plastic surgery in general. That bombardment by the media into everybody's lives, and that this gets talked about, literally weekly, it's just become acceptable. It's part of our society now, so more people are willing to have it done.

With the economic impact of American growth over the decades, more people have the cash to have it done. The growth of facial plastic surgery continues every year.

I seldom see anybody who's horribly concerned about letting anybody know. I've had patients who were in their 30s—I'm thinking about a young lady who had a skin resurfacing procedure, so the skin was damaged and she looked absolutely awful for about five to seven days. She kept going to college. She was taking classes. She walked on campus with a face that looked like she was in a car accident or something. That's because she didn't care that anybody knew what she had done. Then, once it healed, obviously, there was a great improvement.

And then, on the flip side, you have patients who are extraordinarily concerned that anybody would find out that they would be, quote, so vain, end quote, to have a cosmetic procedure done, when in fact, everybody's vain. That's just the way we are. You want to look good. The extreme is almost comical, sometimes, with people who are so open to the fact that they have this facial plastic surgery and almost brag about it. Then you have other people who would be just mortified if their friends found out they had something done.

What about kids?

With children, the only two procedures that I would do are otoplasty, which is setting the ears back, and rhinoplasty. That's pretty much it for cosmetic. Rhinoplasty gets a little more complicated. You have to wait until they're old enough, which means they've essentially stopped growing.

You want to operate on a nose that's not going to change in the future and then you have to have realistic expectations, not only for the patient, which would be the child, but also the parents. They're self-conscious about the problem with their nose and the parents want this fixed. If they're a good candidate, that surgery's relatively easy.

Otoplasty is typically done at age five or six. They're pretty young and it's the kids who get teased because their ears stick out. That's not so difficult to comprehend, from an ethical standpoint, and go ahead and perform, as long as the parents understand the risks, because obviously the child can't consent to anything.

It's an hour and a half procedure. A lot of them do come in because they're getting teased and when those ears aren't sticking out, they're not going to get teased about it. Children are done under general anesthesia, so they're asleep.

As soon as they take those bandages off the next day, their ears are set back. They have a normal curvature to them. I have them wear a headband at night for a couple of weeks and that's it. You know the scar's behind their ears. They don't see anything. They can go to school two days after surgery.

Adults, I'll do in my office, and I actually do a pretty significant number of adults, compared to the total number of people I do. They've always wanted it done, they're finally financially able to do it, and they come in and ask, can I do it at this late age? Of course, I can. And then we do it in the office under local anesthesia.

What's funny is that I've seen a lot of teenagers come in with what is a relatively minor problem, like an otherwise absolutely beautiful young girl with a small hump on her nose, and they're teasing her about it. I almost question it, whether it's jealousy because she's very pretty, and the only thing that they can tease her about is the small hump on her nose. It's devastating to the person, and so you do the rhinoplasty. Someone I was thinking about that would walk in the office with her head hanging down, very self conscious, very timid. It just destroys their self image, their self-confidence.

After surgery, she was just a completely different person with all the confidence that you could imagine, and that's neat. I can picture this person with a big smile and her head held high. I remember her mom saying that she's just much more outgoing, not only at home, but at school. That's when you get that good feeling about what you're doing.

How important is appearance to us?

You can do line drawings of a face and show subtle changes to the lips, nose, and the symmetry of the face, and virtually everybody will tell you which one is better looking, and they'll be, if you can use the word, right. They'll be right and we'll say that is what beauty is.

America is so inundated with the media, whether it's advertising or the extreme makeover, and all this. We're placing more importance on beauty than we ever have.

Men are becoming a larger percentage of plastic surgery patients than they were, but it's still 85% women. I think because—I have to be careful with my wording—women place more importance on their appearance than men do, for the most part. Men aren't wearing makeup, most of them. Women do. Women are getting their hair done and men, typically, will see a barber. There are a lot of differences in the way we take care of ourselves.

There's also the image of the distinguished gentleman. You can look older, but you can still be attractive, as a man. As a woman gets older, it's unlikely that they're going to be considered a distinguished-looking woman. Either they're attractive or they're not. Either they look young or they don't. That's the reason more women are having it done.

Men, interestingly, our skin, because of our beard, has a better blood supply and does tend to age a little more gracefully than women. They have a little thinner skin, so women will tend to age; get the lines a little earlier, than most men will.

Technologically, things are becoming less invasive. The trend is to have procedures that they don't have to go to the operating room for. They can come in to have it done and go to work the next day or the same day.

What's a typical day like for you?

My day to day is very routine; 7:30 in the morning operating room, until, typically, I'm done at five. I can't remember the last time that I wasn't home for dinner. I try to keep Fridays really light, or I take them off. Now, that's something I choose to do. It's not something that I have to do.

I'm in a relatively small town to do what I do. My lifestyle is fantastic. For one, we have a great emergency room in town I'll tend to see the patient the next day.

Obviously, I have to be on call. This weekend I'm covered by some other ear, nose, and throat doctors in town, and there's a general plastic surgeon in town too, so there's a lot of calls covered. We do get a lot of time off.

How long do you plan on practicing?

I can't even imagine 30 years from now wanting to say, "I don't want to do this anymore." I absolutely love what I do. If I did retire, I'd miss it. I'd do some woodworking. I'd get into carving, start doing more art, true art, sculpture, something that would be three dimensional, so I'd be able to use my hands. I still do some woodworking. I'm sure I'll get back into that with some other projects, working with your hands, creating something. I've always been able to build things, design things. It goes back to the art. That's why those technical aspects of surgery always came easy.

{When I asked about his young kids and whether they might be future doctors, he addressed it briefly by saying one of them has expressed interest, but he's only 11. That somehow triggered this revelation.}

When I was in eighth grade, I was in a car wreck, where I fractured some bones in the right side of my face. An otolaryngologist in Bloomington, Indiana, put 'em back together again. I didn't forget the incident—but I didn't make the connection to the fact that he was an otolaryngologist until I was almost done with my residency program. *Oh my gosh, Dr. White put my face back together again!* It was almost shocking. Maybe subconsciously it was in there, somewhere, but it's one of those where you hit your hand on your forehead, going, I can't believe I never made that connection! Obviously, it isn't on my mind as a reason I went into this specialty, but it happened to me.

We've been talking about your work as a facial plastic surgeon and why you pursued this. And now, after more than two hours, you mention that you were in a car accident as a kid and a doctor put your face back together?

{Broad smile} I haven't brought that up for years.

V

Life on Call

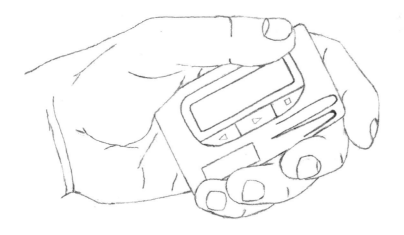

"The person who makes a success of living is the one who sees his goal steadily and aims for it unswervingly. That is dedication."

—Cecil B. DeMille

CHAPTER 17

A CUT ABOVE

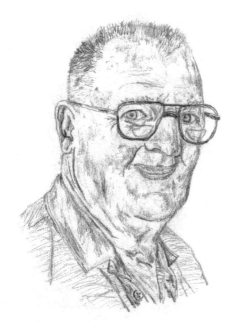

"Rest while you walk."

John Riesch, MD
General Surgeon, Milwaukee

What kind of guy has the cojones to perform his own vasectomy? Well, Dr. John Riesch does lots of amazing things, not the least of which was that bit of self-surgery. When it comes to medicine, nothing seems to scare this guy because he works so hard to get it right.

Doctor Riesch was among the first to try endoscopies–operating through tubes with the aid of a camera, which causes less trauma to the body, enabling a much faster recovery time. Riesch was also among the first to perform lumpectomies, substantially reducing disfigurement in breast cancer patients.

Growing up on a farm, working hard is all he's ever known. He loved that life, but Dr. Riesch never considered becoming a farmer himself. What he gleaned from that agricultural upbringing was a work ethic that puts most of us to shame. But for him, it's not work, per se.

Riesch loves, LOVES, being a doctor. He claims to work 100-hour weeks and denies missing out on anything in life. He somehow manages to play golf occasionally, and has one of the smoothest putting strokes I've ever seen. Chalk it up to the surgeon's touch.

I met Dr. Riesch in 1997, shortly before he became president of the Wisconsin Medical Society. In his mid 70s, Dr. Riesch is full of energy, happy as hell–almost gleeful. When you ask how he's doing, he'll usually reply in a snappy, quiet voice, "Perfect. Perfect."

His newly built, spacious home is exactly as he described–the exterior resembles that of a barn. The interior is anything but barn-like, though the home is unique with its wide open spaces.

In the family room, two massive, round and rustic chandeliers hang from the ceiling by pulleys. Thick ropes wrapped around hooks near the floor hold these monsters in place. The scene resembles something out of an old western, where a bad guy in a saloon slices the rope, crashing the chandelier on top of the cowboys playing poker beneath it.

Doctor Riesch gives me a 20-minute tour of his extraordinary home, which he's obviously proud of, before settling into patio chairs overlooking his serene, backyard prairie, which encompasses dozens of acres. As always, he's eager to chat.

My father graduated from third grade. He had a favorite expression: "You gotta work like hell; rest while you walk." My dad worked all day long. My father and my mother had tremendous stamina. And for years as a kid, I never slept more than four hours per night. It was all I needed.

My father could repair anything from the tiniest wristwatch to the largest thrasher machine, and I would drive him a little bit daffy because he was always trying to get me to learn something about repairing machinery and whatnot, and I had no interest in it. I was constantly watching my chickens hatch, the ducks hatch, a calf being born next door. I was just fascinated by birth.

My mother used to tell me I had such nice hands that I should be a surgeon. It was always kind of a joke of motherly love. She was a high school graduate and she used to tell me I'm not a bad kid, but I never learned to stand on my tongue because I was always talking.

My youngest boy is an oral surgeon. I guess he's a chip off the old block. He's gregarious. At his house, it's almost humming, as everyone is talking at once.

We were always proud of our Swiss heritage. They talk about racial bigotry and what have you. Growing up in a small town—dumb Swiss. And I just accepted that. But of course, instead of getting angry, I just went out to prove them wrong.

I grew up on a farm on Big Cedar Lake—worked the farm in the summertime; lived in Slinger in the winter. We just had a cabin to live in and we carried our water out to our privy. We didn't have electricity until I was about 15-years old.

When I was a little boy, my father was cleansing the cow after having the calf. He had his arm deep in the vagina trying to get the afterbirth. I ran and grabbed his arm, pulling on him, and telling him just to be careful. I'll get help. I thought the cow was eating him.

I just couldn't read enough to understand how two cells could eventually evolve into an animal or a human being. I did enjoy the features of life and death on the farm—you kind of accept them both.

I saved my money and I bought five goose eggs for 25-cents a piece. And at that time, none of our chickens were clucking anymore, so I captured one that was still making a little noise and put her on the nest and then, put a crate over the top of her and would feed her, water her and keep her covered day and night. And then, periodically, she'd get out and I'd have to chase her all over the farmyard and put her back on my eggs. And by gum, I got five goslings out of five eggs.

That fall, my oldest brother was driving a two and a half ton truck that didn't have brakes. Farmers didn't take time to fix their equipment until after the harvest season. As he came around the corner, he hit one of my goslings, a good size, and was killed. My other brother was so angry, he said, "Wait till I tell John," meaning me. And when he told me I said, "Well that's the way it is, life and death on a farm."

To this day, it's a joy to take care of farmers because they're very factual, very pragmatic and very practical. "If it has to come off doc, it has to come off."

So at what point did you seriously consider medicine as a career?

When I was at the University of Wisconsin-Whitewater, the war was coming on now, and I really wanted to get to medical school. I wanted to get an embryology class in there, but there was no way I could get in. Now, the embryology course was a three morning a week course and I only got there once because I had competition from my other class work. I had to be in two places.

Well, at the six-week time, I received a message that I had to meet president Williams. I played major sports. None of the kids that played in major sports were in any scholastic trouble. We won ballgames because we outsmarted them; not outplayed them.

I walked in. He was looking out of a big bay window and he heard me coming. He never turned his head and he said, "Riesch?"

"Yes," I said.

"Sit down!"

I thought, *Oh boy, what did I do? I'm in my last semester. I'm graduat-*

ing. I have to go in the Army. Was it the bonfire we had out at Whitewater Lake?

My mind's going crazy about the party, where the cops said we had better tone it down. We were always at the margin. I always organized a lot of parties, so I could get my class work done and my athletic work done and my studying done, and then my parties. I pulled off a lot of parties.

"Well, how'd you do it?"

I didn't know what to admit to. "What did I do, sir?"

Finally, he turned around and put his face within inches of mine and I could almost feel his spittle, and he said, "I want to know how you did it."

I just fried to death. Thanks goodness, I didn't commit to anything that would have gotten me in deeper trouble.

He said, "I want to know how you signed up for 22 credits?"

Sigh of relief, no big deal. I went in and signed up for 19 and then went right back in and signed up for a three-credit course.

He said, "But you can't do that. You're missing class twice per week."

"Well, Dr. Clark has 3 by 5 cards and he takes your name and calls, and one of my friends calls for me. The notes I get from them. When there's an exam on a day I should be there, I cut another class, try to get coverage and write my stuff."

He flumped around for a while and said, "I don't know what to do. You're getting A's in all your classes in all 22 credits."

Well, the long and the short of it is they allowed it to go through.

Gosh, I look back at classmates who were all so successful in the world. It just blows my mind to think they come from this small school and do so many good things. We had championship teams, smart people.

Do you think athletics had something to do with your success?

No question about it. Athletics teach you how to win. They teach you how to lose. They teach you how to grow up and how to be gracious. You develop friendships and you develop camaraderie. I played high school football and college football. And in all the time I played quarterback in football, I never once, ever, would ball out my offensive lineman if he missed a block and I got creamed.

We had a left tackle, a big rawboned kid from Watertown. He missed a block and I was just clobbered from behind. I got up spitting blood. My nose was bleeding. My teeth were loose. He literally, cried because he had missed a block and I got smacked. I bumped into him about 10 or 15 years later in the Minneapolis airport, and the first thing out of his mouth, he was apologizing again for missing the block.

So you did very well in college. Tell me how medical school went for you.

Oh, it was terrible. I was coming out of the service. I hadn't done any studying to speak of. I went to medical school at the University of Wisconsin. I was accepted, actually off the alternate list because I was in the middle of the Pacific in the Korean War. My other friends were all drafted. I could've gone to Korea and got blown away. I've often wondered if I could ever shoot a man. I imagine if it comes to life or death and someone's attacking you, it's either you or him, I suppose.

I was in the Pacific for a year working as a soldier and a military policeman in a top-secret area. When I came back to school, it was very difficult after being away from any kind of studying activity for two years. I found anatomy just overwhelming. I could not get anatomy, and my mentor took me into my counselor and said he couldn't understand why I was doing so poorly. I had a high D, low C, at the best, and I was studying.

But finally, just beyond the six weeks time after my session with my counselor, it fell together. I was trying to learn the artery, the nerve and the vein separately, not realizing that they all ran together, which just cut my anatomical knowledge by two-thirds, because you learn all three together. When that fell together, I became a very good anatomist and I fell in love with anatomy after being a terrible chore and a bore.

Then, I just loved medical school. I was probably a student that could be pinholed and say, "You know this guy likes every session, every assignment, every rotation." And I did! I loved everything. I just couldn't get enough. As a matter of fact, we had to rotate through a period of time with a dear Dr. {Frank} Weston for doing proctology and do proctoscopic examination. Well, a couple of my colleagues didn't really want to do that, so they paid me.

After the sixth week, Weston looked at me and said, "Riesch, weren't you here for the last few weeks?" and I said, "Yeah." And he didn't pursue it. But these guys were paying me a few dollars to take that rotation in the morning, so they didn't have to go. I would actually just kind of hound the hallways and look for things and experiences.

Speaking of money, I didn't have any money. I would sell my blood. You're supposed to sell it every three months. I sold it every month because I'm AB negative and I'm less than two percent of the population. I get $25, the girls got a two and a half dollar box of candy and I had $22.50 in my pocket.

Four years—finished medical school. It's a long time when you think about it. People don't realize sometimes the years that you give up of your life. Two years in the Army, four years in college, then, a year of internship and four more years of residency.

I am 33 years old and I am working the emergency room in downtown Milwaukee, hot, sunny afternoon. Here I am and all of my friends are out teaching, have a home, two cars. Some of them already have cottages on lakes that they purchased. I'm still making $2.57 an hour as a physician, which was good money, but am I ever going to get caught up materially, financially? That's the only time I was depressed in my life. I was depressed for about 10 minutes. Then, I got up and took care of the next patient.

I wasn't spending any time with my children; I wasn't having a good family life. I was working in my residency—I was working 10 nights a month at an emergency hospital to support my family. I was feeding one of the little children in the middle of the night and falling asleep at the drop of a hat. It's just a long time for all parties, including children.

I don't think it ever affected them because I would never complain to them. My children grew up when I was in private practice and they always knew where I was. I was at the hospital or my office, so they could always find me. I made a point of always attending their activities, be it plays, sporting events, awards. I was there. No matter what, that was first. I would never come and not ask the three children, how was your day? What did you do? I participated in their life as much as I could in that fashion. My rationalization is it wasn't quantity, but quality. To this day, I have a very, very tight relationship with my children.

How did you finally decide to pursue surgery?

I really was in love with OB, and that was my first rotation. I was with a fellow from the South and we were so busy. We had two delivery rooms and the residents were never around and we just delivered all the babies. We used to have to run all the way across the other side of the hospital, where the vaginal bleeders were in order to give them blood, etc. This was a torrid situation. The chasing we had to do.

I had already rotated through general surgery and enjoyed it very much. And this sounds a little bit bravado, but I could see I had good hands in the operating room.

I had two contracts in my pocket at the time. One was to go into surgery and one was to sign up for OB/GYN, and I just didn't know which route to take. But I did decide that evening, that moment...I went into surgery.

I graduated in '58. Vascular surgery was just being born. The first carotid was done in '54, so we were really anxious to do carotid surgery and we did. I can remember the first man I did. He was completely paralyzed, and in the recovery room. He started moving his arm and leg. Wow! What an amazing operation.

Well, we learned a lot. You don't operate on acute strokes. It was just coincidental that this guy got better. But after I did 25 of these and got published, I had people coming to see me from around the state to learn how to do carotids because there was nobody to teach us.

We were doing an endarterectomy,* and we had to take coat hangers and twist them to various sizes. We'd open up an artery that was occluded with arteriosclerosis and push that along, and peel that away from the ves-

* Surgery that involves removing plaque from the main arteries in the neck.

sel. That was so gross. I remember one time we were doing it, and the senior tried it and the junior tried it and the junior said, "I couldn't get it."

I said, "Come on guys. Give me a try."

So they said, "Go ahead, smart ass."

By gum, I put it in and we did get the plug out. We worked on dogs. We worked on cadavers. We just taught ourselves. Vascular surgery was a huge exposure.

I finished my internship. As of the first of July, I became a resident. What the heck? I didn't change over night. First night on call, three o'clock in the morning, I get a call from my chief, senior, fourth year. I'm a first year.

"John?"

"Yeah."

"Ah, we have a perforated ulcer over in the emergency room. Go take care of it."

Boy oh boy, here we go. I had to say to myself, *Man, I'm in it now.*

What made him comfortable enough to know that I could go over, take that patient into the operating room all by myself and take care of him? Well, because I had worked enough with him as an intern. We were on call every third night. Next time on call—same thing. Third night, third time. Three o'clock in the morning. I had gotten into bed for a half hour.

"John, there's perforated ulcer over there."

I was taking care of sick people, I'm getting up, and I put my shoes on. *What am I doing? Do I want to do this the rest of my life?* I took my shoe and I threw across the room and hit the wall.

Well, I thought about it for about 50 seconds. *Yeah, I really want to do this. Get going kid.* I went, and that was the end of it. And ya know something, Steve, I have never complained about a phone call in the morning, at night, on a holiday, on a weekend because I want to be there to help them.

What kind of advancements have you seen since the early days?

When I was a resident, we had penicillin, we had sulfa, and that's about it. We had these burn people who were dying left and right. We would take off dead legs under ice anesthesia because we didn't have antibiotics. We'd put them on ice for a couple of days and take them to the operating room.

It's unfortunate because we're going to get pushed back because of the lack of advancement with new antibiotics. The bugs all develop resistance as we overuse antibiotics, and the public doesn't get it.

Fortunately, God smiled upon me, and allowed me to participate in laparoscopic work. I've done 7,500 hernias or more. I've done close to 5,000 gall bladders. I haven't opened up an appendix in 15 years. I had a guy the other day, who had abscess the size of a softball. I opened him up and got him all cleaned up and he's five days out and he's going to go home tomorrow.

You know who's going to be great, Steve, are the grandchildren, and people with Nintendo games. It's all hand/eye coordination because you're working off a screen.

I enjoy teaching in medicine. It probably comes from my bachelor of education background. I like teaching to be fun. I don't like it to be threatening. I don't like it to be demeaning. I press the students to answer all the questions right. I press them until they can't answer the question because it's a means of letting them know that there's still something they don't know. But it's done softly. I'll give them assignments and I'll say, look it up and talk to me tomorrow.

I detest sarcasm in teaching. I detest the demeaning nature or overtone to make somebody look dumb or bad. What purpose is served by that?

Did you experience that?

Oh, sure. There's always some creep that tries to be the big shot. This is true in life, in general. You don't have to make me out to be an idiot. If I did a dumb thing, teach me so I don't do it dumb again.

And if you're humble, God will recognize you even more. When you know what you're doing and you are satisfied, everything worked out just the way you wanted, you don't need somebody to tell you.

More often than not, you get thanks and things from families. I've given a lot of graduation talks about maturity. Maturity is when you can do something for somebody without any adulation, without recognition and without even a thank you from the person. No slap on the back. Friends, colleagues, relatives, nobody recognizes it, but you know what you've done—the endorphin release, the physical high, the mental high, the emotional high, the adrenalin high. It is something that is immeasurable.

I lived in this community for so long I have come to know a lot of people, just on that basis. But to me, it is not recognition of accomplishment. I get tomatoes. I get poultry. A guy clean plucked and gave me a turkey—wild turkey. We're going to have it for New Year's Day. I like cooking during the Holidays. I told my wife, I want to make it like the regular Thanksgiving turkey. It is a reward that is unending.

When I was a resident, I used to get the biggest kick out of this. I don't really smoke, but they'd bring me cigars.

Do patients recognize you in public?

Oh, yeah. My wife gets such a kick out of it because I make no bones about it. I'm always pretty cordial and love to greet them. We chat and I try to make small talk. The most embarrassing part is that you see so many people that you recognize. You can't think of their names or anything. You probably recognize the operation you did—you can remember that.

I would never have made it as a politician because I can't remember names. I get my kids' names mixed up at times, and dates. I don't know my own social security number. Why clog up my brain with something I can look up in my wallet?

I love to tell people about books and authors and it's so embarrassing when I do that and I can't remember the author of the book. It's like looking at a painting and not knowing who the artist was. It's a terrible weakness, and it's laziness, pure laziness.

I oftentimes call staff members sweetheart, pleasant names. I can't remember everybody's names, but it's a terrible feature in my character. A lot of the patients understand and say, "I know you don't remember me, but my name is Jane Doe. Thank you." It's enjoyable, but it doesn't make me feel macho.

Your cup runneth over. It's self-indulgent. I just love taking care of people. I love being able to help guide them. That is such a thrill. It's not egotistical. It's just knowing that you can do things to help people, and I guess that's what led me into medicine.

Most of us can't imagine taking a knife, cutting somebody open and then repairing a problem. Can you remember the first time you did that and how it went?

It went very well because I haunted the operating rooms. I haunted these places just to see and help and do anything I can do. But surgeons in surgical specialties have to have an element of confidence, ego, if you wish. Some of them are quote, unquote, prima donnas, and I don't cotton to that.

But I think you have to have a personality, as such, that you can believe in yourself and believe you can do things. But this speaks to something about surgeons' personality that is somewhat intimidating to other people because they have confidence in themselves.

We've learned a lot during my period of training. Fortunately, my curiosity has kept me on the cutting edge. I'm the second guy in the Milwaukee area to do laparoscopic work. I was the first in the whole Midwest to do conservative breast surgery. I've had my finger on the pulse, so to speak, because I have an innate curiosity and because I probably have such an egotistical feature in my body, that I'm not afraid to try something new.

To take somebody and do an aortic aneurysm, and literally cut them in half, and cut off their blood supply and repair it, put it back together, you have to believe in yourself. Nobody really understands—the patients, the family, even non-surgical doctors—the responsibility you are assuming. The risks are astronomical. It weighs on you. But you go into anything and everything doing the best you can do, and that's all you can do.

When students or staff or nurses or techs say, "I'm sorry…" I must have heard it a million times over my lifetime, No, there's no room for sorry in medicine. You only have one chance. No sorry. Just do your job. Don't apologize, especially if it's not going right. Just do it right.

I don't know that this confidence or this bravado carries over in my individual life. My wife loves cars. I hate cars. I hate to drive. If my life depended on telling you how a car worked, I'd be dead meat. No knowledge. I don't want to know about it. When they don't work, I get out and kick the tire and walk off and swear and look for somebody to help.

I'm a-mechanical—I really am. I'm afraid of electricity. I don't even know about a faucet. If it doesn't work, I talk to my wife because she's got all the tools.

The only thing that makes you nervous is when you know that you have—a huge aneurysm, for example, and somebody with severe COPD {chronic obstructive pulmonary disease}. If it ruptures, and it's an emergency, you're not going to survive. You've got to try to do this before the emergency sets in. You have to do it so you have everything in place.

These elderly patients are precarious. They cannot tolerate one complication, no matter how small or how big because they are not going to survive. That makes you a little tense. And I've always had a thing in the operating room that—I've never thrown an instrument in my life. I've never screamed or hollered or lost my head in the operating room. I become tense, curt, when I find that things are tight. I want everybody to pay attention. And if I find that my techs or my nurse is not focusing to the degree I want them to be, I will tell them, "pay attention."

I also have a rule that the levity doesn't start until everything is complete and comfortable. Then, the surgeon exposes the levity. Now, you can tell the jokes, now you can laugh, now you can start talking about what you did over the weekend. That's my philosophy, and I try to pass that on to the students who work in the operating room.

I try to always make a point of thanking staff. Every time I leave that operating room, I thank every member in that room for helping. I teach this to the students. We allow them to do certain things, endoscopy, and handle the machinery, which prolongs the nursing staff because it takes more time.

But as much as you try to explain the risks, patients don't really know the degree of risk that you know. "The doctors never told me anything." My immediate response is, if I was involved, I say, "Now, wait a minute. Here are my notes. Here's what I told you."

It's the families who are just totally resistant and they want to kill the messenger. You have no bedside manner because you had to tell them the truth. There's nothing more we can really do for mom, dad, and it's in God's hands. And however soft you put it, they distort it. People like to be angry with somebody who gives them information they don't like to hear. And this isn't just true in medicine. Your car doesn't work. The guy tells you what has to be done, so you're angry with that guy. So you go to another guy and finally go to three or four, whatever it is, until you realize, hey, there is something wrong with the car.

They become obnoxious, accusatory; challenge your integrity, your character. That hurts me. And you have to really bite your tongue, not to lose your temper. There are situations that I've gone through over the years where I will just say to the patient, "Look, I've really tried hard to help you, but I really think you have to get other opinions. You have to get care where you can trust people because medicine and the care of a patient is a team."

I don't mind being chewed out, if I have not complied with their wishes, but I'm so compulsive about that, it is not a problem. I will try to work through it. Be satisfactory to them. You don't have to go through that torture.

Let's stay with patient issues. How often do you have trouble getting them to do what they need to do to heal?

I could sue 100 patients a month because they aren't compliant. They won't take their medicines. Boy, would that shut off lawsuits in a hurry. You know, if we would quit suing, not just physicians, just quit suing everybody, there'd be much more money available to further develop care.

I make tapes of all my surgeries, and I give the patient the tape. But some say, "Ah, you're really exposing yourself to lawsuits." The hospital went nuts when I started doing it. But I said, "Come on, it's their operation." So they sign some kind of a sheet.

I say, "No. If they're going to sue me, they're going to sue with or without a tape." Every patient—"Man, Doc. Wow! What talent."

I say, "No, this is something that's been accomplished, technically."

Well, they rave about it. And it gives the patient a greater understanding of the improvement that has come down the pike.

It's great because if something goes awry, you have a reference point to go back and say, "Listen, is there something that I saw that I can use as a reference point?" We learn by experience. We learn by reading, and we learn by discussion. It leaves three imprints on the brain. Then, you don't have to memorize because you've learned it three different ways, so it sticks with you.

But medicine isn't always so fascinating, is it?

I don't like to do hemorrhoids, but I make a game out of it. Make a challenge out of the things you don't enjoy doing—the redundant things, the awkward things, things you find obnoxious.

When I was a little boy, I had to pound the carpets. Everybody had throw rugs. I hated it. I would get sweaty, and I was all dirty. My mother would take me aside and hug me.

"Ya know, Johnny. In your lifetime you're going to have to do a lot of things you don't like. Make a game of it. Make it a challenge. Do it well and get enjoyment out of it." I would run up, hit the carpet and run away before the cloud of dust could settle upon me. I've thought so many times about that.

I was sewing up a drunk one time who was lying underneath a train—just all chopped up. Fortunately, he never got his arm or leg or anything underneath the wheels, but got beaten up by the undercarriage. He was stoned out of his mind. I must have put a thousand stitches in the various areas.

A friend of mine came in. He was talking to me and I kept talking to the drunk, and got it all sewn up. He said, "You don't get mad at drunks?"

I said, "No. I quit getting angry with drunks years ago because it serves no purpose. They're not going to help you. But if you talk to them, play silly talk and games, make it fun for him and for me, we both get done and neither one's angry."

Even vasectomies, I got so tired of them. I would try to make a game by trying to do it in so much time. I did my own.

You actually performed a vasectomy on yourself?

I had a wonderful, beautiful family and I really wasn't planning on having any more children. We were sending many vasectomy patients into Illinois, because it wasn't truly, completely legal in the State of Wisconsin. Since there was no one else doing it, I decided it wouldn't really be very difficult to do this upon myself. Because I had a vague history of having a possible allergy to the local anesthetic, I really didn't want to do it without someone in attendance, in case I'd have a reaction.

Interestingly, one of my colleagues had requested for me to do a vasectomy on him, so we set up on a Saturday to do this in our office. I had it all set up and the colleague was on the tilt table. I prepped him and made the injection of the lidocaine. Within moments, he was having a seizure. Well, he wasn't in any trouble. He was exchanging his air quite nicely, so I just proceeded and went ahead with the operation. It takes me about 10 to 15 minutes to do this. By the time I was finished, he awakened and I said, "What is this seizure activity?"

He very embarrassingly, responded, "I was afraid to tell you this, but every time I have an injection, I always pass out. It's been that way all my life."

So we kind of laughed about that for a little bit. I went on and he was sitting on the stool and the chair in a corner and I set up my own tray to do this. Shaved my skin and prepped it and put the injection in and I heard this noise. After I injected myself, I turned over toward the chair where he was sitting and here he was, having another seizure. Well, there wasn't much I wanted to do with him and could do with him at that moment without breaking my sterile set up. I just kind of watched him for a moment or two, and he was okay. He wasn't slipping or falling, and he was breathing fine, so I proceeded and did my own vasectomy.

As I was closing the skin, he awakened and we started chatting about this again as I finished. I said, "What is this? I certainly can understand that there are some people who pass out when they have an injection, but you're passing out when someone else gets an injection."

"Yeah," he says. "Every time I see somebody get injected, I pass out and have a seizure."

"But what do you do in your practice?" He's a fellow physician.

"Oh, when I have to give somebody an injection? I never do. Give it to my nurse and I walk out of the room, so I never have to witness it."

It's a loving friend and a true, loving story.

Weren't you nervous about doing this on yourself by yourself?
Not really. I'm a little crazy.

Isn't the perspective totally different, hovering over somebody and hovering over yourself?
It was rather awkward, but what I did was shave myself and tape my donniker up against my abdominal wall. I was standing up so I could see and work. It really was rather simple. I didn't have any problems at all. I followed myself and followed my sperm. I was free of sperm. It worked.

Twelve years ago, I did a self-diagnosis on me of prostatic cancer, and had surgery. I was back to work in 10 days.

I had four bypasses. Honest to God. I walked from the hospital to the car, from the car to Usinger's. I thought I died and gone to heaven. "We have to stop at Usinger's. I want a piece of smoked sausage."

Speaking of heaven, how much of medicine is out of a doctor's control?
With medicine, people think it's a science. It's not. There are so many things we don't know that it boggles my mind. You learn that you are not all in control. You see people come back from death's bed, not from me. I may push a button here or there to make sure they get the electrolytes correct, blood counts, but man... I've participated in resuscitating patients who were dead. And stories I can tell, and I will relay one.

A patient. We get him going. He gets straight-lined. Finally, we get sugar into him, to correct his potassium because of poor kidney function, and we brought him back.

"Do you remember anything?"

He says, "You really hurt my chest."

I said, "Yeah, I'm sorry about that."

But he says, "I had the nicest visit with Tommy."

"Tommy. Who's that?"

"You don't know him. That was before you were taking care of us. We lost our son some many years ago."

I said, "Really."

He said, "'Dad, I've been waiting for you for so long. It's nice to see you.'"

He had an out of body experience, and I've had a lot of patients who've had that. That's exciting and that really makes you believe. But beyond anything else I can tell you, yes, I'm a Christian, proud of it. No matter how smart you become in your field of medicine or whatever, there's something else controlling all of this.

One of the best remarks I ever heard about dying was a personal friend we went to visit who said, "John, I'm ready for a new body." I thought, *My goodness, that says it all.* It literally brings tears to your eyes. {It does and he pauses}

But there's an interesting feature in death, as I try to console the family. We are selfish. We don't want to give up that loved one. No matter how much pain they're having, no matter how bad the outlook is, I mean, they have a terminal situation, somebody's looking for that straw, something magical.

I always make a point of calling the family and extending my sympathies. Patients become more than patients. They become friends, dear friends, to the point that you'll lay down and die for them. I oftentimes go to the wakes. The funerals, I think, should be a little more private for families.

Is there an emotional line a physician needs to draw?

The emotional line has to take place that you make the right mechanical decision in the operating room. As you make a decision that is most safe, most appropriate for the patient, not for your love of a patient. That's a tough line at times, and one has to be careful of that. But that runs pretty much standards for all the decisions you make. You make all these decisions on the basis of statistics, experience, background, patients' tolerance. You have to keep yourself in those confines if you're dealing with a patient you're very fond of.

When you have a case that goes badly, how does that affect you emotionally?

Destructive. Each and every fellow who cares for people, whether it be surgical, non-surgical, any entity, you build into your training that you look back and you reflect on anything I did or didn't do or should have done.

We're never, ever above learning. At my age and stage in life, man, I learn something every day. If you don't do that, you're not going to get better.

I read three to four books per month. I love to be well versed. I love to read both sides. I'm such a conservative. As I grew up, one of the most exciting things in my life as a little boy—was Sunday afternoon dinners. It was a time of talk and discussion and we would all sit around the table and talk. When I reached the age that I could enter in the discussion with respect, I was thrilled to death. That's one of the things that led me to believe that I could read and participate and offer information. I remember that almost to the day that I was accepted in the family now and I could make statements and that they would say, "Well look, he's done his homework. He's read his material. He knows what's going on. What he's offering is substantial."

You love learning, but that doesn't mean you have to keep working. Do you have any plans to retire?

No, not really. I quit working the emergency room about a year and a half ago. I miss it. I enjoyed the challenge of working on your feet and thinking on your feet. I wouldn't want to do it all the time because you don't see the end result I work about 100 hours per week. Well, I can sleep at the drop of a hat. I get a 15-minute sleep, and I feel pretty good.

To tell the truth, there are times, like today, in the middle a church, I get a phone call from the pharmacist to tell me that a patient can't have codeine. That could've waited until lunch time. I wasn't testy, but you know, that bothers me. We are humans and could use some rest.

But it doesn't sound like rest is a top priority for you.

I have a lust for life. I'm not afraid of death, per se. I don't want to die until I accomplish some more things in my life. I have the grandchildren that I want to see grow up. But there are features of my life I still want to experience. I don't know that I really planned on retiring as long as I have my faculties, and I'm still pretty quick. I do my operations as fast as anybody else. Ideally, I'd like to die after ending a case, after walking out of the operating room to write my order.

CHAPTER 18

IT'S THE RELATIONSHIP, BABY

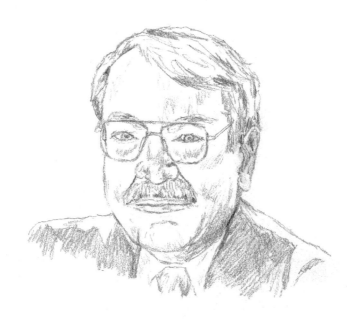

"What could you possibly do with your life that could begin to be more rewarding than what we do?"

Robert Jaeger, MD
Obstetrician/Gynecologist, Stevens Point

I'm positive that Dr. Robert Jaeger was born with a smirk on his face. Jaeger once showed me his business card, which described him as an "Infertity" specialist. The typo wasn't that far off, given his medical specialty, and he roared with laughter when he showed it to me.

Then, there was an AMA meeting we attended together in Chicago, where Dr. Jaeger was passing out long stem silk roses at a campaign event. When I pointed my camera in his direction, he immediately grabbed a stem and put it between his teeth like a tango dancer. In my news reporting days, Dr. Jaeger was my go-to source on just about anything related to obstetrics. It seemed he was always the president or some other officer in his specialty society. That was in addition to his volunteer activities at the state level, where I really got to know him in recent years. I once remarked to him how amazed I was that he could so frequently attend medical meetings over so many years.

"I could never give back to the profession as much as it's given to me," he replied, solemnly. No smile. No goofing around.

I caught up with him following yet another meeting he attended at the Wisconsin Medical Society. Doctor Jaeger had an important physician role model in the family who shaped his professional interest early in his life, though I have no idea where he developed his sense of humor.

My grandfather was a country doc in Columbus, Wisconsin. He actually had his name on 25,000 birth certificates when he died. At his funeral, they couldn't get all the people in the church. He had a tremendous rapport with people. He loved practicing medicine and taking care of people. His patients loved him.

He had a tremendous influence on me. If you're going to pick something to do with your life, that seemed like a really good thing to do. I knew that was exactly what I wanted to do with my life by the time I was 12.

I started out wanting to be a family practitioner, general practice. I realized, relatively early, it was not going to be possible to keep up on all areas for all time. Eventually, you were going to fall behind and the last thing I wanted to be was a poor physician.

In medical school, they always throw a good deal more at you than you can possibly absorb. You try to get as much in as you can and hope that you got the important things. It was tremendously more work than anything I'd ever done before or since. The stress is significant.

Looking at the specialties was a process of elimination. I enjoyed surgery, but I didn't want to be in the operating room all day, every day. I enjoyed taking care of people and I wanted to have a longer-term relationship with them than surgeons have with their patients.

I like kids. But boy, when kids get sick, they get really sick. It is scary and they can't tell you where it hurts, sometimes. Obstetrics is fun, delivering babies. I ended up sort of backing into it—some surgery, some obstetrics, and a lot of primary care.

For most women, we're the only physicians they see between the ages of 15 and 60. If they need other medical care, we're usually the ones who make the diagnosis and refer them. We have tremendous rapport with our patients. I'm not sure you could call a physician/patient relationship a friendship, but it's certainly much more than a business relationship you have with your banker or lawyer. What could you possibly do with your life that could begin to be more rewarding than what we do?

We're being paid for helping people and we're privileged to see people when they're most stressed, when all their guards are down. We get a view of humanity that very few people see. You develop a tremendous respect, in my case, for young women. What they do in having children and raising those families, it's just tremendously gratifying.

But every specialty has its downside. Ours is the hours. On an average day, I usually start in surgery at 7:30, which means making rounds between 7 and 7:30 and catching a little bit more in between. I finish surgery usually by 10, and I'm in the clinic by 10:30. I don't have time for lunch. I usually work straight through until 5:30 or 6, then review the lab reports, and catch up on some paperwork and make rounds again. I'm usually home by 7:30 or so.

When I first started practice it was every other day, but for many years, it was every third day on call. Those days we never leave the hospital. We spent the night there, and then we went back the next day.

The current situation now—I have seven partners, so it's only once in every seven nights, which is much more doable. I don't think I'd be able to practice obstetrics now, at my age, if I wasn't in that kind of relationship.

Can you remember the first baby you ever delivered?

I was a third year medical student, and it was at St. Mary's Hospital. The first year resident was there and the attending physician wasn't going to make the delivery. The resident walked me through it. I was so worried I was going to do something wrong that the emotional impact of the delivery was pretty much lost until afterwards. Actually, it was probably well into the second or third year residency before I was able to relax enough with the delivery and not worry about what I was doing enough to enjoy what happened with the delivery and the parents.

Did that first one go okay?

Yes, it did. Fortunately, most babies do well in spite of me. {Laughs} Essentially, what an obstetrician is, is an insurance policy. Easily, 75 or 80% of babies could be born at home or in a taxi and do well. The problem is the other 10-15% who can get into serious trouble, and that's what we're there for.

Nationally now, the cesarean section rate is approaching 26%. Some of that is the result of changes in medical liability situation. Some of it's patient demand. Now, at least, we're very active participants in those deliveries.

How concerned are you about that c-section rate going up?

I don't know the right answer. There've actually been studies done in other parts of the world that have shown, in spite of what we used to think, that cesarean sections may be equally safe for mom. They're always safer for the baby.

In some parts of South America, the cesarean section rates are 90%

and the maternal death rate has actually gone down with that. Some of that may reflect the availability of health care professionals in rural areas, where these people are coming in to the cities to have their babies born by c-section in daylight hours and get good treatment and care.

In any event, there's a lot of controversy right now about whether vaginal delivery affects the supporting tissues that frequently get us into trouble later in a woman's life with urinary incontinence, pressure from her uterus, actually coming out prolapsed.*

Interestingly, there was a study published just this month, comparing the rates of those kinds of problems in women who've had children with women who've never had children. And after menopause, it's about the same.

What is the risk for women?

Some of it you can identify ahead of time. Some have high blood pressure or diabetes, where you know you're going to have problems with the baby. Some have abnormal presentations, like a breech, where you can get into serious problems with entrapment of the head. You can lose a baby in that situation.

Occasionally, in labor we'll find, all of a sudden the baby's heart rate drops way down, indicating the baby is not getting enough oxygen, frequently from an umbilical cord that wraps several times around the infant's neck or entrapped in some way or even prolapsing of the cord. Without an emergency c-section, those babies would be lost.

What's it like to lose a patient in pregnancy, or lose the baby? It's probably happened in your long career, right?

Unfortunately, yes. There are times, especially with a baby where you really don't have a chance, the patient will present and say the baby hasn't moved for the past 24 hours. The reason the baby hasn't is, for instance, a knot in the cord was pulled tight and there was no way to predict or prevent that.

I've only had one situation where we lost the mother. She presented in our emergency room with seizures. She had a condition called eclampsia,† which resulted in the herniation of the brain stem and death. We ended up doing a cesarean section a week later without anesthesia to deliver a viable infant. That is truly a devastating experience for everybody present. But losing a baby is devastating. You see nurses cry. We don't talk about it, but that's when doctors cry.

It took a long time to learn—it's not something I learned in medical school—you can be more help to those patients than to those patients who have a normal, healthy child. Patients who have an emotional disaster like

* Prolapse is condition where an organ falls down or slips out of place.

† Eclampsia is a life-threatening condition for the pregnant mother and fetus characterized by high blood pressure.

that can get tremendous benefit from someone who just listens, empathizes, and tries to help keep things in perspective and offers sympathy.

When that happens, I kind of go into the patient's room and sit there until the patient wakes up, if she's been under an anesthetic, or until all the patient's questions are answered, and I'm comfortable she's grieving appropriately.

Do you remember deliveries or do they all just blur after a while?

The hard ones, you remember every single one. And the disasters—you remember every one of those, too. They're always with you. And then, there are some patients who you just never forget. They're just special people. I remember one. We had a misfortune. We lost a baby. By the time she got to the hospital, the baby was gone. That's every parent's nightmare, to lose a baby. But this young lady adjusted to it like no one I had ever seen before. Her first comment after it was all over was, "I know you did everything you possibly could, Doc, and I don't want you to feel bad, because it wasn't your fault." She was more concerned about me than herself.

Do some patients have a hard time accepting a bad outcome and blame the doctor?

Not initially, but over time and for some, it may depend on their relationship with their physician. For instance, if you get a baby who has brain damage, a year or two or three years later, Uncle Joe is gonna ask who is going to take care of him when you're gone? That starts the thought process going that there ought to be some way to compensate these youngsters or at least arrange for appropriate care for them. Our system has no way to help these little ones.

They end up as suits, and juries are tremendously sympathetic. It doesn't make a difference whether or not the doctor could have prevented that. They see the doctor as a source of deep pockets. He has malpractice insurance, and of course that's what it must be for, to take care of these little ones. That's not at all what it is for, but that's the way the juries read it and they're helped by lawyers.

Ultimately, it's got to get better. There has to be some reason brought to the courts. Unfortunately, it seems there are two types of lawyers right now: those who sue us and those who make money defending us. Neither has an interest in changing the system. Of course, any changes in the system have to survive challenges by the Supreme Court, who will push it back into the same disastrously failed system where justice takes a back seat.

But every physician has to make an effort to see a patient, not as a potential litigant, knowing that if something goes wrong, you probably will be sued. You may lose, even if you've done everything correctly.

On the opposite side of that, there are times, looking back, there are things I could have done a whole lot better and those patients haven't sued. I've always told the students, "If you walk out of the operating room and you don't find yourself asking yourself what you could have done better, then it's time to quit."

We're continually looking for better ways to do things. I can't tell you how many hours I spend attending lectures and reading journals every year. Things change, and it takes a certain amount of experience and judgment to know what changes are significant and which are not.

It's very easy to adopt a new surgical technique, for instance, that looks real good, without there being enough national experience with it to know if it really is as good as it says. I can name a number of surgical procedures that have turned out not to be of benefit and actually increase risk. But it wasn't known until they were done for a decade.

A word of advice to anybody who's considering medicine as a career: Ignore the liability problem because it has to go away. It will get better. Eventually, we will prevail. Ignore all of the griping about insurance companies, HMOs, and government reimbursement. The system doesn't operate without physicians.

If you feel in your heart, what you want to do is what I've just described, there is no better thing you can do with your life, and I would encourage you to pursue it.

I sense you feel people are going to be turned off by medicine because of these problems.

They certainly are. We're getting fewer applicants to medical schools, and for a while there was worry about them not being as qualified. The only reason they're qualified now is that 50% of this class is now female. Back when I was in medical school, out of a hundred of us, there were three women. I was probably more uncomfortable than the patients, at least initially, doing pelvic exams, especially on young women. I have two female associates. There are some patients who prefer a female and there are some who don't.

What's it like to preside over the vast majority of these births that go well?

A big part is actually seeing the father and the mother, and the joy they have from a little one. To hold a little, breathing human being, and to know this is going to grow into an active member of society, is a very special feeling. My part may be relatively small, but even when it's easy, it's tremendously exhilarating. I still have trouble getting to sleep after a delivery. It's a real high, and that's why it's hard for me to retire now.

Do you have any adult patients you delivered as babies?

Oh, yeah, quite a few. It's not unusual for a patient to come in, and at the end she says, "Oh, by the way, my mom says you delivered me."

How many deliveries have you presided over? Have you kept count?

No. I think I stopped counting after 3,000, and that was over 20 years ago. It's probably about 10,000, but I honestly don't know. Each one is special. It's never routine. To be able to hand the baby to the mom is just a spectacular feeling that nothing else is ever going to replace.

What's different about delivering babies today?

Most women are waiting to start their families today. Most don't start in their late teens, early 20s anymore. Twenty-five is probably much more average. We do see the younger ones, too. But mainly it's the later age groups and they tend to be a little bit more mature, a little bit more knowledgeable, and more frightened.

Over your long career, you've also been extremely active in professional medical societies. Why?

I always felt that you had to give something back, and early on a friend got me involved in what was then the maternal child welfare commission at the State Medical Society. From there, I ended up being appointed to a subcommittee on maternal mortality. Because I gave reports from that group to the State OB/GYN society, I got to be known there and was ultimately asked to put together several meetings, which we did, and fortunately, they were successful.

When I first got active in the State Medical Society, we couldn't get insurance at any price, and we had to find solutions. I became active in my county Society, which elected me to the Board of Directors of the State Medical Society, for three three-year terms—nine years.

You just can't sit back and complain if you don't try to do something, so I ran for the AMA Delegation and was elected. I've been on that for 12 years now. It comes from a congenital inability to say "no," coupled with the desire to give something back.

What do you consider one of the bigger accomplishments related to your professional involvement in medicine?

My annual premium for medical liability insurance is about $55,000. It's been static at that for at least about the last decade. That is, if you compare it with the rest of the country, about average. It's not spectacularly low, but it's been static. That's made insurance available in the state, and with the availability of insurance in the state, we've been able to retain physicians. That's the key to Wisconsin providing outstanding medical care.

Do these outside activities complicate your family life?

Yeah, it does. My wife ended up raising three kids, pretty much alone. You try to make sure the time you have with them is quality time. When I was home on weekends, after I finished the chores, the boys and I would go to property we have and bow hunt or futz around out there.

On Sunday morning, we'd get up early and drive up and do some musky fishing. There weren't too many problems you couldn't solve sitting in a boat all day. They still come home to hunt and fish with me. It was a little more challenging with my daughter, who figure skated competitively. I ended up sitting in an awful lot of cold ice rinks.

My wife's been an absolute jewel. I can't say enough nice things about my wife. That's true of every person I've met who's done the same sort of things that I have. We're all supported by unbelievable spouses.

If they have one fault, it's that they and the federal government are the only ones who can operate without a budget. But otherwise, they're spectacular people who tolerate us being late for dinner, traveling incessantly, and living out of suitcase. We keep four suitcases in the bedroom because I end up traveling so much, mainly to meetings. They get unpacked, but you pack 'em again because you'll be going again in two weeks.

So how long can you keep up a pace like this? Aren't you exhausted?

I've been practicing for 30 years in July. You can't just stay up all night. It's harder and harder to recover the next day. But there's going to come a time, it's probably going to come within the next two years, when I'm going to have to hang it up. There is no provision for part-time docs.

The question then, is how do you go from full speed to kind of dead in the water? That's going to be a difficult adjustment, because I still haven't been able to find anything that gives me the kind of charge I get out of delivering a baby or successfully completing an operation, or even seeing a patient I've seen in the clinic for three decades and delivered her children.

When you're not working, how do you relax?

I go to meetings. My wife says I'm a meetings junkie. I like to fish. We have a beautiful home on a nice lake, chock full of a whole lot of fish that need my attention. I have a number of boats that get neglected, and some day I'd like to spend some time with all those things.

What will you miss when you do slow down?

The voice on the phone at two in the morning from somebody who didn't identify herself, saying, "the condom broke," to the elderly patient who looked up as I was doing a pelvic exam and said, "Does your mom know what you do all day?"

What do you say to that?

Exactly! {Laughs} This kind of thing happens every week, if not every day. The patients have a wonderful sense of humor.

CHAPTER NINETEEN

QUARTER POUNDER WITH THIGHS

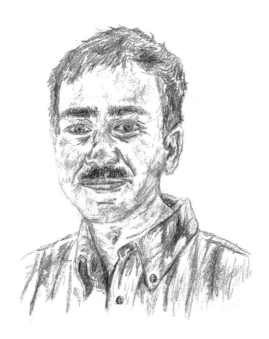

"We saved eight lives the first year for 50-cents a blood test."

Dennis Costakos, MD
Neonatologist, La Crosse

Dennis Costakos was ahead of his time, even in high school, when he discovered a superior treatment for eyelid cancer that would later become common practice.

"This paper proposed to use hot hafnium {Hf182}, which undergoes dual disintegration, emitting gammas as well as betas," wrote Costakos at age 16. The paper not only earned him a Physics Honorable Mention in the 1975 Borough Science Fair, but a letter of recommendation that helped get him into medical school.

Costakos became a neonatologist—a highly trained pediatrician who treats premature babies. He practices at Franciscan Skemp Healthcare, which is part of the Mayo Health System. Costakos is an assistant professor of pediatrcs at the Mayo Clinic College of Medicine. I met him for the first time in

2000 at a medical conference, oddly enough, while in a hotel swimming pool. After hearing about my work at the Wisconsin Medical Society, he expressed genuine interest in the organization and immediately pledged to join. Within a few weeks, he did just that–becoming the first and only physician I've ever inadvertently recruited while wearing a swimming suit!

If Dr. Costakos is anything, he's a joiner. To his core, he believes each of us has a responsibility to help make our communities better. Professionally, that means doctors with specialized knowledge have a duty to disseminate it to colleagues through membership in professional associations, so more patients may benefit. In his rapidly advancing specialty, this is critically important.

The doctor's own mother suffered the anguish of multiple miscarriages, though he only states this as a matter of fact and not as a reason for his becoming a physician who routinely saves infant lives.

I have no trouble finding the path to his home, as the e-mailed directions are precise. "Go 0.9 miles on..." My car begins an ascent on a winding dirt road in La Crosse, a charming city on the banks of the Mississippi River that borders Minnesota. As I approach his driveway, two boisterous dogs run out to greet me. I slow to a crawl, worried I might run over them. A smiling Dr. Costakos waves me up.

We begin the discussion in the living room, facing a large picture window which boasts a panoramic view of the hillside farm field across the road. A lone farmer is on his tractor in the distance, as sunshine streams into the room.

I can still remember my mother, Pauline Costakos, getting breast cancer. She decided to be treated at Cornell New York Hospital. They had state of the art stuff at Sloan Kettering and they were able to cure my mother, basically, with surgery. I was a young teenager. I was very impressed that they were able to treat her and save her life. The only thing that stuck in my mind, though, is the cure was surgery. In this case, a small-sized tumor. In the mid to late 1960s, that meant a lot of surgery on the body. Not surprisingly, they used words like "radical."

My mother would go on to get cancer in her other breast almost 20 years later. The second time around, my mother remarked how different the anesthesia was, how small the surgery was, how it had changed and progressed. But I became interested in healing people without resorting to radical procedures, without extensive removals of tissue.

I was working as a patient transporter at Albert Einstein Hospital while in high school. There was one particular eye cancer, that to cure the cancer, they just remove the person's eye—called malignant melanoma of the conjunctiva. It's just a little cancer of your eyelid, so I became interested in using physics or chemistry to try to treat the person with that surgery—the first paper I ever wrote.

I used an isotope, a radioactive chemical that nobody had thought of using. Hafnium 182 has a very long half life, so if a hospital purchased it, it's a one-time purchase for the hospital's existence. Basically, I had figured out that this isotope put out two different types of radiation, within a magnetic field. I could curve the one that I wanted to the patient's eye and let the other one go into the wall. I wrote all the physics equations.

I didn't have to treat any patients. Doctors had worked out the biology of the tumor and they already knew what radiation worked. But with the current radiation techniques in the '70s, they had to use surgery. I used an electric field to give the medical team the radiation they wanted, but not the radiation that would hurt the patient.

Of course, I put it in various science fairs, and I presented it to some of the physicians at Albert Einstein. I remember David Milstein, MD, the director of radiation or nuclear medicine reading it and saying, "No, this would not be something we would do." He said to me three or four years later, "I held your paper. That idea now is not so far fetched."

Well, maybe 6-8 years later, I went back to get a recommendation for medical school. He told me everything I had foreseen in that article went on to get done. To me, it just seemed so obvious, in the sense that I was really approaching the problem as somebody who was not a physician. I was 15 or 16 years old. My interest was chemistry and physics, but I wanted to be a physician. I put at the front of the journal that I wanted to be some kind of a medical scientist. I knew where I wanted to go and what I wanted to do.

In those days, the science folks in physics and chemistry, and the math and biology folks, really were in different circles. The groups basically did not really talk to each other. Everybody sort of went off in their own direction. I wanted to be a physician before I was ten. My grandmother Felicia said, "If he wants to be, don't discourage him. It's a good profession." After my mother's experience with cancer, even though for a little while I was moving more toward engineering or physics, that revitalized my interest in using physics and chemistry to heal people.

What was it like growing up in New York?

We lived in a brick house that would be 45 minutes from Time Square by car. While my existence was fairly sheltered—in the sense that I lived in this little suburb as I became a teenager and even through my life— Manhattan was never very far way.

My mother would go on to have five pregnancies with my dad, and three were miscarriages. My sister Olivia and I were the children in the family.

My father, Nicholas, had done some work as a dental technician, but ended up enlisting in the U.S. Air Force. Even though we lived in New York State, my father worked in Connecticut, which was not too far away.

In some ways, my background was atypical in the sense that even though we grew up not far from New York, our summers were spent either in New York State, which was much more rural, which later would become an advantage for me when I looked at practicing in Wisconsin. But I didn't feel like a fish out of water when I went to Dartmouth.

I felt just as comfortable in my medical school years, when I did some research and had to go to London {England} to help with a talk. I felt equally comfortable riding around in taxis or reading a city map.

How I got into the whole idea of becoming a physician was—like any other family—you have your legends. My father's brother was a medical person when he died at Pearl Harbor. He was a medic who was studying to be a physician, taking time out to serve his country.

I also had thought about a life more in public service. When I was a teenager, I did go to Washington, and was a volunteer page. I lived in Mt. Vernon, in a dorm. I got to meet Senator Edward Kennedy. The number of camera flashes when Senator Kennedy spoke was just absolutely blinding.

But I realized, as a page, that if you went to law school or business school, and went on the hill, you probably carried people's lunch before you got to do a lot. That was grunt work. There were going to be folks better than I, but most of them had an aversion to science. I thought, *Gee, the large majority are not going to go into the sciences, or medicine necessarily. Maybe that's where I should go, because I can do this.* I was about 17 at that point.

If I'm going to spend a lot of time studying, I might as well return something to society. What does society need? It needs political freedom. It needs public health. It needs individual health. Medicine seemed to have a lot of that.

I realized that once you became a physician, you can deal one-on-one with people's mental health as a psychiatrist. By the time I went to medical school, even with a degree in biochemistry from Columbia College, I thought I was going to be a psychiatrist; at the minimum, a neurologist.

I went to Dartmouth for medical school. Dartmouth was always sort of known as a place that had the biggest gym of the Ivy League and the smallest library. I remember {pauses}, there was a little bit of a nerd in us. I had a briefcase going to class, and I was very well prepared. I took a lot of math. I took linear algebra, differential equations—things that you really don't use as a physician all the time. But I took no computer courses, even though I do a lot of computing now. Some things, I thought, I can learn later, or they'll improve.

We had two half days per week of no classes, so that was always the time to go get your groceries or go work out. There was the every Thursday night party that one of my friends threw. I was almost constantly invited to dinners because I made sure that every two weeks, I had six or seven medical students over, where I barbecued or cooked. No matter how much studying we did, there was an awful lot of socializing.

Everybody {at Dartmouth} was very different. I remember meeting one woman whose father was a state senator from Alaska, and her experience of growing up was not something I knew much about. There was a fella whose parents were professors, who retired in Maine. I was one of only two or three New Yorkers in Dartmouth's class, and there were two other folks of Greek American extraction.

It's such an intense experience in medical school, it was very {pauses} different. There were Bostonians who came from long lines of going to Harvard, and they had a certain attitude. I remember them always talking to us about how we should join groups of physicians against any nuclear weapons.

And of course, just before I got to my clinical years, I was lucky that I got a summer fellowship to go to the National Institutes of Health, where I worked with a very good neuroscientist, Esa Korpi, an MD PhD from Finland. We wrote some papers together, but I worked in his lab. It was very physical and fairly long hours, and as we probed the brain using chemicals and drugs, mostly animal models, or samples from humans from brain surgery, or even autopsy. I came out still thinking I was still going to do psychiatry. I went into clinical psychiatry and I realized it wasn't for me. As I looked at the different rotations, the ones that I found myself enjoying most, were obstetrics, because they were generally a happy group.

Psychiatry, it seemed, people had weeks to figure things out. It was too slow for me. I thought if I'm going to do anything, I'm going to do obstetrics. Then pediatrics was the best of all the worlds, especially neonatology. Neonatology was basically a surgical sub-specialty of pediatrics.

On the other hand, there was the side that you had to talk with parents. You almost were working as a psychiatrist would work. Part of the day, you might have been a surgeon or an anesthesiologist. You got to go to the deliveries, so you had the obstetrical excitement of it. There were happy stories. In addition, there were some babies, because they weighed one, two, three, or four pounds, I might have to counsel those parents for months, so I thought, This is for me.

I did my first rotation in neonatology at one of Brown University's Hospitals. Then, as a fourth year rotation, I went to Yale. I was able to finish my entire medical degree in three years, and that gave me a year to practice medicine and do other things.

I did a rotation in southern California, in obstetrics, so I could see my grandmother. I also got to do a rotation in very inner city New York, and Dartmouth had wonderful rotations in rural New Hampshire, as well as big academic medical centers in New England, which we did. By the time

I got out of medical school, I wanted to practice in a quieter community. It's even more important to do a residency and a fellowship in a rural community.

One of the things that attracted me to medicine was that there are days—most days—when we're sort of unsung heroes. We go in and do a lot of things for the baby. The mother's still drowsy from the anesthetic. Nobody really knows what went on, but you made that baby better and they're going to stay a couple of days in the hospital and then they go home.

On the other hand, one of the other things I enjoy about medicine is when we figure out that something like folic acid can decrease birth defects, then it becomes like we're almost like public health folks. When we go out, it's not just to tell our own patients, but to try to be clever and get the word out further. We can say breast feeding is important, and folic acid, you should be taking it, even if you're sexually active and you're not even thinking you want to be pregnant. You have to take this, because if anything happens, you could be left with a child who's gonna be in a wheel chair versus totally healthy.

Medicine does afford you those two different hats, where you can have the satisfaction of curing a rash, or somebody's dehydrated and you re-hydrate them. It can be done in hours or it can be done in days, depending on what's going on.

Sometimes we do things that are not as satisfying. It can be hard at the bedside. There are children who die. There are children who survive, but are not perfect. There are times we make a diagnosis and part of the diagnosis is that the child will be mentally retarded.

On the other hand, there are instances when we take a spot of blood from folks because we pick up patterns in the blood, we can give them a vitamin and they're normal. If they don't get the vitamin, they're not normal.

I felt pretty good in the early '90s that Jon Wolff * and I pushed for Wisconsin to check every child for biotinidase.† At the time, that was very radical. We were one of 19 states that started doing it. Now, I think everybody does it. It was because I had gotten a patient from another state transferred, where I figured it out. And I said, "This has got to be happening to Wisconsin kids, too." And after a long struggle, including with legislators in Madison, we got it put on the state screen. We found one or two kids the first year, and then we were able to treat family members. We saved eight lives the first year for 50-cents a blood test.

You always keep in mind that science and medicine builds on itself. In this case, the biotinidase discovery was made in the early 40s, but nobody

---

* University of Wisconsin pediatrician and researcher

† Enzyme that prevents seizures, developmental delay, eczema, and hearing loss.

thought it was worth anything. They just put it on the shelf. It was sort of a forgotten idea.

Then in the '80s, somebody said this enzyme that they knew from cattle, does it have a human purpose? Once they found it in humans, they were able to correlate it with an infant disease. Once they found it was a disease that kills, they were able to develop a screening test.

But one state had the screening test—Virginia—because of one doctor's long struggle. What I helped to do was to take that lesson in Virginia and say, "Wisconsin needs to get on this. We're not going to wait until we're the 49th state to get it." If you have a patient for whom an idea that you found works, don't you almost have almost a moral obligation to get it published, or get it out at a medical meeting?

It seemed that when I was back East, if I wanted to get involved in the medical society or church or anything, it was almost exclusionary. There were more people who wanted to do it than they wanted to let do it. It just seemed like the same people did it. If they needed anyone, they would get someone else they knew.

When I came to Wisconsin, it was almost totally the opposite. There wasn't any remuneration for doing it. You did it because you liked it. But you could do as much as you wanted. You could be a member one year and ten years later, you were the president or on the board. It was unbelievable.

When I say exclusionary, I mean even the medical societies were exclusionary when I was back East. They wanted to keep it a small nucleus of people. Maybe you didn't even know they existed. Nobody talked about them—just the people who went. You heard about them later.

"You went to what? You went where? Did what? That sounds great. What did it cost?"

"Fifteen dollars to join."

"Why isn't everybody a member?"

"I don't know."

"How often do they do it?"

"I don't know."

"How do I join?"

"You call so and so."

"Yeah, we can't let you in unless we speak to your boss. Speak to your boss. Speak to your boss."

"Na, I don't want you to join that. I already got somebody in that."

That's how it was. You come to Wisconsin and it's not like that at all. Even at the level of non-medical stuff, helping out with volunteer stuff at the Heritage Night in La Crosse, or Octoberfest, or with church. If you want to help, they'll find a role for you. I did not find that at all in New York or New England, or in the years I lived in Virginia, when I was at NIH—totally the opposite.

It gets back to prevention is worth a pound of cure. You have to keep in mind what you're building, that some of the things you do will help people in 20 or 30 years. Usually, you do that in a work setting and you probably even get paid for it.

A lot of research comes out of Wisconsin. There are things that are used all over the world. Whenever we've had a great idea in Wisconsin, or we'd want to move along our state, I was always told, never say what Minnesota's doing. That's the best way for it not to get done. Sometimes you find with state bureaucracies, it's not to your advantage to quote a neighboring state. But if you do a comparison to somewhere halfway across the country, that's okay. That's a legitimate comparison.

Tell me what your training after med school was like.

When I went to this hospital in New York, everybody was going into pediatrics. If I was up at seven, in the emergency room, and home at nine {p.m.}, and I did that four, five nights in a row, I finally was going to have a day and a half off before I started my neonatology rotation. That would be 24 hour, 30 hour, days. I was young, and I was single, and I was living in Manhattan.

When I was a resident, we were on call every third night, so you'd be in the hospital 24 hours, 30 hours, and then you'd be exhausted. You'd eat; do a little bit of studying, maybe. I had no TV. I didn't need a TV. I felt it was probably better to jog or walk or go to the library.

The next day, you'd be back in the hospital in the morning and you would work until, if you're lucky, five or seven o'clock. Between then and bedtime, because you were on call the next day, you could do something. You were always on call one Friday, one Saturday, one Sunday. You had one weekend a month off.

The way it worked is, day one you would come in at eight, let's say, and you were on call eight to eight. The next day started, and you were still working, so 8 a.m. to 8 p.m.

The new day started; you're not going. The others are coming, but you're still there. If you were really lucky, you were out that night between five to seven o'clock. You've been there since 8 a.m. that previous morning and you were busy treating cancer patients, neonates that couldn't breathe…you were busy.

And then that night, you could do what you wanted now. But after 36 hours, if you didn't get any sleep at all, you probably had to go to sleep. If you had even two or three hours of sleep—and remember, you're in your young 20s, you would probably change and go out. Then, you had the whole New York City nightlife—anything you wanted—ahead of you. The next night, though, you had to be in bed by midnight or 11. You'll be tired because the next morning, you'd be back in the hospital by eight.

Did you ever feel that level of fatigue was affecting your judgment or decision making skills?

When I was on call in Manhattan, you would do one night as a fellow, and you would be so exhausted. They wouldn't ask you to do another night on call for six or seven nights. Here, I found I had fewer patients and more to do, more to do on each patient. The challenge became doing more nights in a row.

If you get zero sleep, it really blows the next day totally to do anything. I learned that, in New York. If you had one or two hours sleep, you could easily be fresh, lifting weights that day, or driving. You could do about anything with two hours of sleep.

Zero sleep, you were finished by the time 8 a.m. came. With zero sleep, you couldn't leave at 8. You had to work until 5. Well, now you're up 36 hours in a row. You didn't even want to eat at that point. You wanted to just sleep.

But working that level of hours, can you say in good faith that you gave your patients everything they needed? You could think? You could make decisions?

No, you're not as awake or clear. But I'll tell you this. One thing I've learned about myself, because of the way I've been trained and just through practice, if I've been up 30 hours in a row, multiple times over four or five weeks, I'm very tired.

Only a year ago, I was doing two, three weeks in a row on call, and sometimes a whole week up at night. I sometimes will tell my wife, "I'm not safe to drive, but I could resuscitate a patient because it's rote." It's so built in, so automatic. Your hands are doing it, and you're dictating, and you know the drug dosages, and it's just done because of the training I've had.

With a practice that's growing, I'm basically on call 15 days a month. Do you want a situation where the people in training never do more than a 14-hour day and the minute they graduate you ask them to do a week {of 14-hour days} in a row?

When you, say the first time, place an intravenous or help somebody into a wheel chair, the first time you learned to do something, you've learned to do it. But you're going to be doing it hundreds of times and you're not learning any more. But you're beginning to pay back, and that's why federal and state government will always subsidize medical school education.

By the time you become an intern and a resident, you're not going to get paid anywhere near what an attending physician makes. The word resident comes from reside. You reside in the hospital. It was only 50 years ago people used to say they worked six days a week in hospital greens and whites, and on the Sunday, they walked outside with family for a bit. They did this every week for five or six years and became neurosurgeons.

When I was a resident, we were expected to give our all for our patients, and we would have a list that we would have to get done. We had to check certain blood cultures or draw certain bloods, and get patients examined, and make sure they get their chemotherapy. Then, because we were in a program, we would be expected to take a patient and present them, tell something new about the science or the treatment of the disease.

You could socialize all you wanted at that wonderful Irish bar, but at the end of the day, you better not drink too much because you had a lot of reading to do and a lot of work to do. If you met someone that you really liked—I met my future wife, Anne Meredith, in Manhattan—you could go on a date and stuff, but still had to squeeze this all in somewhere along the way. It did get done. But I think that you quickly realized by the time you were a resident, you're in a teaching program and you're learning.

When you go to college, all the work you do is for you. The more I put in the more I get out of it. When you go to medical school, it's a little bit the same thing. You're paying tuition to be there for the first two years. The more you open the book or listen to the professor or read, or watch the DVD or CD, that's for you.

By the time you get to the second year of medical school, things are now changing. You're already entering the wards, so that you might spend a few hours each day, if not all of it, beginning to do things now. You're paying to be there and you're learning by doing it. But it's not for you.

After my residency, I wanted to do a fellowship. You're sort of a super resident in terms of techniques. But now you're the fellow, and you're going to start producing some research. I did and it got published.

The patient was a young teenager whose temperature went very low. All the textbooks causes for temperature going low were not there, except there were three other papers that a certain disease could do it. Everybody's patient had different characteristics. Everybody speculated why the temperature went low. I had a fourth case with the same disease, but speculated a different reason.

I would later learn that there were a lot of these patients. When I became a fellow, I went to Cornell and I remember telling somebody about the patient and he said, "We see 50 patients a week with that."

I asked, "Why don't you publish it?"

I guess he said because it was so common. Then I realized, he had the biggest practice in New York and everybody with that disease came to him. He never bothered to tell the rest of the world. I told him about the patient I saw as a resident. He said, send it to such and such journal, which had offices in Toronto, and they ended up publishing it.

I was going to become a fellow now. I was really a New Yorker now. Now, I was leaving the gentle world of pediatrics with New Yorkers and was a fellow. If you will, it was more funneled and bottlenecked.

I was in a fellowship program where everybody trained as a pediatrician, but they're not going to do pediatrics. They're going to do high-powered intensive care, and they were coming from not only all over the country, but from all over the world. I realized, as I was with these folks, that there were a few native Americans there—native, being New Yorkers, in this case.

I would meet a woman who was just, very confident and an excellent physician. She was from Brazil. Spoke beautiful English. She was pretty much all business. She was our senior fellow. There wasn't a single thing this woman couldn't figure out or couldn't do. But basically, after she helped you, she was like a wisp of smoke, gone.

There was another woman, Isabelle Dieudonne, MD, from Belgium, who spoke beautiful French. She showed up, as our senior fellow, dressed to kill. I could never understand how she could get her hands into surgeries, in intensive care and want to come in dressed in designer clothes all the time.

One day, there was a baby that had a history of surgery. I was just going to be covering for the night. Literally, for 12 hours, I would be covering as a fellow, this is phenomenal to me—90 intensive care patients. The only reason we could get it done, I had never seen a computer system like that before in a hospital. Even 25 years later, I am still awed that this one hospital had a set up that made it so efficient. The rest of the world is catching on to that. They were way ahead of their time, largely the work and vision of William Frayer, MD. I was there for about two years, and I remember their attitude was, make believe that wherever you go, you will be the only one doing it.

Sure enough, my first job, in La Crosse, I was the only neonatologist. That training was very good because when I was at New York Hospital with 90 patients, no matter how difficult a patient was, if you called the senior physician once every six months that was probably fine on a night call. If you called more than once, like in a month, you'd be told, "You're really not doing your job if you're calling me." Even though you'd be doing the 90 patients and they were all critically ill, and you had some nurses to help you and a few interns, basically, they expected you to figure it out.

There were a couple of physicians who were able to function as neonatologists, so if I did three weeks of on call, every once in a while, I could have some help from one of them. I had worked almost 40 days in a row on call here. My patients were having good outcomes. The hospital only had one physician to pay, whether you work here or in Manhattan, where there are 90 patients, and 15 doctors.

If you were to look at most practices, with the exception of some academic medical fields, the residents are not doing such long hours. Do you want a system where all the training has never let anybody work more than 14 hours? Because the way the health system is set up, I don't think there's a practice in the world—unless it is a totally clinic job—that you are not going to be on call and work long hours. So how do you train for that?

Two things are vivid: When I was at Dartmouth, my first rotation was internal medicine. I remember our first night on call. First of all, this is how the medical system works, just to show you how disorganized it is in ways.

Every time I ever started a job in medicine, they never tell you whether you're on call or not the day before. If you've ever started a new job or anything, you're a little nervous the night before. You don't sleep well.

Every time I've ever started a new service, I had no idea whether I was on call the first night or not. I learned the morning I got there. You don't know what to pack. You don't know what to tell friends or relatives. You don't know anything. The large majority, I was on call the first day I got there.

The first day in medical school, I learned I was on call that day. I was one of these kids who liked to stay up late and still was able to get up for school. I was on call and it was about four, five in the morning and I was starting to get tired now. We had been up all day. We had just put our last patient to bed and I remember our chief resident said we are not going to go to bed until we look at the microscope pictures of the people's sputum, deep lung secretions, under the microscope. We're going to gram stain it, like they would have done a hundred years ago. By the time we got done doing that, and it wasn't anything that great to see, it was 6 a.m. Rounds started at 7. The chief resident said, "Okay, let's all meet at 7." He literally, took two steps in the door and was going to go to sleep for an hour, and the two of us, myself and the other medical student...the interns' little bed was down the hall.

I said, "Where do we sleep?" We didn't even know, so we called the operator. "You've got to go to the medical student call rooms."

I said, "Where are they?"

"They're on the other side of campus."

We got to the other side of the campus at 6:25. Then, we realized we had to get back. When we got to the room, there was no phone and no alarm clock, and we realized if we fall asleep for one second, we'll never get up.

When we got back at seven, the new day started. The chief resident signed out. He was gone by 8. The intern said he was going to try not to do admissions that day because he wanted to be out by three. We, the medical students, had duties with people until 3 o'clock, so I did my first spinal tap that day at 3 o'clock, after being up all night.

They selected a patient for me. I remember the poor woman was in a coma. She had spiked a fever and they had to know whether it was meningitis or not. I did her spinal tap. That was my first rotation in medical school.

Weren't there moments when you said to yourself, what have I got myself into here?

I definitely said it my first night because I had never stayed up like that. I began to train myself to stay up all night and still function when I did my obstetrics rotation. I did that rotation in California, so I was assisting with 40 deliveries a day. I would help, obviously, more than one obstetrician. It would be from eight to eight, and California was much more progressive. They said, "You're going to work eight to eight, and by nine you're home in bed. We'll see you the next day."

Three months into my internship, I had made rounds and I was just doing the routine work by myself. I went in to see a baby who had bad pneumonia, who also had heart disease. The nurse came out and said, "He stopped breathing." I did CPR. In those days, the mouth to mouth on this baby, with chest compressions, and I did bring him back. It was the most amazing feeling. He had died, and I brought him back. That was the first time I had ever seen a patient die in front of me, and I was the only doctor there.

I can still remember the first patient I ever saw dying of cancer. {Pauses} could remember how brave those children were in my training. You also never forget patients you see who you thought a little bit of intervention or prevention would have saved them.

Once in a while I would encounter a patient where a person who could have saved their life easily, couldn't get there any quicker than they did. It might have been a situation where one of the physicians became ill, and so they immediately called for emergency backup, but the backup was an hour away.

This one doctor drove an hour with traffic and probably got there about two minutes too late. It reinforced for me that—and we've done it in our own system—it's great to have the doctors who know how to do every single thing, but the nurses have to know, also.

You have to have people who are always available who know what to do in the first five, ten, fifteen, twenty minutes, an hour. We've certainly strived in our system for that, and it's worked very well. We just made sure to say, "Okay, everybody's got to know this portion of it. And you keep doing it until you know it. If you can't figure it out, you're probably in the wrong place." Most people have risen to the challenge and have been able to do it.

Sometimes, situations don't happen well. Even though I didn't personally give {pauses}... A baby was born without intestines or intestinal coverings, and was in shock. I gave plenty of fluid to the baby. But the insensible loss[‡] was very high. When I brought the baby back in by ambu-

---

‡ Insensible loss refers to non kidney water losses, such as through the skin or breathing.

lance, even though I put a central line in the baby out in the field, the baby needed additional fluid. I remember this one physician saying, "Let's give a rapid amount of salt water to the baby now," and wrote the order correctly, but unfortunately, picked up the wrong vial and it was a high concentrated salt.

Now, they had only a 50% chance of living from their condition. But one never knew then, when the baby died a day later from seizures, what was what. That definitely had influenced me. You learn from repetition. The best thing that we can do is work as safely as possible, standardize, build in redundancies, so that there becomes reliability. If it's important that X gets done, and something doesn't happen by a month, then Y gets done, you need more than one person to remember Y.

Also, if I can pick up the wrong solution, as in this case this physician did, then it's best that that solution not be available. Let it be in a locked box off the floor. Let somebody need to go get it. We've done that now. Basically, our hospital, we've moved on to say, that if this should never be given by accident, let's just not have it available. Medical errors are something that, humans being humans, we will make.

Some days you have to be a counselor, other days it's more hands-on and you're sewing somebody up or cleaning a wound, or you're taping something in. But there are other days where you have to think more like an engineer. How do I make this process reliable? Everything's so expensive in medicine. Can I really afford to let five different people do it five different ways? Is there one superior way? Should I talk the doctors into one superior way, if I think I've got it? Should I drop the way I've done it for 20 years, if that way's better?

I do think we try to have a clean competition, almost like the Olympics. Stand in line. Strip off your clothes and your egos. Leave your weapons at the door. When we sit down at the table to improve health care, we're all physicians. We get together and talk as physicians and, in some cases, for the best collaborations we bring nurses to the table, social workers, hospital administrators, and the other folks. If you don't sit them at the table, you're not going to get it done right.

All of us, including medicine, have to not only think about efficiency and learning to do things in new ways, but to use old ways and continue to improve them and conserve things. One of the most exciting things is the idea that for flu shots, maybe you can give a smaller dose and get the same benefit. That's one of the great strengths of the American medical system.

Is America leading the way, in terms of innovation, in saving premature babies?

When I was a medical student at Dartmouth, somebody said that the fellow who was coming on rounds with us is the preeminent Italian pediatric surgeon. He said, "I've heard Americans can save babies under two pounds, two ounces in a reliable way, and I want to see it done and take it back to Italy."

That was very, very inflating, but at that point in America, it was very difficult to take care of babies. Below 26 weeks it was almost impossible. And 26-28 weeks, they had a lot of disabilities. So that's where we were in 1980. We had not had a single death at Franciscan Skemp of any baby that was 22, 23 weeks and above, between 1996 and 2003.

By 1991, I remember leaving New York, and I had never seen a 24-week baby live without major disabilities. Most of the time, it seemed like we could save the babies with reasonable outcomes at 25 weeks and above.

By the time I got to La Crosse, four or five months later, with the introduction of surfactant,[§] within the year, we were reliably saving babies at 24 weeks, and 23-week babies, a third to a half of them with big disabilities. By the year 2000, we were not only saving these babies, but they were out of the hospital much quicker with much less disability. And it's even improved further by 2004.

What's going on? What's changed?

We see less neural tube defects because of folic acid. I think the biggest advance in obstetrics was antenatal steroids.[¶] The idea that a woman who's in labor can't be stopped is not a new one. We've had tocolytic agents {drugs} to try to slow labor for 25-30 years. They will slow labor a few days, but they don't stop pre-term labor. What's fantastic are the antenatal steroids, which decrease morbidity and mortality in the baby, without adversely affecting the mother in any major way.

The biggest advance that has affected neonatology is definitely being able to put surfactant in a bottle. This is the missing ingredient. It took 50 years to actually get it in a bottle. By itself, I don't think would be enough. It's the combination.

The second major thing, of course, is the growth of information systems and the Internet. I used to have a beeper and no cell phone. So if I got beeped, I had to drive around with my car if I was on my way home, and find a phone to call from. With the Internet, the time for an idea to get into practice has been shortened by at least a year or two because of all the efficiencies the computer can help you do.

Of the biggest advances that I know coming is injecting women with a very cheap steroid during their pregnancy. That reduces prematurity by 30%. Many of these women don't even have premature babies, and the ones that do, the babies are a lot less premature. What baffles American physicians is that women don't seem to be short of this steroid, so why should it work?

§ Substance that helps premature infants breathe.

¶ Given to the mother before birth to help the child's lungs mature and to prevent respiratory problems.

Timing of the delivery is affected by progesterone/estrogen and corticotropin-releasing factor {CRF}. Animal models are showing that if sheep are put on a diet, and then get pregnant, they have premature babies, and then their progesterone/estrogen levels are thrown off. This is going to be one of the biggest things for perinatal medicine.

When I started training in this field, nine out of 100 babies were born premature. By the time I went to residency it was 10. By the time I came to La Crosse, it was 11. And this year, it hit over 12. So, American society continues to have more and more premature babies. You can be in a hospital where the number of births is decreasing every year, fewer births and the number of premature babies is staying the same.

Why?

Well, part of it is that American lifestyle. Maybe part of it could be diet. There is a lot of activity about the importance of getting the right oils in your diet, fish oils or omega-3 oils in your diet. What determines how many premature babies there are and what are premature babies like when they come out? We realize now it's how well we take care of that whole family and that patient for all of their life. And that includes, if you're having constantly a diet on the run, you're not getting enough exercise.

If you think about children with their Gameboys and Internet, and their TV and their beautiful homes, why go outside and play? And, are we going to run and jump? Are we going to dance? Are we going to run with the dog? These things affect whether you have a premature baby.

Also, we know that if a woman is pregnant, she should not be on her feet for more than 10 hours. If she's on her feet for more than 10 hours—there are longitudinal studies of nurses who got pregnant—and if you go and look at who delivers prematurely, it's the nurse who does two shifts.

So much of this is preventable?

A lot of this is preventable. It is partly our genes, but environment also interplays. For every hour in front of the TV, I can guarantee you the child's cholesterol will be higher, and I can guarantee you they will be heavier.

To give you a feeling of the cost, understanding that any costs I can give a feel for in La Crosse are going to be much less than other parts of the country. For example, we already know for the same disease when they're treated in the upper Midwest, it's double the price at Duke. It's triple the price of the Midwest Mayo area in Boston. It's six times in New York.

Part of it has to do with the fact that the people taking care of you cost more to employ and support with living wages. It depends on how much it costs of them to feed themselves and park their car. I've never paid for parking at Franciscan Skemp. When I was at New York Hospital {late 1980s}, they said that as a staff person, if I wanted to park for 12 hours, that's a thousand a month. If I wanted to leave the car overnight, it was two thousand. Nurses are in the same boat as the cleaning person. If they don't take public transportation, they have a car. It's going to cost to park, right?

To give you some idea, I have a patient who is tiny, born in a small town, within an hour of here, who has had a clinical course that is very straightforward for a baby that weighs less than two pounds. Not including the physician billing, the hospital bill alone, a third of the hospital stay is already way over a $100,000. By the time the baby leaves, I'm sure the bill will be a quarter million, not including neonatology billing, only because that's submitted late, so I don't know what that's going to be. That same baby, if they were in New York, that bill would be closer to eight or nine hundred thousand dollars.

What's the prognosis for such a baby?

This person will probably be fairly productive. I'd say the chances of any major disabilities will probably be less than 3%. This child could go on to live 70 or 80 years. Then, if you take $250,000 and divide it by 80, it's about two and a half thousand a year. And if that person goes on to become a chef or a physician or anything, they'll earn back two and a half thousand dollars in tax money for society pretty easily with the way the dollar deflates.

A child that I saw in the same time period as the child I just told you about, was treated for a disease where the baby would die, but was home within seven days. That hospital bill will be less than 25,000.

On the other hand, in the same time period that these children were born, a normal vaginal birth costs less than two or three thousand. Even if there's a week of severe disease—a disease that would kill you—if we can fix it without complications in a week, it's 10 times the cost.

Once you start talking babies under two pounds, you're already at one 100 times the cost. All the technologies we've developed to save premature babies and make them better are fantastic! And the rest of the world adopts them pretty quickly.

A lot of the best minds in the Netherlands trained in the U.S. in neonatology. But they will not try to save any babies below 25 weeks. I'm routinely saving babies with good outcomes below 25 weeks in La Crosse. But in the Netherlands, if you're born even one day below 25 weeks, there's no care given. You're allowed to die. What they say is, We think we can get a reasonably reliable outcome at 25 weeks and above. But everything below that is not reliable, therefore we will not do it. Therefore, we will not advance, but we will wait until the U.S. perfects it, and then we'll put it in if it makes sense.

I've looked at babies for given weights and gestations from different parts of the country and compared them to La Crosse. A lot of times I've seen the La Crosse patients do a little better, if not a lot better. Part of it gets down to, how well do we treat our neighbors?

For example, I can go out in La Crosse and there are beautiful parks and places to play, and the air is fairly clean. Is that true everywhere in America? There are parts of California, I'm told, that if you grow up in one section, there are beautiful parks and places to go. And if you grow up in another section, it's not available. I can tell you who's going to have more premature babies, babies that are going to have worse outcomes.

But I think that what it gets down to is that every home in America really has to know, are there enough fresh fruits on the table? What oil are you using to cook your food? Do you really have to work two shifts when you're pregnant? Do you smoke tobacco, chew tobacco? Did you understand why drugs, certain drugs are illicit, and society has banned them? That is crucial.

In addition to television, and its effective cause of a sedentary state, we have to watch what food is marketed to kids. The amount of money that advertisers spend selling cereal with a lot of sugar, and other bad foods, is way beyond any expenses paid in the United States for health care. Is it wise? It's probably not. We need a government that helps business thrive and we also need a government that protects the rights of workers, that pushes prevention. Without government, if you leave it all to the private sector, there will be too much short-range thinking, the environment suffers, the emphasis is the bottom line in the next six months.

The way {many health insurance} contracts work, they don't want to test the hearing of baby X if their rival HMO does not. Well, that's short sighted. That's where physicians can get together and say, Look, we believe that parents have to have car seats when they move their kids, and let's remove the obstacles to car seats.

Let's make it that we want all children's hearing checked before they leave the hospital. We don't care what HMO they're in. We don't care who the payer is. It needs to be checked. We feel certain illnesses should be screened in the newborn period. We're going to pick illnesses that, if their caught early, we have a cure for.

Let's not just screen for things if we have bad news for the parents. If I were to tell you your child had X at day four of life, and by the way, if I can't do anything about it, I just ruined your life and theirs. Maybe I should just let them get sick at age 40 or 30 and they lived their life with whatever dreams they've had.

Finally, if you see a pregnant woman on a subway or public transportation, do you get up from your seat for her? When you buy your beautiful house with all the things in it, do you worry about your neighbor two miles away who doesn't have access to a park, in some cities? There is less income disparity in the upper Midwest. There is more neighbor caring about neighbor in Wisconsin, which is probably part of the reason I stayed in Wisconsin.

Describe what it's like when it goes well and you can save these preemies.

One father, he and his wife actually made a mural of their child's progress. That child was born at 24 weeks, probably around 800 grams {1.76 pounds}. Their child did well. The mom was in her 40s, and had lost every other pregnancy. We saved this little girl for them, and basically, that girl also needed heart surgery. That woman went on to have a second full term healthy child. I can't tell you how excited that family is. Imagine being 39 or 40 and you've lost seven pregnancies and at 44, you have two normal children.

I remember one grandmother who brought me a little hand-carved rocking horse when my daughter Chloe was born, because I had saved their little granddaughter at about two pounds.

I can get phone calls where I can help people because we've done some studies or helped people and not expect a single penny to flow to myself or our system and still feel good about that.

There's the public health, there's the individual counseling, there's the hands-on where it is the nitty gritty, draw their blood, intubate them, sew their surgical catheters in, do their spinal tap, control their pain, give them morphine or whatever is needed, control their seizure disorder, whatever the case may be. But the other part of it is the counseling and the public health dimension.

We've got pretty good perinatal statistical data. I've been here 16 years and we admit 100 to 140 patients to the N-I-C-U.** I've treated several thousand patients, here in La Crosse. One day it kind of dawned on me that a good 40% of them would not be alive in the early '60s. Just coming here, I remember being told that at a certain week of age, the babies were just allowed to {die}—didn't even necessarily get a neonatology consult.

The minute I rode into town, I moved that line back several weeks. I have one patient where he was a little baby this big {gestures as if holding a small loaf of bread} and he had a bump on his spine. A few weeks later when the baby was bigger, we had surgery done at our hospital and removed a tumor that was half the size of the baby. That child is now a healthy teenager.

We have a formal follow-up clinic. I can follow up easily for two or three years. We also have the neonatal follow-up where patients that were born even before I came to La Crosse are treated.

You've met some of your neonates?

Oh, yes. The gathering occurs yearly. Anybody who's graduated the neonatal unit is invited, and we keep good records of all the graduates.

** Neonatal Intensive Care Unit

It takes one year to plan it. The hospital is really good about providing the hot dogs and savings bonds for the kids. And I get to see some families I took care of. Some families, I took care of two or three of their premature babies.

It's also good to see how kids cope with disabilities when they have them. I have one little girl I see at the picnic who was born with a brain disorder and an open spine lesion and automatic paralysis at birth, at a time when we didn't know that more folic acid prevents it.

It is amazing to see how children and their families deal with disabilities. The most impressive thing that I've seen in Wisconsin is that if a family had a disabled child, the child we knew from the get-go would not be normal, almost universally here, everybody takes the child home. I can remember only once or twice that didn't happen.

I found in a lot of other places, they institutionalized the child right away. I was told very early by the parents, if the child's going to be mentally retarded or disabled, we're not taking the child home—early in the game, sometimes even before we knew how the child was going to do.

While I was on the East Coast, very often if some of the families would be so affluent, so intelligent, everything perfect, they couldn't accept any imperfection. We were told those children were adopted. That was routine.

In this area, I haven't seen a lot of what we call boarder babies—babies who were born to mothers that were not going to take care of them. I haven't seen babies born with nowhere to go, and they're fine anyway.

Or, I see babies incredibly disabled and the parents say we're going to try to take him home and do our best. Some die fairly quickly. Some seem to do quite well for a long time. I'm amazed, whether the parents are young or old, rich or poor, married or not, even alternative families—how they take these children home and do fine with them.

The other thing that's amazed me is that there've been actually lawsuits about wrongful life—a premature baby is saved by neonatologist and the parents sue that they should have been allowed to die. That has not come up in La Crosse.

"Do you want everything done, understanding that in the best hands, 50% of the time the child may not make it?"

Everyone in La Crosse says, "Please, do everything."

CHAPTER TWENTY

DON'T SHOW ME THE MONEY

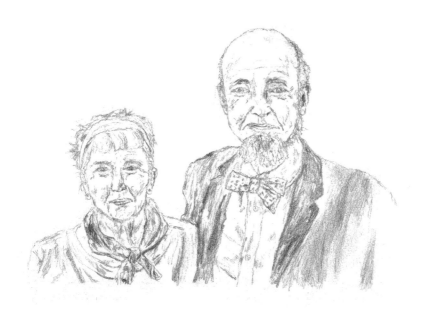

"I don't want to work for five dollars an hour. But I have no choice."

John Frantz, MD
Internist, Monroe

Mary Frantz, MD
Internist, Monroe

It's amazing what kind of talent can be had for minimum wage. John and Mary Frantz have more than a century of medical expertise between them, and they're both still practicing, for about five bucks an hour.

They fell in love with medicine and each other a long time ago, and they must be pretty fond of the Badger State, too, because they've lived and practiced in rural, southern Wisconsin for most of their lives.

Although both are in their 80s, the word "retirement" isn't in their vocabulary. "By the time you've been a doctor for 50 years, you wouldn't know who you were if you didn't do a little of it," says John. Neither ever imagined practicing medicine for minimum wage.

~~~~~~~~~~~~~~~~~~

John: When we got old enough, we were compelled to take our retirement income or pay a 50% penalty on what we should have taken. We decided that we might as well work for fringe benefits only.

So you're not getting paid?

John: The insurance carrier complained that we were fraudulently getting insurance because we weren't on the payroll, and the solution was to pay us minimum wage.

Mary: I kicked and screamed about that. I don't mind working for nothing, but I don't want to work for five dollars an hour. But I have no choice. We want our health insurance benefits.

You have to be the only two doctors in America working for minimum wage.

John: Well, there are a lot of doctors working for nothing. There are many volunteers after retirement.

You're not doing it for the money.

Mary: No. Having been depression-raised kids and being by instinct, prudent, if not miserly, we have no shortage of financial resources to manage our retirement.

Mary, tell me a little about where you grew up.

I grew up on Long Island, near New York City. My father worked in the city. He was a publisher. My parents were both college educated. I grew up in a family that valued learning. I had an older brother and a younger brother. I went to an excellent public school system that was very progressive in the '30s.

I went to Antioch College in Ohio. My father was very much in favor of that. It wasn't until the end of my college career that I decided to go to medical school. Before that, I was thinking more of going into science, as a research chemist. I actually had rather a prolonged time in medical school because of getting married and my teaching being interrupted.

It was during the war, and 85% of the places in medical school were taken by men from the armed forces. But then, by the time I finished, I was in a class with about 15-20% women.

John, where did you grow up?

I grew up in Indianapolis, and I went to high school there. I went to Haverford College, in a suburb of Philadelphia, it's probably the most Quaker of the Quaker schools. The Quakers are very good role models because they witness more their actions than their words.

I have three older sisters. My father was a clergyman in the Presbyterian Church from 1926 till his retirement in the '60s.

How did your parents react to your interest in medicine?

The next best thing to being a preacher, because they're service professions.

Where did you go to medical school?

Rochester {New York} was a very good choice because they kind of showed the way about how to organize a medical school without promulgating grades. If you wanted to know your grades, you'd have to transfer to another school and sneak a look at the transcript in the Dean's office. They didn't want us to be competitive. We were all fellow scholars helping each other learn. Twice during the pre-clinical years, they cancelled the final exam at the last minute with an announcement that we all mastered the material, so what's the use of going through the charade?

Really? Never heard of that.

Well, nobody has, except people who know about Rochester.

How did you two meet?

Mary: My first year and a half in Rochester, I couldn't get into the {medical} school and so I worked in a research lab in physiology. I worked in a high altitude lab with a noted physician physiologist, and John was one of the guinea pigs we would put in this high altitude chamber and monitor him. I was the technician who monitored him.

We often joked that he had so much brain power to start with because otherwise in those days, they might not have been as careful about monitoring how low the oxygen got. But he came out okay. We found out we enjoyed the same things and went on some bike trips together and some concerts.

John: The physiology department was quite congenial. One of my main assignments was trying to figure out how aircrew on a B-29, say, could stay conscious if the oxygen system was shot up. There was myself and one of the other students who managed to stay conscious at 25,000 feet for 30 minutes on acute exposure. I've always felt as though if you didn't pass out, you could hardly have killed many brain cells. I wasn't as worried as she was.

Mary: I wasn't all that worried at the time, either. In retrospect though, we should have been worried. I was only one and a half years into medical school when we got married.

Tell me a little about medical school.

Mary: I dropped out for two years and had a couple of children and went to the University of Colorado. Oh, I loved going to school. The work load wasn't as alarming as medical students find it today. We worked hard, but we enjoyed our work and maybe it was partly that Rochester ethos that you were all enjoying your work. You don't have to beat out on anybody else. When I went back to Colorado, it was a little overwhelming with two children, but John did a great deal of child care in the evenings and we had good child care.

John: We went together through the West to look for a place for her to be a student and for me to be a resident in training. And we ended up at Colorado because the head of the medical department was also the chairman of the admissions committee, and he was in a position to assure us that our application would be considered as a unit.

Mary: I was somewhat oriented towards general practice, but he persuaded me to go into internal medicine, instead. When we left Colorado, we did student health work at the University of Missouri in Columbia, as kind of a base of operations to look for a multi specialty clinic that was big enough to absorb both of us.

John: I had a disappointing experience in Washington State. They were very interested in me, but when they found out about Mary, all kinds of red nepotism flags went up. And so we figured we needed a bigger group to avoid that problem.

Mary: When we came to Monroe, why, it was a specialty clinic. They didn't have any family doctors at that time. I ended up telling them I'd go into pediatrics, internal medicine, wherever they wanted me. Internal medicine is where I turned out to be. I worked at getting my specialty examination just on the basis of years of experience and examination, rather than having to go back and do a residency—an option which is no longer open. I went into general practice after medical school in an internship. We practiced in Western Colorado, for a few years. We really liked the practice—John was already a specialist in internal medicine. But I did family practice and delivered babies and took care of kids.

The other physicians were nice enough people, but they were not very high class, ethical physicians and we felt uncomfortable. We couldn't both be out of town at the same time because we didn't know who to tell our patients to go to.

Do any patient experiences stand out?

I was just a year out of practice. I had a very sad OB patient—a woman in her 40s who had never had any children and she finally got pregnant. She was so excited. She did everything right all through her pregnancy, but her baby died shortly before it was born. It was a still birth. I felt just awful. She knew how bad I felt and said, "Don't feel bad. It's okay. It just wasn't meant to be." How she comforted me.

I'm very emotionally involved with my patients and I've learned how not to let it interfere with my work. And also, doctors are very emotionally involved in their own success. They feel very responsible, so it's a lot of ego thing, too. It's not just worrying about the other person.

The track record?

Mary: Yeah. When we first came to Monroe, I wasn't ready to be a full-time physician, in any case. I had, by then, three children and another one on the way. I was happy to work part-time in whatever capacity they wanted me. By the time I might have been considered for a full partner, the whole structure of the clinic changed and everybody was employees anyway, so it didn't matter.

John: I graduated in March of 1946, one month after my 23rd birthday. I was quite an introvert. I had an aunt and uncle on my mother's side with schizophrenia and perhaps I was vulnerable to that sort of thing. That's one of the reasons I went into medicine, instead of astrophysics because it would permit me to be a scientist and still be compelled to deal with people. I looked at myself later on when I heard that salesmen were the worst suckers for other salesmen and I realized that that's because they relate to each other more properly. It's a two way street. In spite of my extrovert facade, my sales resistance is in tact, and deep down inside, I'm still a mad scientist, introvert.

It's hard to think of you as an introvert.

Mary: He disguises it well.

John: You want to know what our biggest mistake was? Getting married before she got her degree. She ends up with my name and we can't tell whose mail is which.

Does it get confusing when people call and ask for Dr. Frantz?

John: By now, our patients know us. We've been here 50 years.

Mary: You {interviewer} met me at my 50th reunion in 2001 and I graduated in '51.

After all these years, isn't it challenging to keep up on medical developments?

Mary: It's very challenging and it's also very interesting, because I've always been interested in the science of medicine.I don't use the computer for extensive knowledge purposes. It's putzy stuff. You get one letter wrong and it doesn't work. I'm used to using the encyclopedia, talking to people who know.

We're about to go to an electronic medical record. We're going to be forced to do this thing. We already have to dictate our medical records, but it means that instead of being typed up and put in a paper folder, they're going to be e-filed, electronically. In order to review them, we'll have to pull them up. This is not going to be easy for me. If anything is going to force me to retire, it might be that. This is the sort of thing that's difficult for us old timers. They sort of expect us to use a template and just fill in the blanks. But that isn't the kind of medical history I take. I take a narrative history and I can dictate it. If I want to correct it, then I end up typing it myself.

John: The typists all seem to have personal ambiguities about what to capitalize and I can't resist fixing that.

What's it like to cater to a small community over such an extended time?

Mary: Well actually, the Monroe Clinic is not your typical small town practice. There are 60 doctors at our clinic, so our patients come from all over Northern Illinois, Eastern, Western, Southern Wisconsin. I have patients who I see socially and I know them from what they do in the community.

John: I talk quite a bit compared to other doctors. If somebody who I've only seen once or twice decades ago, remembers details of those conversations, that's quite a compliment, especially when it's extraneous to a health problem.

I had a lady with a railroad widow's pension that would self destruct—back before women's lib back in the '60s, if she remarried. She met this soulmate and she couldn't afford to marry him and lose her pension. She was too straight to do any obvious solution and it was a trumped up tragedy.

I got on the phone and called up her priest, and told him the problem and asked if there wasn't any way to marry her in the eyes of God, but not use any paperwork from the courthouse? And he says, "Oh, that's no problem." So, that's what happened. In the eyes of God, she was married and in the eyes of the railroad retirement board, she was living in sin and therefore, entitled to her pension. That served 'em right.

Does she know that you made that happen?

John: Oh yeah, she was right there when I called the priest. She was remonstrating, "Don't call him. He won't go for it."

Do you tell each other about your patients? How far do you carry patient confidentiality?

Mary: I often wouldn't tell him the name, especially if it's someone we both knew. But I might talk about a case or a problem. We still had a lot of interesting stuff to talk about. We both are pretty well aware of the fence around what we learn professionally and what we learn personally. In fact, there was a lady in town—her boss came to me for some other problem and said, "But I understand you've seen so and so.. ." I said, "Well, isn't this a nice day today."

He went back to her. "You're doctor wouldn't tell me that she'd seen you." So both he and she got a very high opinion of me.

John: You want to hear the most ridiculous one? Technically, you can't give the patient a copy of his own record without him signing a permit.

Mary: Like many directives that come down from above, they aren't necessarily thought out in all their repercussions. It used to be in my own case at the clinic, that if I sent a patient to a psychiatrist, I got a report back. Now, the psychiatrist can't send us a report. If we want to see one, we have to go over to the psychiatry department and ask to see their closed files.

For your own patient?

Mary: For my own patients. And sometimes there isn't even a note in there that they saw the psychiatrist because that would be breaking confidentiality. But there are notes that they saw a gynecologist, orthopedist or whatever. It sometimes really does affect the patients, but if it interferes with proper and adequate care and safety, then it's definitely gone too far.

John: Well, yeah. Remember David Satcher—the surgeon general, the black guy, who's son of a sharecropper in Mississippi? He kind of put the insurance companies in their place by telling them the brain is just one more disease like heart or kidneys, and you shouldn't act like people are only entitled to 90 days of treatment for brain disease. It's like cutting them off digitalis for heart trouble. And he made it stick. This differentiation of psychiatry compared to other confidential things is quite artificial. David Satcher was correct.

Mary: The psychiatric medications have made a big difference. We both had the experience of working at the county mental hospital and now they don't have a county mental hospital. Unfortunately, we don't have adequate community provision for the few people who should have that protected environment. But I have patients with schizophrenia who are gainfully employed and running their own lives on medication.

How did your work affect your family life?

John: We weren't overburdened with call schedules and we had time off to do things together as a family. And we took trips together and went to meetings and so I would say that we were more blessed than most of humanity in those regards and not afflicted like most doctors are.

Mary: That's true. We shared the same interests. We read the same medical journals, go to the same meetings. We may go to different sessions at the same meeting and share. We both understand what the demands are. We don't take formal call now, but if either of us has a patient in the hospital, you say, "Oops, I have to go. Dinner will be in an hour or two."

But wasn't it difficult for both of you to have such demanding jobs while raising a family?

Mary: We had five children. Working part-time, living in a small town, it was easy to walk home for lunch, be with the kids after school. Our children were brought up with responsibilities for helping around the house. The oldest was eleven when the baby was born, so they had child care responsibilities, too. I don't think we overburdened them, but we certainly expected them to be responsible for one another.

John: We did pretty well by our kids. We took the older kids on quote, adult, unquote, vacations mostly backpacking or canoeing. The younger ones had gone to stay on a farm or something while we were doing these things with the older ones. They were very anxious to run with the herd and they were doing adult type things at quite a young age. Our youngest daughter climbed Mount Marana, in the Tetons, when she was only seven or eight.

Somehow, you two found time to be Peace Corps volunteers in Afghanistan. How did that happen?

Mary: Our children were all home in school, so they had been in on our conversations and one of us came home said, "Hey, we saw in the AMA journal that doctors can bring their children if they go into the Peace Corps," and one of them said, "Let's go, then."

It took us about a year or so to get geared up and apply to Afghanistan. That was in 1968. By then, our oldest child had died in an accident when she was at the university. Our next oldest was in college and she didn't go with us, but she came to join us toward the end of our time there, so we had the three younger ones who were school age.

We like to travel and here was a way to travel at government expense and live and be part of another culture. Our kids' enthusiasm had a lot to do with it. We would not have wanted to have whining teenagers along.

Our assignment was to teach and we thought that would be pretty interesting, teaching in a medical school, and it was. It was a very good time for us. We taught in English. The medical school was a small school in Jalalabad, Afghanistan, east of the Capital, which was set up with the coop-eration of Peace Corps. Supposedly all of the students were supposed to be fluent in English before they were accepted into the school, but of course that didn't happen because this is one of those cultures where influence gets you anywhere—influence and a little bit of baksheesh.*

We were assigned doctors who were sort of in late stages of training who had been through residency training in English speaking countries. They were our translators.

Did this experience change how you practiced medicine?

It certainly changed how we practiced over there. Half the time, the electricity wasn't working. They didn't have films, so you couldn't take an x-ray. If the patient had pleural effusion† and couldn't breathe, you had to figure out how to put the needle in and get the fluid out without an x-ray picture. But I was never tempted to do that over here. Why take a chance?

Mary: Our Afghan colleagues were expert at physical diagnosis be-cause they didn't have sophisticated lab and x-ray facilities, so I think we probably learned some things from them. You try to keep people comfort-

---

* Bakshees is a bribe in some Near-Eastern countries.

†Pleural effusion refers to the abnormal accumulation of fluid around the lungs.

able and take care of the major problems. You don't have as many of the worried well, as in the practice here.

John: We had kind of an aphorism for ourselves, that if it could be tuberculosis, it probably was. All kinds of oddball tuberculosis, like tuberculosis of tendon sheaths that you never see over here. It kept turning up over there. Tuberculous meningitis was a major problem. Backaches were frequently TB of the spine. The main reason why it was so prevalent was because of socio-economic conditions and a little bit of malnutrition.

Mary: When we were in medical school 50 or 60 years ago, tuberculosis was very common here, too. It just had been better controlled through isolation of patients. It's not necessary any longer. But before the tuberculosis drugs, it was the only way from keeping it from spreading throughout the community. The TB drugs were just coming into use when we were in school.

John: When we were dealing with tuberculosis in Jalalabad, it became apparent that a major problem was people just taking the treatment until they felt better. They really needed to be sold on taking it for the best part of a year, at least, so we organized group therapy for the TB patients. All the Afghans carry their own x-rays around and we'd have a group of eight, ten, twelve TB patients showing their x-rays and they would say, "Yeah, that's where I quit taking my medicine." It's really quite dramatic.

People came out of the woodwork for the American treatment for tuberculosis, but our group therapy was the only difference. That was quite a triumph because our compliance rate was comparable to the rate dealing with literate, educated people here. Illiterate, uneducated people are not stupid. All you have to do is take the trouble to get through to them. What we were particularly proud of is that we rose above our prejudices about confidentiality. They couldn't have cared less and they enjoyed the group therapy.

What was it like to come back? Was there culture shock?

John: The worst culture shock was the pet aisle at the supermarket.

Mary: The grocery store—our kids just couldn't get over that. They developed a new appreciation. It made us very close as a family by shared experience and very appreciative of many of the things. We also discovered that just as we were frustrated by bureaucratic hurdles there, we got home and found there are bureaucratic hurdles here.

Another interesting thing in Afghanistan, there were more women who had emphysema than men, even though women practically never smoked. But in the little houses with no ventilation and the stoves that weren't vented, they were sitting over the little fire cooking half the day. They had smoke exposure for hours every day.

The children had more bronchitis also. When they got older and were running around outside, they didn't. But the babies tied to the mother's back got the same dose of smoke that she did. Inhaling a lot of smoke is an irritant. The emphysema doesn't have anything to do with the nicotine in cigarettes; it has to do with the pollution.

Let's talk about smoking…

Mary: Well, I'll be personal, first. When I went to college, I was a real prissy kid in school. At home, my parents smoked. I very much disapproved of it. When I went to college along about my third year, I was really cutting loose a little bit, so I learned how to smoke. I became addicted, but not in a way that most people were addicted. My idea of addiction was five or six cigarettes a day, but I still expected to have those. If I ran out, I'd go out and get some.

John: Even if it was raining.

Mary: John didn't smoke at that time, though he did so later. He was so determined to be tolerant and tactful, that he gave me a silver cigarette case for a wedding present. I quit smoking every time I got pregnant and then I'd start in again. And then by the fourth pregnancy, I decided, I don't have to start afterwards. I'd been off it for six, eight months of the year, and I didn't. I smoked a total of less than 10 years, about a quarter of a pack of cigarettes a day.

How difficult was it for you to quit completely?

Mary: It wasn't hard. Now, I couldn't conceive of smoking. But in a way, I'm not sorry that I did because I can tell people, "Yes, I gave up smoking. I understand you enjoy it, but look at everything else."

John: I never smoked very much, either. I quit when the Surgeon General was writing his first report before it was published, probably in the 1950s. At the time, I didn't think I had any health problems from smoking. A few years later, I noticed that I got over my colds quicker than I did before.

Mary: Most of the people who find it easy to give up smoking have already given it up. The ones still out there and should quit are hard core. The best hope is to get children not to try it. They don't realize how addicting it is. I get very angry at the tobacco companies targeting young people with glamorous advertisements about smoking. Now, they're sneaking it into movies and stuff, not as an advertisement, but as an accepted thing to do if you're smart and sophisticated.

John: Not that they weren't doing that before. They got away from it for a while. But the food industry is beginning to act a little like the tobacco industry because they've got people hooked on more food than they need.

Mary: Especially children.

John: They can't face the stockholders if they suddenly start behaving properly.

Mary: It's not unusual at all to see teenagers who are probably 40 pounds over weight.

John: And so called adult onset diabetes, which seldom occurred before the age of 30, now occurs in children.

Mary: Some of it is the heavy promotion in advertising of sugar containing drinks and candy.

Kids hardly ever just drink plain water. They want soda. The parents assume, well, if they don't drink milk, maybe they'll have a glass of Coke with dinner. I am a one person campaign when I go to all my various school board meetings. If I don't have milk and water handy, I balk. These are the adults. What kind of example are you setting for kids?

John: Sugar is the most habit forming food because it gives a bigger rush and a more sudden withdrawal, especially if you take it on an empty stomach. Even diet pop stimulates the taste buds and the body has such a good anticipation, that the taste of sugar stimulates some insulin production, so that drinking diet soda makes you hungrier a half an hour or so later than if you hadn't had the sweet taste. Diet pop is for people who have diabetes to be as normal as possible.

Mary: If they want to drink at a party or something.

John: About the only pop I drink is tonic water when I'm the designated driver at a party and you can't tell whether it's got vodka in it or not, so it still seems like a party.

You don't drink soda at all, Mary?

Mary: Very reluctantly. I drink water. I drink a lot of milk. I drink coffee and tea. We don't use any salt in our home either, but we don't hesitate to eat out. We were on an elder hostel trip for five weeks and we were getting salty food all the time. We come home and within a few days, we're used to our salt free food.

John: We have salt shakers and we give them to guests, but we don't have ash trays. I learned something about salt. Mary had to give up salt during pregnancy. It was kind of unfair from her point of view because it was our baby and she had to give up the salt. And so, with the first one, I just plain quit eating salt. Within two or three weeks, I couldn't care less and I haven't eaten salt since then.

When it comes to dealing with old people with heart trouble who can't eat salt without getting into more trouble with congestive heart failure, I have a better pitch than the rest of the doctors. I know if they really do it, it won't be like a drug, where you know the reformed alcoholic has one drink and he's got to hang one on. They'll just say this food is salty and go to a different restaurant next time.

I was talking to the dietician about it a few weeks ago and we were talking about morbid obesity, and I suggested maybe we should call it morbid inactivity instead, because these obese kids don't eat more than people such as ourselves when we were children. It's just too much TV and too much computer games.

Mary: There's less physical activity for a variety of reasons, some of which are social. I have almost an addiction for physical activity. Well, this meshes nicely with my concern about energy usage. We just don't drive our car unless we're going off somewhere for a period of time or unless we have a huge grocery list.

John: We're the only elderly grown ups riding bicycles.

Mary: We walk or ride our bicycles—another advantage of living in a small town. If I've had a day of mostly sitting around in the office—the office is only three blocks away—I have to go for a walk before I go to bed at night. I just can't feel comfortable unless I've had some exercise. We usually choose active vacations where we might spend five to six hours a day in physical activity.

John: My parents were both heavy. I found out before I went to medical school that I preferred to be more active and it wasn't a matter of going out for athletics, it was a matter of walking and bicycling. And my particular bias is to do something useful for exercise, instead of just going to work out.

I'm really grateful to the Y for their existence. I went there consistently for about a year after I had my hips replaced in 1996 because I had trouble with weakness of the gluteus medias muscles. And regular workouts there got me to where I could walk 10 or 12 miles without trekking poles. But last year for the Grand Canyon, I took transcendental training poles—the kind that hitches you in the forearm. We went down the Kaibob and up the Bright Angel trails.

Mary: We were both 81 when we did it.

John: We were the oldest people.

Mary: We were neither the slowest nor the fastest in the group. We just plugged along. We've done mountain climbing and back country exploration all our married lives.

John: Our first trip to the Grand Canyon, we did on abandoned prospectors' trails. It was 12 miles along the river. The second one was hardly ever used. The rangers will give you a mimeographed proof sheet, if they think you aren't going to have to be rescued. They tell you landmarks, so you can identify the route. It's not really a trail.

We were really acting our age last year.

Mary: …to go on a trail.

John: Really, the Grand Canyon is rather modest compared to some of what we've done. At one point, we climbed and descended 9,500 feet in one day—in Colorado.

How long ago?

John: Oh, 30 years. When I was 64 or 65, I climbed the east face of Long's Peak {Rocky Mountain National Park}, which is something the Europeans come here to do. When I was 44, I climbed Mt. McKinley.

We've been on the fringe of a lot of cults, but mountaineering, we've been closer to the hard core than any of the other ones.

Like in the early '60s, I made a kayak out of a kit and we've done quite a bit of kayaking in the Great Lakes, camping on islands and in Alaska, in Glacier Bay and Icy Bay.

What are your vacations like now?

Mary: We just got back from a hiking trip in New Zealand, which was day hikes. We didn't camp out. But they were some very strenuous hikes. We'd be 6-8 hours a day, hiking. We were five weeks vacation in February and March and now during the summer, we like working in our garden and we have plenty of days to do that. We can take all of the vacation we want.

So what happens to all of your patients?

Mary: Well if you plan a vacation ahead of time—if they're the kind of patients you see every few months anyway, why you just schedule around that. If you have somebody in the middle of a crisis, you arrange for a specific doctor to cover and know about that patient. Otherwise, they just take whoever's on call. That's the advantage of being in a big clinic—the records are available.

Do any of your fellow colleagues resent the kind of schedule that you have?

Mary: There may be some doctors who resent it a little bit. Even though we're only seeing maybe 15 patients a week, those are patients somebody else doesn't have to take care of, and we still make referrals. Our patients go to other specialists, and so we bring in a lot more income than that to the clinic than just what they've paid to see us.

We've been fortunate not to have great economic hardship and not to have major health problems.

John: Well, speak for yourself.

Mary: His father became bedridden in his late 80s and 90s because he had bad hips and didn't have surgery, so John seized the bull by the horns.

John: The year before I had my hips replaced, I got my spine fixed, so I wouldn't end up like my dad. I had to talk the surgeon into doing it. Well, I had to explain to him how strong my legs were before they got weaker because he was comparing me to a normal standard. When he finished, he realized getting that much weaker was a problem, so doctors aren't always poor patients.

You two are healthy enough to remain active in the community. You're on the School Board, Mary. How did you get interested in the School Board when your kids are grown?

In fact, I wonder why I didn't do it years ago, it's so great. About four years ago, we heard there were three vacancies on the School Board, and we had reason to be a little concerned about a certain character in Monroe who has been very active and has persecuted us, personally, as well as the community, as a whole. We were worried that this was the time that these forces might be ready to co-opt the School Board, as they've done in other communities. So John said, "You ought a run for School Board." I say, "Oh no. I'm too old." But he kept after me and I thought, *Maybe I'll give it a try.* Well, I did run, but I didn't get elected. I was really disappointed. *Nobody likes me. They think I'm too old.*

So later the same year, two more people resigned or moved out of the area and couldn't be on the Board, so the School Board was going to have to appoint two people to fill in terms. I applied at that time too, but so did seven other people. I didn't get one of those spots. Then, the next election came around with two vacancies. I'll give it one more try and then I did get in. I was just re-elected. I just served one term.

John: So she was 79 when she started.

Mary: 78.

Was age an issue in the previous campaigns?

Mary: I don't know. The two people who were selected by the Board are wonderful people and they're still on the Board. I can't regret that they got the spot.

John: When I was an alderman, I was chairman of the Board of Health.

So you were on the City Council?

John: Yeah, for four years. Mary was the Medical Society's representative on the County Board of Health for many years and last year when she got so busy with the School Board, they replaced her with me. I think she might have influenced the events somehow—one of those nepotism things. {Laughs}

Everybody in town must know you two.

Mary: There are people in Monroe who don't know us, of course. But I like that feature. When we think of being forced to quit working and act our age, and wonder, well, if we needed a more supportive living arrangement, what would we do? We've looked at nice places in Madison, but we think how would they get along in Monroe without us here? It's hard. But we also face our mortality. We'll have to get off the main stage, too.

But not yet.

Mary: Not yet.

What is the plan?

John: Well, how could we have a plan because we don't know the events that are going to determine the plan?

Did you ever envision practicing this long?

Mary: It just sort of happens. I don't envision retiring, as long as we can write our own ticket about how many hours, how many weeks, how many months. I probably work 20 hours a week on paper—sometimes it's more. But if I'm behind, I'll go in and sit at the computer and do charts and stuff. If I have patients in the hospital, then that's extra.

John: I work about 30 hours a week. Early in my career I discovered that retirement is frequently a health hazard, less so for women than men. And so, it seemed as though it was best to arrange not to retire abruptly. In my case, I volunteered to do nursing home work that the other doctors weren't quite so enthusiastic about. You can't exactly make yourself indispensable, but you can make a pretty good attempt if you pick something the other people don't like to do.

My experience in the nursing home is that you can do a lot for the patients. Even if the patients don't appreciate you, you can do a lot for the relatives, so it's perfectly satisfactory entry into being constructive.

Mary: I tell my patients I won't retire unless I have to, and that's true. The clinic has been good to us and we're not pushing into the procrustean mold to see six patients an hour. I usually see probably about eight patients in a day.

John: Well, I have a system for not getting retired prematurely because of Alzheimer's disease. I talk extra complicated while I still can and they look it up to make sure it's true. Then, later on after they get tired of looking it up, I'll get a couple of extra years when they're too lazy to look it up any more.

Don't you want a time when you don't have to work anymore, where you can just play every day?

John: But it's more fun to be on vacation, if you're escaping from work.

VI

Frayed Net

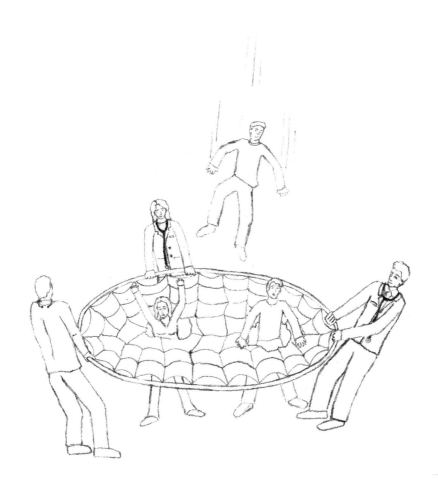

"Law and order are the medicine of the body politic and when the body politic gets sick, medicine must be administered."

—B. R. Ambedkar

CHAPTER TWENTY-ONE

"DR DTOX"

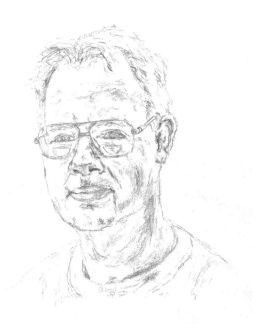

"The total cost of addiction care—3% of it goes to addiction treatment; 97% of it goes to treating the complications of substance use."

Michael M. Miller, MD
Psychiatry, Addiction Medicine, Madison

I had just filled my gas tank and was heading inside to pay, when a high school girl stopped me. Showing me the bills clenched in her fist, she asked whether I would buy her a pack of cigarettes. I was in my mid 30s at the time, but I didn't feel much older than she was until I heard myself respond.

"I'm a health reporter, and I get information every single day about the latest illness cigarettes cause. I want you to live a long, healthy life."

She smiled, looked down and walked away. Sometimes, strangers have more influence than family, so I don't regret refusing to "help" her. In fact, nicotine addiction is the most lethal, in terms of the sheer number of deaths. Addiction, generally, is so pervasive that we as a society don't really notice it. We give lip service to the notion that preventing kids from smoking is the right thing to do, but there's not much money devoted to prevention, especially compared to tobacco marketing budgets.

Why are we so afraid to confront nicotine and other drug addictions? It really comes down to stigma, double standards, and "absurd" expectations, according to one of the nation's most prominent authorities on addiction medicine, Michael Miller, MD. Miller, whose license plate reads DR DTOX, is president of the American Society of Addiction Medicine.

I first met him in the late 1980s, when I was a news reporter. I had never heard of an addiction medicine specialist before then.

Miller, in his early 50s, is intense, intellectual, and focused, yet he's affable and approachable. His mother "was disabled by mental illness," but he says he doesn't think that had much or anything to do with him becoming a psychiatrist.

He's off work today, relaxed, wearing a sweatshirt and tennis shoes, spending his morning teaching yet another interested person about addiction. Doctor Miller starts by telling me about one patient's long battle against depression and alcoholism.

There was a lady I worked with in town. I certainly was attached to her and she was attached to me. We were very close in age, a few weeks apart. Our life paths had been different. She had grown up with a lot of addiction in her family. She had 15 years of very productive work. Her alcoholism was profound, and her mental illness was profound. I knew her when her kids were little and her kids, on numerous occasions, would come into the living room and find her nearly dead, either from an overdose or suicide attempt, or both. I knew these kids were getting affected by this.

I detoxed her a million times. It was one of those cases where you can't help but be humbled because you know it isn't up to you. It's up to God. God was keeping this lady alive. She should have died a million times.

She really appreciated that I cared about her, and would always be willing to see her. She had some real periods of recovery, both from mental illness and her alcoholism. But oh, she had deep wounds and she couldn't eventually see herself as successful. There were years when she wasn't my patient any more. She was getting her health care services in the public sector, terribly disabled. I would hear of her on occasion. I detoxed her children at different points, as they grew up into their own addictions.

Well, eventually, she died. She had developed a variety of other medical conditions. I don't think her bipolar depression killed her. I'm not sure that her alcoholism killed her. It was something else. She was in a lot of pain.

I saw her obit in the paper, so I went to her funeral. This thing can take your breath away at times. But what really had the most impact on me, was these girls, now in their 30s, whom I'd met when they were in their teens. They were really shocked to see me at their mother's funeral. They hadn't seen me in years. They didn't know at first, who I was.

I was just there to pay my respects. I sat in the back of the church, where I had been to Mass many times. At the receiving line, I realized that all of the girls were drunk. They were certainly embarrassed because I could smell their breath. This was probably all they knew how to do. The loss of their mom was so hard for them and all they knew to cope with it was to be drunk. This isn't just learned behavior. It's also their genetics. It was so sad for me to see that they couldn't experience their mother's death, go through normal grieving. It was just sad that these women weren't able to handle this normal human event without being loaded.

When you look back at this patient, what was it that she wasn't able to accomplish to turn her life around?

She could not identify herself as a winner, even though she had successes. But in our most intensive work in therapy, it was like, here it is. You can have it. Go grab it. She just couldn't.

When you have a case like that, is there anything you learn from it that you try to bring to subsequent patients?

All of us in medicine need to be very grateful for the experience and the opportunity, and also very humbled and to realize what we can do and what we can't do. There is stuff that's bigger than us. A lot of people get well or not get well, but not by all the training and experience and skill we bring to bear and all the compassion we bring to bear. A lot of them get better or worse, probably to use a phrase that sounds right, according to "God's plan."

You have integrity. You don't take responsibility for either the successes or the losses. You try to distance yourself from that and realize that if you can be a facilitator and healer to some extent, that's great, and you can help people on their own recovery path.

I'm considered an expert in this. I'm a national leader. People look at me and think I have some intellectual mastery over this thing and I understand it. On many levels, I do, but I have to accept the limits. You're a fool to be cocky in this business.

Tell me more about the treatment. How do you help transform these people?

What happens in standard treatment in America is that group therapy is used. In a group session, fascinating things happen. There are other patients who've been there, done that, and they see this rookie come in and say their story and the other patients go, "I said that when I was in your chair." The feedback can be useful, but it's not just confrontational. It's not just, "How can you be so foolish to believe that we're going to believe you?" It's, "Hey look at me. I'm at a new place. You have hope and you can come to where I am." The group experience is extremely powerful.

Most people in addiction suppress their feelings. They deny them. It's easier for them to short-circuit life by popping a pill, or even shooting up, than it is to feel what life has—the ups and downs.

The group therapy process is to help the person endorse the belief that, "I want a different life and I really believe I can get there. I'm going to make changes in my thinking, in my feeling, in my relationships, in my daily behavior, so that I function better. I'm going to develop personal responsibility. I will tell the truth to my spouse, and my kids, and my employer."

One of the key aspects of recovery that my fellowship director at the University of Minnesota taught me is that one of the things that happen for people in treatment is re-popleization.

What does that mean?

Re-peopleization means the person gets connected to other people again. The person begins to be a fully functioning, emotional organism and a member of their social community. You become a human being. You leave your island. You stop being a rock. You come out from behind the door. You re-engage. You join clubs. You volunteer. You take off the cloak of shame. You remove the bandages of the leper. You re-engage the world and you become efficacious again.

But it's part of being a social person and being a whole person and getting out of this network of other drinkers and drug users that you were in, and hanging out with average folks, and re-adopting a conventional lifestyle. Don't stay up all night. Don't go out until dawn on the weekends. Have a normal sleep/wake cycle. Do the things your neighbors do.

The life of an addict had really evolved away from conventionality. Repeopleization means getting out there and being a "normie" again. Some people have chosen to be unconventional, but others have lost a lot of capacity, and have lost the confidence that they can get it back. So yep, I can get up in the morning, brush my teeth and go to breakfast.

In treatment, I can show up at eight in the morning, and I can make a promise to my family and keep it. I can engage with my neighbors and not just be isolated in my house in my basement in front of the television, sucking beers.

From an academic standpoint, Steve, I can say that there are cognitive changes people have to go through. They have to reevaluate their substance use. Addicts tend to overvalue the positive effects of use and undervalue the negative aspects. "It's not that bad. My job isn't really affected. My spouse isn't really going to leave me. My kids haven't been hurt. It's a fun thing. It allows me to talk better and be more sociable. I'm less shy. Sex is more enjoyable. Music is better."

You have to get people to take their balance sheet and reevaluate it, and take some of those pluses off and emphasize some of those minuses. That's a cognitive process and an emotional change. People have to be willing to feel. They have to be willing to cry. They have to be willing to be sad. They have to grieve things they haven't grieved. They have to grieve their own losses that addiction has caused in their lives. They have to hang in there on bad days and not run away and get drunk or high when they feel bad. That's a real change, okay? They've gotta do things differently. They've gotta, gotta act responsibly.

They have to engage and change their relationships, so it's on a cognitive level, an emotional level, a behavioral level, a relational level and, finally, on a spiritual level. They have to be led to a place out of their dungeon of hopelessness. They have to build their self-esteem. You have to help them get past their self-loathing. For a lot of people, getting re-connected to the transcendent is real part of recovery. For many people, it's considered an essential, core element. Most people, in the depths of addiction, have stopped praying. They think that God doesn't care about them anymore. They think that they're unhealable. But the spiritual aspect is getting connected to something bigger than me and really letting that part of you grow again.

In many areas of health care, we're understanding the role of prayer in recovery and the role of spirit in healing from cancer, heart disease, and other things. The behavioral aspects of juvenile diabetes, coronary artery disease, asthma, and a variety of conditions, like Crohn's disease,* have been known for centuries.

Most physicians and nurses are more comfortable with the bio, and maybe with the psycho, but the spiritual and the social haven't been mainstream medicine. Addiction may lead the rest of medicine in this regard.

Tell me some success stories.
I have many patients that will call me up on their anniversary and say, "You were there for me."

Anniversary of what?
Of being clean. AA recognizes sober dates and gives medallions for three-months, six-months, 12-months and every year. These people go to get their pin at AA meetings to get recognized for accumulation of sober time and recovery time. Patients remember that and call me. These are folks from different walks of life.

What they remember is being accepted for who they were, and somebody would sort of take them under their wing and guide them toward a path for hope that they didn't have for themselves.

I have patients now who are taking a brand new treatment. It's a new medication called buprenorphine that's similar to methadone, but it's prescribed through the doctor's office and through the neighborhood phar-

_____
* Crohn's disease is a disorder that causes inflammation of the digestive tract.

macy, rather than through some special methadone clinic in a far corner of town. I have some patients who were really down and out; people who had been through every treatment system and had been rejected by everybody, who talk about how grateful they are for being accepted as people. This medicine is really effective. And the gratification you get as a clinician, seeing people be well is just great. In my 50s, with this new treatment that just got approved a few years ago, it's extremely rewarding.

There seems to be a particularly strong physician/patient relationship here, perhaps more so, than in other specialties.

It's a huge part of what I do. There are people who practice addiction medicine who don't emphasize it as much. A big part is not just to collect information from them, but to build a relationship and a comfort level so they'll feel comfortable coming back. You've gotta get somebody to come back. Making that bond, so they won't be a dropout, is a key to eventual successful outcomes.

It would be hard to be effective if you're not honest with patients and you're not genuine yourself. I don't do a lot of self-disclosure, but it's pretty clear to patients that I'm genuine. They can tell that I'm really listening to them, and I try to get to know them as a person, and not just as a case.

But the rewards—the personal rewards are so tremendous. It would really be draining if all it did was take from you, but I'm in a line of work that feeds me every day. It fills me up emotionally. It helps me grow spiritually, which also makes it rather odd that I'm paid to do it. It's certainly wonderful that I am, but this helps me because it keeps me grounded and it helps me be real and genuine and helps me not fool myself.

Did you ever have any qualms or reservations about pursuing a specialty where it's not always all that clear whether you've been successful? It's not like there's a cancerous tumor and you remove it, or somebody breaks his leg and you reset it. It's a different game, isn't it?

Well Steve, your question betrays commonly held misconceptions. People with addiction get well. In fact, one of the reasons I did choose this is because I really like the patients, and saw how much they got well and how grateful they were when they did get well.

In surgery, you see results quickly. But in internal medicine, you don't. When you're managing hypertension, diabetes, rheumatoid arthritis, or emphysema, you don't see people have complete remissions for the rest of their lives. You manage them chronically over time. You get to know them. You help them improve their functioning over time, if they can, over the coming decades. The same thing happens when you treat major depression, and the same thing happens when you treat schizophrenia, alcoholism, and drug addiction. It's chronic disease management.

But I never had any qualms about addiction with regard to efficacy, outcomes, and success. When you sit as a group at a big treatment center, you see how peoples' lives have changed, and you see how grateful they are. Back in medical school, when I sat with these married couples in therapy for six months, and saw the changes they had gone through, and you could compare in one group, the six-monthers, the four-monthers, the two-monthers, the rookies, and see the changes people go through, I knew people got well from this disease.

The outpatient group I developed with the help of some superb counselors at the Midelfort Clinic in Eau Claire, where the HMO sent 80% of cases to outpatient, had a success rate of 82%. You can have wonderful success with this treatment, if you can provide enough resources and you provide enough continuity of care. Successful outcomes? Not a question.

The question I thought you were going to ask was about going into a field that was stigmatized, that nobody else went into, where the patients aren't liked and aren't understood, where the condition is baffling, to even most people in medicine, where you marginalize yourself in the medical community by choosing to be with unattractive patients.

Then, answer your own question.

I didn't consciously decide to do it. But I am sure, unconsciously, the part of me who has always cared about the downtrodden, who has always cared about the marginalized members of our society, me, who was a protester walking picket lines in Louisiana, and was called a "Communist" for doing so when I was a kid. There was a part of me that cared for the person who nobody else cared for. It wasn't a conscious awareness, but I'm sure I was drawn to the opportunity. It really is a way that I act out my faith. You can be extremely humanitarian working with people who don't have a lot of opportunities.

If indeed the treatment is as effective as you suggest, why aren't we treating these people?

Well, denial in our culture, for some reason, is pervasive. We don't want to believe how big of an issue it is. Those who work in this field know it's not just the patients who have denial, it's the culture that doesn't want to face up to it and it's more comfortable to stigmatize it than to embrace it and come to solutions. Part of the reason that people believe the treatment doesn't work is that the standards for measuring outcomes for addictive treatment are so different than for other chronic diseases.

Basically, if you have a medicine that reduces symptoms when the medicine is there, you take the medicine away and the symptoms come back. My goodness, it looks like it got better, and it wasn't just by chance, and the medicine really works.

In the treatment phase, the patient functions much better. But in pre and post treatment, my God, they're sick. We have a treatment for hypertension or diabetes that works. You know what happens in addiction treatment? You measure how much somebody drinks and send them to treatment, and a year later, you say, "Are they drinking?" And they are.

People go, "See, treatment failed."

Well, treatment was stopped a year ago. What would you expect in a chronic disease? Would you expect the symptoms to return? Doesn't it show that the treatment really worked? That during the in-treatment phase, substance use decreased 80%, functionality improved 80%. You withdraw the treatment and the symptoms return? That's not rocket science, but our culture calls that a failed treatment system. But for hypertension, we call it a successful treatment.

So how long does treatment need to last until it's more permanent?

Applying treatment over two years really gives the best results. What would happen if every addict in the country had the opportunity to have access to the treatment that doctors and airline pilots receive? Do you know the treatment success for treating airline pilots is 92%? The treatment for treating physicians is from the mid 70s {percentages} to the mid 80s. Why? Because they're followed very carefully, they're followed for at least two years. They have to do regular urines; they're in group therapy for months.

Is the total cost of that treatment the cost of one open heart surgery for that chronic illness? No. Do you have return of the illness, like you have reocclusion of the coronary artery? Heck, no.

When you've treated intensely for two years, this is a very treatable illness, if you apply enough treatment. Nobody wants to, because people haven't figured out the treatment models that are so effective, what the numbers are, what the costs are, and what the cost of not treating people is.

Have we made progress? We've made tremendous progress. We understand a heck of a lot more about how the brain works, how addictive drugs work on the brain, what recovery is, the aspects of recovery that we need to aim for, how to structure treatment, what duration to apply, what monitoring to use, what sort of behavioral contracts to include. We know how to do this. It's disappointing we don't have the opportunity.

I'll run into people at a neighborhood party or at a family reunion or even sitting around with other soccer parents and they'll say, "What do you do for a living?"

And I'll say, "Oh, I practice addiction medicine."

A few times people will recoil, as if there is something weird about that and chuckle in an embarrassing way. But most of the time they say, "That must be very interesting and very challenging, and I'm sure you're really busy."

What I say to them is, "I'm busy. But there's a lot of difference between a case and a patient. And in my business, there are a lot of cases but there aren't that many patients." To be a patient, you have to define that you have a need, but you have to seek service and have an ability to pay for it. In our culture, the number of people who have cases of addiction who then get treatment is anywhere from 5 and 20%.

It's this huge public health problem. It costs our nation more than $700 billion per year. It's the number four cause of death in Wisconsin. It's the root of a third of all Medicare and Medicaid expenditures. It's the medical fallout from substance use and addiction.

There's not a single department of addiction medicine in any medical school in the country, okay? We don't pay for treatment. The total cost of addiction care—3% of it goes to addiction treatment; 97% of it goes to treating the complications of substance use. I'd love to have more patients, because I know the cases are out there and they're choking our communities.

If eight of ten are not getting the help they need. Who are the two that are getting it?

Like in the early days of psychiatry, a lot of the treatment was given to self-pay people who could afford it—upper middle class people. The irony is that CEOs of corporations have benefits for their employees that limit their addiction treatment benefits. They can have wonderful benefits through reputable insurance companies for their hearts, lungs, and abdomens, and for every other area of their brain, for their Parkinson's and their strokes. But if it's addiction, the benefits are very limited. If the CEO's child has a problem, the CEO writes a check and goes to private treatment. The employees can't go.

In America, the other thing that's terribly, tragically, ironic is that the people who get help now are prisoners. There's a tremendous amount of addiction in prison populations and a tremendous amount of people in prison who do not have their addiction adequately treated. But they are people who are getting treatment. In this country, in many ways, it's easier to get treatment if you're in jail than if you're in the community, because community-based resources are so sparse.

Another thing that's scandalous about this…a huge percentage of treatment in America, is public sector based. Of the people who do get addiction treatment in our country, 75% of the funding is public sector based; not through private health insurance. We don't stand for that for hearts and lungs. We have community health centers for the uninsured, and if you don't have employer-based health insurance, there's a public safety net. But the public safety net for mental health and addiction care has really allowed the private sector not to feel guilty.

The private sector can turn its back on people with mental illness and addiction and say, "Oh, if there's a problem, you can go to the public clinic." The public clinics have filled the gaps in the private sector and in addiction far more than for psychiatry. If you need methadone, if you need residential treatment, and sometimes if you just need general outpatient counseling, the treatment is provided through public sector delivery systems, even with public funds, whereas, for other health conditions, that would never be the case. That's who's getting help.

If indeed we could save so much money, helping these people avoid all these problems, how come the private insurance companies are unwilling to make the investment and prevent more expensive problems later on?

There is still a broad belief that people bring their problems on themselves when it comes to substance use disorders: that it's self-imposed. The concept of impairment and control over substance use, which is the core feature that distinguishes addicted substance users from casual substance users, that concept is very poorly understood and it's counter-intuitive.

Only 10% of the public has addiction; 90% don't. The vast majority of people who use substances can use with complete control. You can choose how many drinks you'll have. You can choose how many joints you'll smoke, and you can even choose how many lines of cocaine you'll snort. You don't lose control, and your life doesn't fall apart. It truly is a social behavior, and it can be, as the phrase goes, recreational.

Loss of control happens to a small percentage of the population. It's a very real phenomenon that the majority says, "That's a copout. You're making this up. You could control it if you wanted to. You don't have enough willpower. You brought this on yourself."

There's a hesitancy to provide medical care for a condition that is thought to be self-imposed. We see a few lines of thinking comparable to this with regard to obesity. You chose to eat a poor diet. You chose to not exercise. We will charge you higher health insurance premiums if you don't meet weight targets. But there's really not the scorn toward the obese like there is toward the addicted.

When I teach medical students, I always try to teach that addiction is not a desired state; that people who develop addiction desire to use. They wanted to get a buzz. They wanted to be like anybody else on their block who chose to go to a social event and be under the influence of something.

They didn't choose to lose control. They didn't choose to lose their jobs. They didn't choose to lose their spouse or their organ function. They didn't choose to get HIV from injection drug use, or get hepatitis C. They didn't choose to carry a tank of oxygen through the mall because of their nicotine addiction. They didn't think it could happen to them. Addiction is not a desired state.

People choose to use recreationally, but for a genetically exposed subset of our population, regular exposure to these chemicals can lead to loss of control and a potentially fatal illness. I wonder if part of the reason for why the public doesn't embrace addiction treatment is that we don't really understand what it is. Pull the veil off and explain what it involves.

Addiction treatment did not grow up in America through the original health care system, and professionals didn't learn how to be addiction counselors through academic channels. There are bachelors and masters, and even associate degree training programs for addiction counselors now, and there are fellowships for physicians in addiction medicine, like I had the opportunity to take over 20 years ago.

But a lot of the counseling came up through on the job training, and you learned to be a counselor at a treatment center. Addiction treatment is not integrated into general hospitals, or even general mental health systems. It's a separate delivery system, in separate locations. We know that Betty Ford is out of town and somewhere else. But every community should have a program in their community hospital.

I work at Meriter in Madison. It's one of the few hospitals that has the mission and the courage to offer these services instead of saying, "It's not our problem." Because the delivery system is in different locations, the funding systems are separate, and the professionals often don't interact with other doctors and nurses, addiction treatment is more mysterious, less well-understood, and less embraced.

What happens in treatment is that people need to understand that this did not happen to them because they're bad or weak. Most people enter treatment with a tremendous amount of shame and guilt and low self-esteem, and have internalized most of society's messages that you're a loser, you have only yourself to blame. They need to understand what the general public, which is them, didn't understand before they got into treatment, which is how the brains of addicts are different, how the brains of addicts react to these chemicals differently, how the chemicals change the brain of the addict to function differently than before they were early users. The main thing we have to do is give the person hope.

We live in a world in which there is tremendous therapeutic pessimism about addiction. One of the biggest barriers I need to overcome in my professional life, every day, is the therapeutic pessimism of physicians. Physicians don't believe that addicts can get well. Physicians believe this is a hopeless revolving door. Physicians, in their training and their practices, don't get exposure to and the experience of people getting well, and seeing how people do recover.

The public has this therapeutic pessimism, and patients have it. What happens is that they've tried to stop. They've developed problems in their lives, and they've tried to stop. They were able to stop—for a month, for three months, or six months. Then, they returned to use and their problems returned or got worse. They've been over this cycle for a period of months or years where they really, really try, and they can't do it by themselves and develop a sense of hopelessness. Many of them don't approach treatment because they don't believe it will be able to turn them around. They haven't been able to have success through their own efforts, and don't see anything else on the other side of the hill.

I had an insight one day. I was going to teach a roomful of residents and medical students and I thought, *What do you want the bullet points to be? What do you want the take-home messages to be?*

I walked into this room. They've never seen an addiction medicine specialist in their lives; they have no idea why they were asked to come to this lecture. I sat down and said, "When you work with a patient who has alcoholism or addiction, the only thing you have to do to be successful with them is to love them. That's what you have to do because nobody else does, and they don't love themselves. They're terribly ashamed, and they're used to people in the health care system getting down on their case, making smart aleck comments, yelling at them, blaming them. They expect the health care system to treat them the way that the rest of society does, if not worse.

"Walk in there and care about them as a person, listen to their story, be non-judgmental, and have them experience you as somebody who cares about them, even with their alcoholism or drug addiction. It will be transforming for them. I see it in my patients every day when I see them realize how I'm interacting with them. You can do the same thing. If you don't do it, if you walk in there with an attitude, if you walk in there and make them feel worse and make them feel still more guilty, and make them feel more self-loathing, you'll be just like the rest of 'em.

"And the patient will clam up and not give you accurate information. You won't make an accurate diagnosis. You won't have a good doctor/patient relationship. They won't do what you ask. They won't come back. You'll have a treatment failure and a self-fulfilling prophecy. The first thing you need to do with these patients is to love them."

How did they react to that?

Very respectfully, very thoughtfully. Whoa, what's this guy saying? They also know I'm not nuts. When they hear it, they like, mull it around, but it resonates.

I feel good about the opportunity to work with these young people. When you work in psychiatry, it's somewhat out of the mainstream of medicine. You could be looked askance by peers. "Oh, you're just a shrink. You don't practice real medicine."

If you're in addiction, the stigma's worse because the common belief is; well of course, these people brought it on themselves. It's willful misconduct—all of which are inaccurate and biased statements. But they're part of the popular culture and popular stigma, the young doctors in training pick up from the culture we live in.

Within addiction, there's a caste system. Working with alcoholics, the unwell, the unemployed who are neighbors, everybody knows an alcoholic. Everybody has them in their family. We may hate alcoholics, but we know Uncle Joe and Aunt Patty are alcoholics, and we love them, so they're okay.

But junkies? Oh no. Junkies are different than drunks. If you work with drug addicts, you're even more to the marginalized group. And if you're a doctor working in a methadone clinic, obviously, you can't get a job working anywhere else. "Maybe you could get a job in a prison. Maybe you've lost your license."

A doctor who works in addiction with drug addicts in a methadone clinic, which I don't, is the most stigmatized of all! Is there something about me that likes to say, I'm up to that. I'll be different. I don't care what those bastards say. I'm going to go out and take care of these people and do a good job of it. I am sure that is part of it that's drawn me to this line of work. I'm happy to be there when nobody else is willing to be in the fray.

It's such a tremendous opportunity to be a physician to work with people who are in a real time of need in their lives—it's a watershed moment in their lives—and to help them in such a life-changing experience as recovery from addiction is a tremendous opportunity.

Addiction medicine is a fascinating specialty. If people understood it more, more people would come to it because it provides so many opportunities. Addiction affects every organ system.

In my work as a physician, I do my own histories and physicals, which most people with psychiatric training don't do. I function as an internist. I have to know hepatology because of how the liver is involved, and all these chemicals act on or pass through the liver. Neurology is very important for the impact on the brain and the neuropathies that can be caused.

I see patients in the emergency room. I love doing consultation work, where I'm up on the general medicine floor with patients who have every kind of illness in the world, where an alcohol problem may be a complicating factor. I get to work with every age group. I get to work with both genders. Many physicians don't have those opportunities.

I get to use psychiatry, and the psychiatric aspects of addiction are tremendous. I do individual therapy. I do family therapy. I do group therapy. I do medication management. Almost every aspect of psychiatry comes into play, including forensics. I testify in commitment proceedings, and I testify as an expert witness.

My work in organized medicine is so extremely varied, and I work at the county, state, and AMA level, as well as in my specialty, so my biggest hobby is volunteering for organized medicine.

And within that, my sub hobby is public policy within medicine. I might spend my day hanging out with legislators, with physician leaders from throughout the country, with hospital administrators, with journalists, or with community-based organizations. These are things that are very different than being in an exam room with a patient or at a bedside, so my life is incredibly rewarding.

How did you get here?

It's all evolved. It wasn't by design. The public policy stuff came really naturally to me. It's a passion of mine. I won the civics award in ninth grade! I understood how government worked from an early age. When I was 10-years old, I spent three weeks in Washington, DC, living with my cousin and being on my own, touring every government building and understanding every government department as a really geeky little kid.

In 11th grade, I was in the first class of something called Presidential Classroom for Young Americans, which is a fascinating leadership development program where you live in a hotel in DC for a week and spend time visiting all three branches of government. The cool thing is interviewing leaders. An ambassador, a cabinet secretary, a senator would speak in front of a ballroom of 150 of us, and then we'd go to microphones in the aisles and ask them questions. I'm a political junkie.

You're a Southerner, too, right?

I grew up in a city called Alexandria, Louisiana, which is directly in the middle of the state. It was my dad's hometown. I'm the youngest of three boys.

My dad was a practicing physician in that community. He was the chief resident at the teaching hospital for the Tulane faculty. The story he told countless times was, "I made about $10 per week and spent $2.50 on cigarettes."

Even though he was technically an OB/GYN, he really loved to operate and was a wonderful surgeon. He really was a Renaissance physician. He delivered tens of thousands of the babies. He went into practice in 1942—with a medical deferment from the service—and joined a man who had just built a six-bed hospital.

Soon after my dad joined the practice, his partner was drafted, so my dad was one of the few physicians left in the community to take care of all the families in the town. Husbands had gone off to war, and he ran the hospital doing general surgery, orthopedics, primary care, and OB/GYN by himself for three years, including his own anesthesia and radiology. People who knew him say it almost killed him. He never really was the same after that, and he seemed to move a little slower and was a little calmer.

He would sometimes go make rounds and come home to have breakfast with us as we were getting ready for school. He came home for lunch every day. He had a huge practice, and he was extremely productive. When I was a kid, he'd sometimes come pick me up after he'd left the office and I would ride with him to the hospital and I would make his p.m. rounds with his OB and surgical cases.

How old were you?

Oh, six through nine.

Was this when you started thinking you might like to be in this profession?

Absolutely not. I had no interest in doing it. When I got older and saw his office practice, I realized what a grind I thought it was. I thought it would be actually kind of dulling to do the repetitive thing of seeing a patient and then another, just go from one exam room to the other. I didn't appreciate the doctor/patient relationship and the emotional attachments you have to your patients. I thought it was more like shift work, where he was running through a huge volume. I knew he had worked a lot of hours, and so I thought I could do other things. I had a lot of different interests. I could actually do something more interesting. Boy, was I wrong.

At what stage did you start thinking that medicine might actually be for you?

I was taking a liberal arts curriculum at a Jesuit university. What happened was I really fell in love with philosophy, and an area of philosophy I found interesting was epistemology. I recognized that it was extremely interesting to try to understand how we know things. What is knowledge, and how can humans grasp it? But I realized that philosophers can't make a living, and they sit around and contemplate. I thought, *How do you apply epistemology?*

Well, you can do it through psychology. I remember my father saying, so many times, "When you're a physician. You have the right to do anything. With a medical license, society gives you the right to teach without a PhD, to work in the pharmaceutical industry without pharmacy training, to be anything you want to be."

I thought, the people who do clinical trials on medications on the brain are psychiatrists; psychologists don't have that license to use medications. If I really want to pursue applied epistemology, I gotta take it the whole route and be an MD psychiatrist. And so, in a relatively short time, I decided that, and decided to become a psychology premed. I went home on Christmas vacation and I told my dad, "Guess, what? I've decided to do psychology premed."

He didn't lift his eyes from the journal he was reading and said, "Okay."

Okay? He certainly deadpanned it. Everybody knew what a huge deal it was for him, because his first two sons had not gone into medicine.

You had an interest in psychiatry. Your mother had mental health issues. Did she have anything to do with your decision to become a psychiatrist?

Well, I never thought she did, but any good psychoanalyst would say, of course.

Are you saying that, too?

I really don't think so, but it's not in my awareness.

Tell me what medical school was like.

I hated it. In fact, I dropped out. I went into medicine thinking it would be a really interesting, intellectual pursuit. I found that the experience was extremely anti-intellectual, that it was a trade school, that it was cramming facts that you would accumulate by rote memory, and that inquiry was not a part of any of it. I was absolutely miserable. I made the decision in March of my freshman year to drop out. When I did, I felt wonderful. It was such a relief. I felt I had kind of been released from prison.

The medical school had a policy then that required you to actually get a psychological examination to make sure you weren't making some terrible mistake, so I had several interviews with senior faculty and had a psychological evaluation done to make sure I wasn't kind of doing something crazy, and everybody said, "This is definitely the right thing for you to do, so go take a leave of absence or whatever..."

It was a wonderful feeling when I realized I was sort of freed from this. When I was applying for my leave of absence, I had to meet with a number of people, one of whom was the Dean of the medical school.

He wrote me a letter. It said, "Dear Mr. Miller. You are hereby granted a leave of absence to Tulane Medical School At such time as you feel it would be in your best interest to return, please notify this office and you will be readmitted."

What I learned later, soon thereafter, was a small public scandal. He had interviewed to become Dean at another medical school and had accepted the position without telling Tulane. He was a lame duck when he wrote that letter, so he would not have to live with the results of it.

I was very young when I was accepted to medical school. I was 19.

Medical school at 19?

Yes. I got my acceptance letter four months after I turned 18.

Tell me how you pulled that off.

Well, my birthday's late, so I wasn't 18 when I got to Georgetown. And I had 30 credits by the time I showed up for my freshman year by doing various things to earn college credits. My sophomore year, I went to school for 12 months and completed 52 credits in 12 months at Georgetown. Then I realized that I had enough credits to graduate. So I was only at Georgetown for two and a half years, and then I applied to medical school. That's when I learned how flawed the whole selection process is.

I am named after my Godfather, who was one of my dad's classmates in medical school. He was on the admissions committee for the medical school. He was a loyal member of the Surgery Department.

I hadn't taken chemistry or biology until my second year at Georgetown. I took the M-CAT during my third year at Georgetown, which was my last. So I sat for the M-CAT six weeks into organic chemistry, six weeks into physics—with no other biology classes beyond freshman biology. I was up against biology and chemistry majors, and I made like a 760 out of 800 on science on the M-CAT. I knew at that point that standardized tests were unfair, that this process isn't right.

At that time, it was very hard to get into medical school. People were going to medical school in the Caribbean. I saw people slaving away to get 3.8 GPAs, who couldn't get into medical school. I had no knowledge of science. It measured my ability to take the M-CAT.

When I got to medical school, my lack of preparation made me almost flunk out because I didn't know science. I was completely unprepared, academically. All the classes in histology, microbiology, and biochemistry were review classes for my classmates—they'd taken these as undergraduate courses in college. I had no idea what was going on. I was completely lost.

But, I decided to apply to medical school because you could apply without a degree, after three years. I had all of the requirements, and so I applied. I didn't want to go to Tulane. I didn't want to follow in my father's footsteps—at least, I didn't want to be in his shadow.

I went through the interview process and at the end of the day, I had a meeting with the Dean of Admissions and he said, "Mike, do you want to come to Tulane?"

I said, "It's not my first choice. I'd rather go to Dartmouth."

He said, "Well, what do you want to do with your application?"

I said, "I submitted it and I came here to interview."

He said, "Well, let me just tell you what's going on. Your Godfather is breathing down my neck and if you tell me to process this application, it will be brought to the admissions committee on Tuesday and you'll get a call the next day, telling you you are accepted to Tulane Medical School. You have to tell me whether you want it processed or not."

I said, "I'm really sorry, sir. I am not responsible for the pressures you're facing. You have to do what you're gonna do. I'm not going to tell you to throw out my application. Submit it and we'll see what happens."

Next Wednesday, I got a phone call saying, "You're accepted to Tulane Medical School." I went with no science background, except freshman level courses.

But it doesn't end there. I went back and taught high school at my Alma mater and had a wonderful time. I learned how much I loved teaching. I taught ninth grade general science. I taught speech and drama in my second year of teaching. I taught a second-year biology class for the seniors.

This was a Catholic high school in my hometown. I really had a wonderful time and I had to take six credits every year in pursuit of a bachelor's in education in order to keep my provisional license or teaching license. I had to take education classes. That's how I came to Wisconsin because I didn't want to deal with the heat of Louisiana for summer school.

Then, I decided that to really be a high school teacher, I would have to take two years of classes to get a bachelor's of education. To teach college with psychology, I'd have to take probably four or five years for a PhD. As I sat, I was three years away from an MD degree. Now, how does that calculation turn out? To go back to school to get an MD degree, if I wanted to be a teacher the rest of my life, why don't I teach medicine instead of something else? That was a pretty easy decision, and I went back. Two years later when I decided it was in my best interest, I called the new Dean of Admissions.

"Hello. My name is Michael Miller. I have a letter that says, 'when it's in my best interest,' to contact you about reenrolling. Well, it's time."

They were livid. They were so unhappy that I had to jump through no hoops. I said, "I should brush up. I don't think I should just begin my sophomore year. Can I retake some classes for the freshman year? The spring semester starts Monday, doesn't it? I'll see you then." They were really unhappy. But I had the letter!

Do you think that previous dean did this on purpose, knowing he was leaving?

He was very kind and I think he wasn't hugely invested in the issue and it was certainly wonderful for me.

Okay, so you took that semester again. How did that semester go?

It went fine, because then I was like the other kids. I had taken the class before. Not as an undergrad, but two years before as a med school freshman. The material was like a refresher and an expansion, and I could actually study and learn things and do some independent research and some extra projects and sort of embellish it, because I had a foundation. That was fine. That was fun.

So you didn't hate medical school that semester?

I did not hate medical school. It was challenging. People now would not believe my academic record in medical school. It was far less stellar than one would expect. My career's been successful enough that people would probably think I was near the top of my class, when I was far from it. I had my struggles. I didn't feel like I really had things down pat until I'd been in practice for maybe a year. By then, I felt like I measured up with my peers. I had finally closed the gap, but it had taken a long time to feel like I was on the same lap on the race course as they were.

Did you ever feel you had an advantage growing up with a doctor, sort of learning things by osmosis?

Absolutely not. What I learned from my father was not taught to me directly, but I passively absorbed it and it shaped my career. We all know stories about people who go to law school without ever intending to practice law, because it opens so many doors. People don't appreciate that a medical degree does at least that much, as far as opening doors and allowing you to pursue a wide range of interest.

When I grew up—partly because my brothers were older and my mother was disabled with mental illness—my dad and I were best buddies. My identification with him on a personal level was very strong, and we were just incredibly close. Following in his footsteps is something that has been really important to me, but his footsteps were different footsteps than the average doctor.

My dad was a specialist and a generalist. For some reason, I remember two journals he read every month. He read *"Medical Economics."* He loved it. And he read *"Human Sexuality,"* because that's what he did in his profession. He read those in the chair in the living room at night, so he was a student all of his life.

But he did many things. He was the first chief of staff of the first big Catholic hospital in our town when it opened in 1950. He was the president of the state hospital association, as well as a leader of the state medical association and a member of the State Board of Medical Examiners. He was involved in organized medicine. That's what has shaped my career.

I have a very diverse professional life, and that's what prevents burnout. I work really hard, and I do get tired sometimes. But it's so stimulating, because I do so many different things every day.

You chose your specialty based on what reasons?

It was based on fascination. I was interested in neurosciences. That was my favorite basic science course, so neurochemistry, neurophysiology, and neurology were very interesting.

I didn't know anything about preventive medicine and public health. But when I took those classes, I actually thought of doing a residency in preventive medicine. I ended up doing what I came to medical school to do, which was to go into psychiatry. I did not go into it thinking addiction would be my sub-specialty.

I happened to have tremendous good fortune. There was a program in the 1970s that the federal government had called the Career Teacher Program that was administered through the National Institute on Drug Abuse and the National Institute on Alcohol Abuse and Alcoholism. There were 65 faculty members chosen nationwide to learn more, do research, and to teach. I had four of them for my teachers; one in medical school, two in residency, and one in fellowship. That's just a roll of the dice, and it was incredible.

When I was in medical school, I took an elective with a psychiatrist because I thought he was really good and that I would learn psychiatry from him. But I had no idea he worked in addictions. When I took my rotation with him, I tagged along with him as we would drive twice a week across Lake Pontchartrain to Mandeville, Louisiana, to this unit where he had 30 inpatients, who were doctors, nurses, and pharmacists doing group therapy about their addictions. Watching him do intake interviews in a group, three patients would come in together for an interview with him. It was absolutely fascinating. And it was my first exposure to group therapy, and to family therapy and addiction.

When I went into residency again, I was going to be a general psychiatrist. But it happened that there was a rotation in Milwaukee, at the DePaul Hospital, which was an addiction hospital, one floor of which was for impaired professionals. And I sat in on group therapy with the doctors.

I transferred from Milwaukee to Minneapolis to finish my residency, because I wanted to do consultation liaison psychiatry, which is being on the medical wards, seeing medically ill patients with psychiatric problems.

But when I got ready to pick my fellowship, I had a choice between addiction and consultation liaison. I had an opportunity to work with an internationally known psychiatrist who worked with the World Health Organization, to be his first fellow in chemical dependency. He had been one of those career teachers himself, as well. I said, *You know, I'm going to do this.*

My first job at the Midelfort Clinic was as a general psychiatrist. But I said, "I'm going to do addiction on the side because I know how to do it."

They said, "We don't care. We don't know what it is. Be a psychiatrist and that's fine."

I did that for six years at a multi-specialty group. After five years or so, I went to the medical director and said, "There've been times when I've spent 75% of my week in addiction, and I think I can do it a 100%. I can make this work for the clinic. I won't be a financial drag on the group. I want to leave the Psychiatry Department and do addiction, full-time."

He said, "We own our own HMO. We have this huge patient population to take care of. We can't lose workforce potential in psychiatry. You have to do psychiatry, if you're working here. No, you can't do this."

I said, "Thank you very much. I'll find a place that will let me."

I found a job where I could do addiction medicine full-time, and that's how I got to Madison.

As addictions go, is alcohol the name of the game as you divvy them all up?

The legal drugs are the real killers; not the illegal ones. The public health problem is the ones that are socially condoned. The one that kills more than all of them is tobacco. The one that kids start first is tobacco. The gateway drug to all other addictions, without any debate, is tobacco, so nicotine addiction is the biggest public health problem. It kills four times as many people as alcohol. The number one killer of alcoholics is not alcohol. It's not cirrhosis. It's not accidents. It's tobacco. More alcoholics die of tobacco-related cardiovascular disease than of their drinking.

If you take nicotine out of the equation, alcohol's a much bigger killer than all the other drugs combined. It's more prevalent. It causes more organ damage.

Normal people evolving into addiction is probably overblown because your predispositions are largely set. Our constitutional culture and environment play a role, and one of the bits of evidence is that coexisting psychiatric conditions make a big difference in the development of addiction, and even your path of recovery and your prognosis.

A lot of this is not just what you learned growing up, but the genes you were born with. The public health message is to recognize what addiction is, and what the warning signs are, when it begins to show itself in them.

A normal person who develops problems changes his behavior and stops. People who don't stop in the face of problems—there's something unusual about that. And it's really hard for the person experiencing it to recognize that it's happening to them, because they always want to tell themselves, "This isn't happening to me."

If you're a male offspring of a male alcoholic, and you're beginning to use in your teenage years, and you develop blackouts where you are awake and walking and talking and not passed out, but the next day you don't remember all the details, like where you parked the car, how you got home, who you were with, and who you had a phone conversation with. If you're a son of an alcoholic male, and have blackouts when you drink, that's a problem—you may need to not drink. If you're the son or grandson of an alcoholic male, and you can drink your friends under the table when you're young, if you're the one who always drives people home because you didn't get drunk {and they did} with significant amounts, then that's a danger sign.

If you're a parent, try to delay the onset of alcohol and drug use for your kids, because that makes a difference. Early onset of use is not a good prognostic sign.

In the older years, when people respond to losses by filling in the gaps with intoxication, that's a danger sign. After the loss of a spouse, after retirement, people sometimes begin drinking more out of boredom, out of whatever, to deal with the pain of the loss. That's not an adaptive response to those normal life events.

But a lot of times you don't recognize it in yourself, and it requires being open to the messages from others. And, again, part of the natural process is to reject those, or blame the messenger, or what have you.

The message in society in general is to be honest. Be honest with yourself and be honest with others. If you have a friend or a loved one who you think is developing problems related to their substance use, don't finesse it, don't ignore it. Be honest and say, "I'm really concerned about you. This doesn't look like a usual pattern. I'm concerned this could be affecting your health. I love you and I want you to have many long years ahead. Would you be willing to talk to your doctor about this?"

We all play a role in it and we're all enablers of people. It's part of the natural course of things. If we can help people and don't cover up for them, and don't deny it's happening, that's important. It goes against natural tendencies.

Well, the person who has three or four or five drinks a day and seems to be fine, may, in fact, be fine. Quantity and frequency don't make the difference. It's the quality. It's the relationship with the drug. It's the role the drug plays in their lives. It's the central position it takes. It's the way it's used as a coping mechanism.

I notice how your personality changes. I notice how your speech changes, how your demeanor changes, how your relationship changes. I notice the centrality, how this is taking an important part of your life. I notice that you make a choice to let this go, but you stay attached to your substance. You'd rather smoke pot than be at your kid's ballgame. That doesn't seem okay. It was fun for all of us when we were 19 and 21, but that's not the way it goes when you're 31 and 41.

"This looks to me like this might be interference. It's getting in your way."

Doctors in general, and there's tons of literature on dysfunctional workplaces by physicians, which comes from not being open and honest and just saying something. Doctors are very hesitant to say something to their peers about anything. We bury it. We try to finesse it. I recognize that it's natural. I'm not too critical of people trying to finesse it. But I know the outcome of trying to finesse it, when it's past the point of finessing.

You see some follow in their parents' footsteps and do what they saw, who actually began using in their teen years because the parents weren't parenting effectively. They don't give their kids the message that it's not okay. Part of the reason that it's transmitted in the family is that the addicted parent is not an effective parent, and the kids develop their own use patterns. Part of why kids acquire it is because it's normative. They heard yelling, so they yell. All these sorts of things are learned behaviors.

But Steve, what I see are tons of people who grow up in these families and say, "God, it was hell for me and I never want to be there." And genetics takes over, and when I work with my patients, so often it happens and you really have to work with this problem. We get to the point in the therapy—"This is really tough because you see yourself becoming your mom, don't you? And you hate that, and didn't want that."

To accept that you have this problem means you have to accept that you have your parents' disease. That's the last thing in the world you want to accept. In my experience, a lot of times, genetics overcomes the social psychology and the person who never drank, or never used drugs who never wanted to be like mom or dad, or even aunt Sally {long sigh}, finds themselves in that situation.

Young early adopters aren't addicted yet. I will, occasionally, in line at the grocery story, comment to a kid who's buying tobacco. "Is this really what you want?" It's totally socially unacceptable to get in the face of a stranger, but I do that.

But the ones who are addicted, it's just so sad. Even for nicotine addiction, the genetics is trumping the behavioral and social parts. The biology is winning. A lot of what we're finding is that the ones who have stopped are the ones who are able, and the ones who haven't are the ones who can't. This residual population of smokers is largely addicts, and they need help. They need biological treatments. They need medication to stop, and they need a comprehensive long term plan. The percentage rate of smoking in the general population is down to the low 20s.

The interesting thing about nicotine is that as it's becoming more accepted as an addiction, it's also becoming like {other} addictions in that people are made to feel more guilty. A lot of smokers don't want to talk about it because they feel ashamed and they feel like you're just going to bitch at them about it. I look at smoking addicts with compassion. My God, it's so sad to see the power of this.

Our culture loves to demonize drugs and blame the substance and put all our energy on supply and control and interdiction and criminalization. The problem is much more than the illegal drugs. It's alcohol and tobacco.

What's the connection between smoking and drinking?

The connection between smoking and drinking is that both of them give you some euphoria. Tobacco has a little aspect of rule breaking. Kids that begin by being a little iconoclastic, begin with tobacco, and then move to alcohol, and then to marijuana. It's just part of the natural history in our culture.

Speaking of marijuana, what's your take on how society deals with illegal drugs?

I was listening to news radio in Madison. Heroin use is up. Let's interview the chief of police. My thought was, if heroin use is up in Madison, why aren't you interviewing somebody from medicine or public health? It's because we view this through the lens of criminality and anti-social behavior, rather than through the lens of this is a health care problem.

That summarized everything so much. People who talk about this in the schools are the policemen, not the doctors. That's our fault as physicians. We're not more involved in the community, and leaving the office and going out in the community and providing the public health talks ourselves.

I find myself, in my 50s, terribly disappointed that I'm losing some of my idealism and becoming a little more pessimistic. It's very atypical for me. I know the science is on our side. I know the economics is on our side. I know that the evidence of the health reform debates of the early '90s was very clear, with the way you improve the health status of the population, is to do early and effective interventions for alcohol and other drug dependence. That it's cost-effective, and is the way you keep people out of hospitals and emergency rooms. To lower health costs overall is to treat alcohol and drug addiction early and effectively. We can do it.

If we take a public health approach to this and don't overemphasize the criminal justice approach, we can get wonderful results. I have that optimism, but our overall culture has so glorified the free market, and free market approaches to health care.

I'm pessimistic about our ability to have the health system reform we need in this nation, pessimistic that our nation cares about the uninsured. I'm concerned that caring for the needy is something we're moving away from. Because of something the sociologists call downward drift, when you're disabled by severe mental illness or by addiction, your socioeconomic status drops due to the illness. People that weren't destitute become that way because of the illness.

I am discouraged, in this world of evidence-based medicine, when we're told to make choices about what to do based on the evidence. My field, addiction medicine, has tons of evidence. Purchasers of health care plans don't want to look at it. Employers don't want to look at it.

The amount of money you could save by doing treatment in lieu of incarcerations, and reducing the prison population and the taxpayers' expenditures on incarceration, the data are clear. I feel comforted that I work in the world where the evidence is on my side.

There are many who believe we will leave the dark ages of stigma against addiction the way that stigma was addressed for other conditions. When biomedical research understood what cancer was and developed treatments that were effective, stigma dropped. When people had treatments for AIDS and they could work, it stopped being a death sentence to get a diagnosis. Some of the stigma dropped. When epilepsy was understood to be an electrical disturbance in the brain, rather than demonic possession, stigma dropped.

Stigma will go away with addiction probably the way it's gone away with other things—clear evidence of a biological basis, clear evidence of effective treatments and mainstream treatments which involve pharmacologic therapies. Addiction is on the cusp of all those.

New medicines are being developed through basic research every year. Brains of addicts are different, even when they're not under the influence. Scientific understanding is gonna lead our way out of ignorance. Part of the negative attitudes and therapeutic pessimism comes from unique and inappropriate ways that treatment outcomes are judged and evaluated. And, absurd and inappropriate standards for success apply to this treatment, compared to other treatments.

Would I want any of my kids to do this, to practice addiction medicine? You bet. It's just so unique to work with people so personally in their time of need. Over a century ago, they said if you know syphilis, you know medicine. Now, I'd say, if you know alcoholism, if you know addiction, then you know medicine—because it affects everything.

What young people need to know is that if they choose medicine as a profession, financial rewards can come their way—but not as much as in business or in some other areas. Intellectual rewards can come their way that are unparalleled. The personal rewards are unique because of what happens in a doctor/patient relationship—maybe similar to being in the clergy.

Chapter Twenty-Two

Sick, Huddled Masses

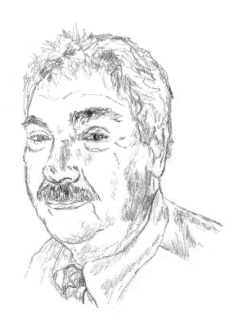

"In the United States, we have a wonderful health care system, but we don't have a fair health care system. The system is crashing, slowly, but inevitably."

George Schneider, MD
Internal Medicine, Milwaukee

Visiting the Greater Milwaukee Free Clinic is like walking back in time. It's as if it was preserved from the 1970s, even though this space had been a private practice doctor's office until the early 1990s.

The carpet is drab, the chairs are worn and the other furnishings are a mish-mash of donated stuff that fills the gap. Even the clock on the wall has a pharmaceutical company name emblazoned on it, as do other free supplies. The office has "crappy file cabinets," according to Dr. George Schneider, the medical director, but he's grateful for them and all of the other donations, because they allow him to help people who are not getting medical care.

When you're sick and have nowhere to go, you probably don't give a damn about these frivolous details. Patients come here in droves twice a week to receive care from the dozens of physicians, nurses and others who volunteer their services.

Although the doors don't open until 5:00 p.m., Dr. Schneider says it's not unusual to have somebody waiting at 3 o'clock. By the time the clinic opens, a crowd is huddled in front of the building.

Schneider, who's in his mid 60s, founded the Free Clinic with his wife, Kathleen, in 1995. He sees its popularity as a bellwether for the failings in our current health care system. When we spoke, his cluttered, private practice office was in the same building, down the hall from the Free Clinic. Kathleen is the receptionist, in addition to being a key player in keeping the Free Clinic alive.

Doctor Schneider, seated behind his wooden desk, looking over piles of paper, tells me about the patients who never get a bill from him and how he's come to help them.

The Free Clinic had been a physician's office. When we were looking for a site 11 years ago, we were looking for a space equipped for a physician's office. It's convenient, being right next door, because I can do things during the day that benefits the clinic and me.

Why were you interested in volunteering your services?

Growing up, the idea of doing something charitable was something that went on in our family. I was born in Milwaukee, and went to Milwaukee Public Schools. I was an only child. My mother stayed at home; didn't work. She was from Northern Wisconsin, from a small farm in a small town, and it seemed to me there were always people coming to the house and staying for a while, who were moving from northern Wisconsin to the city. They heard about her. They stopped in, maybe had a meal. Maybe spent a few nights. I remember my mother giving things away.

"Here are some clothes. Here are some pots and pans and plates and pencils, to help get you started."

My father was a garbage man who worked for the City of Milwaukee, but he also had an interest in real estate and had multiple duplexes in town. Some of his tenants were not always very timely in paying their rent, but he let them stay. He did not evict anybody. There was always that background in our house about doing things for people who were kind of down on their luck. The free clinic maybe was a natural evolution of that.

How did medicine become an interest of yours?

My mother died when I was 13, rather suddenly, so that was always in the back of my mind. In school, I always liked science. Actually, when

I went to college, I was planning to be an engineer, until I took math and calculus courses. I did alright in them, but I really had to work to get a good grade in it. The science part—that came easy. I liked that, so that was another reason I drifted toward medicine. It was science, without all the math. But there were no family members in medicine, no connection with any particular doctor.

I went to Ripon College, a liberal arts college. The classes were small, and PhDs taught them. I started out going to Marquette University School of Medicine, but during the second year, Marquette dropped the medical school. They couldn't afford to keep it open, so that was a somewhat unnerving factor during the rest of medical school. We didn't really know from day to day whether there would be a school there the next day. The doors might be locked. The school stayed open and I graduated from there. They changed their name to the Medical College of Wisconsin.

I had no preconceived notions that I wanted to be a surgeon or I wanted to be an obstetrician or whatever. A lot of it became a process of elimination. Some days I liked surgery as a student and a discipline, but surgeons have long hours and I thought, that's not for me. I always liked internal medicine. I liked the patients we took care of, the challenges, so that's how I ended up in internal medicine.

How did you end up at the free clinic?

At the time, I was on the Board of the State Medical Society and went to the meetings of the Medical Society of Milwaukee County. They had been approached by an out of town benefactor who wanted to donate a large sum of money and build a free clinic in Milwaukee, and was using the medical society as a kind of a spearhead to do that.

I met the clinic director from Roanoke, Virginia. My interest was sort of piqued. The Medical Society was working out the details of the free clinic with the benefactor. They were at the point of advertising for Executive Director, and had narrowed the field down to a dozen or so candidates. We were going to start interviews when the out of town benefactor died unexpectedly, and so the whole project came to a halt because of the question of funding.

A year or two later, the director from Roanoke came to the Society. My wife had just spent some time with a church group with kids from Appalachia, in rural Virginia, and kind of used that as a common ground, talking with this gal. My wife was in the office that day, and I introduced the two of them and they hit it off. Kathy spent the next couple of years working on getting a free clinic set up. Kathy's the one that makes it go. She's the executive director. She can do everything except treat patients. She's a medical technologist. But being married to a doctor, you pick up a lot of medical knowledge by osmosis. I'm just the one with the medical license who helps out.

Twelve years ago, if Kathy hadn't volunteered to do that, I don't think there would be a free clinic. There was no money available at the time, so it was all done by beg, borrow and…I don't want to say steal… The Medical Society helped with donations in kind, putting articles in the newsletter, and helping with mailing lists and stuff.

The estate of the original benefactor did a matching grant of $25,000, so the initial funding was basically from private donations from physicians and the estate of the donor in Virginia.

How many patients to do you see here?

Last year, we saw about 1,930 patients. The volume has probably increased by about 25% a year over the last several years. Volume has increased over the past several years, compared to the first seven years of the clinic.

Does that worry you?

Yeah, it's a concern because the very existence of free clinics is a reflection on the whole health care system. The system is breaking, and it's broken in some areas. So yeah, it's nice to say your numbers are going up, but not at the free clinic.

One of our original goals when we started back 10 years ago was for the clinic to go out of business, but it doesn't look like that's going to happen anytime soon. We see more immigrants who come to the clinic. We see more working people whose employers are making them pay more of the premium and the cost is prohibitive. It's basically, a question of fairness and justness.

The current model based on employment isn't working. In my practice, I see people whose deductibles are going up. The employers' paying less and less their share of the premium, and so more of my patients are raising issues of cost and testing and primary care services, especially drugs.

Covering the uninsured is an issue society has to deal with. That number keeps rising every year, and society—and politicians—sort of dance around the issue and nobody really does anything. The uninsured, that's not really a group of people anybody is looking to take care of and get their support and vote.

Single payer is really the way to go. Whether that's national health or some other model, I don't know. I don't have enough knowledge to answer that question. I feel the current system with private insurance companies—that's a very expensive system. The overhead is high. Their overhead runs anywhere from 15 to 20%. Medicare runs with three or 4% overhead. You could cover all the uninsured on savings from administrative costs alone, so it is worth considering.

Will it happen?

I think, slowly. The system is crashing, slowly, but inevitably. More and more people are complaining about it, everything from the uninsured poor to those who are working, who have insurance. The deductibles are higher, and the co-pays are higher.

We give everybody who comes in an envelope for a totally voluntary contribution. The money we collect from the patients pays the phone bill. The funds go toward rent, and utilities. We have to purchase supplies and some medications, and not everything is donated. A lot of the basics we have to purchase.

Some nights there's nothing. Once in a while, somebody will slip a twenty or a fifty in the envelope, but that doesn't happen often. The average collection each night is maybe twenty dollars.

You're not saying $20 for the whole night, are you?

Twenty dollars for the whole night. There might be a dollar or two in one envelope. One time, I suppose somebody thought it was funny, there was a penny in there, so somebody gave their last red cent! {Smiles}

For donations, what do you need?

It's money or personnel, actual volunteers—medical people, nurses, or non medical people who are willing to come as a receptionist. West Allis Hospital has been very generous in donating services over the years; ancillary services—lab and x-ray. When we've needed somebody to be hospitalized, they've donated the hospitalization. Social workers work with us and the patients to see what program they qualify for, because at that point they're so sick they usually do qualify for some program.

The clinic's open two nights per week. When we first started, we had one physician working. But because of the volume increase over the past two years, I've gone there pretty much two nights per week to work along with the regular physician of the night, and probably working three to three and a half hours a night.

The doors don't open until five, but lots of times there's somebody sitting out there at three. We have 20 chairs in the waiting room and they're usually all filled. We start seeing patients around six and we leave when we're done. An early night, we might get out by 8:30. Some nights we're there until 10 or 11.

I still work in my office on those days in the mornings. In the afternoons, I don't see patients, but lots of times I'm here doing non-patient related jobs. I'm ordering medications. I'm cleaning things up in my practice. Sometimes things just don't go right. It can be very frustrating.

Who are these people who come to the free clinic?

The typical patient we see reflects my practice—an adult with hypertension, diabetes, smoking, bronchitis, or arthritis. It's really the working poor. Our mission statement says that we see low income, working, uninsured people—people who fall through the cracks, those that don't have health insurance, but they make a little more money and they don't quality for other programs.

We see a lot of people who work part-time jobs, who maybe earn $15,000 a year and live on that. Some of them work multiple part-time jobs. Some have full-time jobs, but they can't afford the insurance that's offered, or maybe insurance just isn't offered.

Benefits aren't provided for those who work for a temp agency. We see people who—and this is a situation we've become more aware of recently—who qualify for medical reasons, qualify for disability, and get on social security and disability, so that raises their income, which in turn, disqualifies them from participation in government programs because their income went up. We do see more and more people chronically unemployed, chronically not working.

Have you had cases where there's no way you could handle them at your clinic?

Once in a while, we see patients with fairly far advanced cancers, or chronic diseases like cirrhosis of the liver. We had somebody come in with a newborn baby, just a few weeks old. Fortunately, there was a primary care doc on that night who recognized that this kid was really sick. I'm not sure that an internist or somebody that doesn't deal with kids would have known that. We referred them over to Children's Hospital and got word back that the patient was hospitalized with pneumonia. If they hadn't come to the clinic that night, that child might not have survived.

We've had one or two people walk into the clinic having a heart attack. We've had a couple people come in with acute appendicitis. We had to put him in the back of the car and take him to the emergency room and get him admitted.

We had another lady who came to the clinic and there were 10 steps, and she couldn't make it up the steps. She could only go up two steps. I wasn't working at the clinic that night, but happened to be in my office. My wife asked if I could take a look at this lady, so I was examining her on the stairs and she was obviously, seriously ill. I ended up admitting her to the hospital, much against her wishes. She didn't have any insurance and she knew that hospitals are expensive. She ended up being diagnosed with a very serious problem. She got care, which extended her life, but she eventually died from an incurable condition that could only be cured with a transplant. But she didn't want that.

I saw this patient who had lost his job and noticed some swelling in his abdomen. He went to another physician, and was told, based on the examination, that, "You have cancer. You're going to be dead in two months." So this guy was just going downhill from already being down and depressed. We asked a few questions. Where were you? Who said this? He was a little vague, so we ordered the $800 x-ray.

He didn't seem that ill, just very depressed. He was kind of getting ready to die. We did a CT scan of his abdomen, and there was nothing wrong with him, so we told him that, gave him the good news. It kind of turned his life around. He was ready to cash in his chips and die. He never came back to the clinic, so I assume he went out and got a job.

There are certain things we don't do at the Free Clinic. We don't prescribe narcotics, controlled substances, or Viagra, or those types of products. We don't treat any venereal or sexually transmitted diseases, because the City of Milwaukee has a clinic that we can refer to. We'll screen for veterans, especially if they have any major problems, and will refer them to the VA. That doesn't happen often, but when it does, and you can tell them they're eligible for care, that's great.

People will come in here with kids. Well, they're eligible for Badger Care.* One of the great questions we've found for screening, is, "How much rent do you pay?" The average is probably four or five hundred dollars a month. If somebody's putting down eleven hundred dollars a month, that's a real signal that goes off right away. *Hmm, you pay eleven hundred for rent? You're getting income from some place.*

The receptionists are seeing patients coming to the Free Clinic. They all have a cell phone and a pager. A lot of them have multiple piercings. A lot of the ladies have very nice manicures. Some of them have nice tans. It has to go through your mind. It goes through my mine. And tattoos—let's not forget the tattoos. You have no money for your medical care, but you have money to buy your cigarettes everyday, pay your cell phone bill, and probably your cable bill at home, and get these tattoos.

Once in a while, I'll step back and say, "What's wrong with this picture?" Especially when we have volunteer medical students at the clinic, there have been several times when I've had patients and a medical student in the room observing. It must have been a rough day in medical school that day, she just looked beaten down and worn out, but she came to the clinic. The patient we were seeing was a young woman her age, who basically had a bad cold. She had the tattoos, the cigarettes, the piercings, the all-over tan. Here's one kid killing herself, wracking up debt, and here's another, her contemporary, who's coming to the free clinic, looks like she's having a good time. You try not to be judgmental and sometimes it's hard, but you keep trying.

Your daughter's a doctor. Is she following in your footsteps?

She's an anesthesiology resident—a resident at the Medical College of Wisconsin. As she was growing up, we never discouraged her from going into medicine. Probably from junior high on, she said she wanted to go into medicine.

At dinner once, she said, "Dad, I don't know how you do it. You see

---

* BadgerCare is Wisconsin government program that provides healthcare for the working poor.

these patients. They weigh 300 pounds. They smoke. Their blood sugar is 300. They don't take their medicines. They're not complying. How can you do that day after day, month after month?"

Anesthesia was a good choice for her. It's a quick concentrated experience with a patient, and she realized that. If she decided in medical school she wanted to do primary care, I might have discouraged that. By the time you spend all that money for tuition and supplies, books, and kind of deny yourself income from another job, medical students have a high debt burden when they graduate. Then primary care, the reimbursement, the rewards, are probably not commensurate with the amount of effort, time and debt that's been put into doing that.

Part of the problem with family practice is the hassle factor, the outside influences. Everybody wants to get a piece of the doctor. Everybody wants medical care provided and nobody wants to pay for it, or pay as little as possible for it. I really worry about the future of medicine with the influence of outside forces—businesses, insurance companies, these third party payers, government intrusion.

Despite all these problems, you still provide free care. How much satisfaction do you derive from that?

It's a great feeling to see somebody who comes in who's not feeling well, who's not doing well, who is sick—and you're able, with just an examination and some testing and interpretation of the results, to cheer them up, and get them feeling better. You get a real high from that.

By and large, most patients are appreciative. We had a patient who was new to this country. She was from Russia; a lady in her 50s who came to the clinic with a lump in her breast. She had mammograms and was diagnosed with cancer. She was referred to a surgeon, who volunteered his services for the clinic and did a mastectomy. She got into the system, as far as follow up with an oncologist and radiation therapy. We hadn't seen in her in a while, but she came back nine months, maybe a year later, with a bouquet of flowers for Kathy and me and a big thank you note.

They're grateful, but we've noticed an attitude develop over the past few years, kind of an entitlement mentality. You give somebody something and they want more. That's very discouraging for volunteers, and being at the free clinic it gives us a little freedom to say, "No, we don't have it. That's all you get." Some people we've kind of told, "We don't want you to come back here anymore. Go someplace else." We might be free, but we're not stupid. That's just a small minority, but it only takes one a night to ruin the whole night for everybody.

We've fired patients from the clinic just because we don't want one bad apple to ruin it for everybody else. The volunteers see that, and it typically happens with a new volunteer, and it's easy to say, "I don't need this. I'm not coming back here. These people are abusive. I could be doing other things."

Everybody who works at the Free Clinic donates their time. There are about 45 physicians who volunteer directly at the clinic, and another probably 20 or 30 specialists who've agreed to see people over the years. All the specialists have donated their services over the years—surgeons, oncologists, gastroenterologists, cardiologists.

Do you recruit them?

Some are recruited, but it's mostly word of mouth. They pretty much come from all over the area. The physicians who have come to the clinic over the years have had very high retention rates. Those who've left have basically done so for health reasons or age; they retired or they died.

Over half the people we see are ongoing care. One of the drawbacks of the clinic is they may see a different physician when they come back. But in some ways, that's a benefit because another physician may look at it differently and say, "That's not working, so let's just try…"

Even if you have free staff, how can you afford to pay for drugs?

One of the things that I do outside clinic hours is order medications from the pharmaceutical companies for poor patients. They do supply meds, usually a 90-day supply of medications, but it takes a little effort to fill out the forms and have somebody fax them in. I probably spend several hours per month doing that.

We probably get at least $50,000 to $75,000 in medications per year, and probably end up with another $75,000 a year worth of medications from samples.

How do patients know about the Free Clinic?

It started out as word of mouth. We always had patients, except the first night we were open. Social service agencies find out about us. Local emergency rooms routinely give out a list of free clinic names and addresses to patients who don't have insurance who need to go somewhere for follow up.

Probably 20 or 30% come from this area, but we've seen people from all over. Kathy has helped mentor nine other free clinics in the area, and we've met with these people over the years. In Oconomowoc,† you wouldn't think there'd be a need for a free clinic, but they have a lot of new immigrants there, especially in the summer. They have a lot of migrant workers in farm areas, so they have a need.

Is the demand going to keep increasing?

I think so, until something is done. In the United States, we have a wonderful health care system, but we don't have a fair health care system.

† Oconomowoc is an upscale southern Wisconsin city with a population of 12,400.

The resources aren't going to the people that need them. You see the people who need it the most, but can't get it because they don't have insurance. It's a fairness issue more than anything.

Given such obstacles, how long can you keep this up?

I probably could retire now if I really wanted to. But I would not be happy out on the golf course three days a week, or sailing my boat. If I retired tomorrow, I'd probably spend more time volunteering at the Free Clinic or some other similar place.

Editor's note: To make a contribution to the Free Clinic, see the links section at www.white-coatwisdom.com.

Chapter Twenty-Three

Bleeding Money

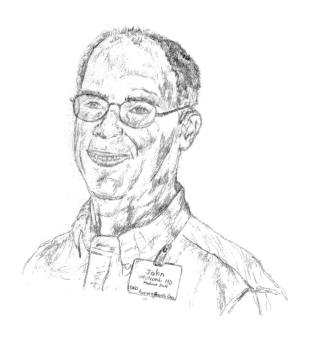

"I made a gamble and came to a hospital that was losing $32 million {per year}. Two years ago, we lost $16 million. Last year, we're slated to have lost 12, but we had a variance and we only lost 9."

John Whitcomb, MD
Emergency Medicine/Internal Medicine, Milwaukee

The world of ER medicine is rather bizarre from an economics standpoint, as well as downright wasteful. Anybody can go there for any reason, whether he or she can pay the bill or not. It's the law. Such is the dynamic doctors like John Whitcomb must deal with in Milwaukee's inner city, and everywhere else.

This afternoon, Dr. Whitcomb's ER is not the bustling place typical of most emergency rooms. In fact, it's rather quiet here and there are plenty of empty seats when he strolls out to the waiting room to welcome me. Whitcomb, in his mid 50s, is a passionate guy at work and at play. "I have, oh, 500 different kinds of Hosta, each of them are labeled," he tells me. "You

begin to understand obsessive compulsive when you come into my yard."
We talk in one of the exams rooms about the innovative and controversial
approach he spearheaded to more effectively save lives and money.

In the inner city, we're doing health care the most expensive way possible because we allow young people to go without primary health care, never get their diabetes cared for, or never get their hypertension treated. Instead of being a mild hypertensive who's taking one pill a day for years and years, your blood pressure spirals out of control and you find yourself on dialysis by age 30.

We have an epidemic of dialysis in the inner city. I can't tell you how many cases I see of the young folks who are coming to the ER as their site to get dialysis. When somebody comes to the ER with renal failure, he has to be admitted to an intensive care unit. It can cost hundreds of thousands of dollars a year, when it could have been $500 a year on hypertensive medication. Society won't pay for the antihypertensive, so now it has to pay for the dialysis. This is insane.

The parody is what television makes of ER, and what really happens in the ER. I've been waiting for 30 years, and I've yet to have a beautiful nurse jump out of a closet and kiss me on the lips! The sexually charged office clearly is just a way of drawing an audience. Nurses, as a general rule, are just the sweetest people on earth. We have fun talking about our families. We're like a family ourselves, so you're working with people you really like to work with. You have a common bond because you're on the team together.

Just before you came in, for example, I was having all the staff in the ER celebrating with me because they had gotten a heart attack patient in and out and to the cath lab* in under 20 minutes. The American Heart Association's goal is under 90 minutes.

We used to look at our processes from the perspective of reviewing failures. "Why did it take you two hours to get this patient there?" When human beings get a query like that, it's sort of like when the police stop you and ask, "How come you were going 80?" You really want to flip the police the bird, because you're just so mad you got caught and you're irritated. You don't change your behavior by negatively oriented queries. You don't improve significantly by chasing your failures.

What we've done in our ER is only track the best, and we post it. We post the name of the tech, the secretary, the nurse, the doctor and say,

---

* Catheterization involves inserting a thin, flexible tube, or catheter, into an artery or vein in the patient's arm or leg. It can help determine what is wrong with a patient's cardiovascular system or be used as a form of treatment for coronary artery disease.

"Tell me how you did it? And congratulations, you were the very best this month." We have about 12 diagnoses, and if you get a best in any one of those, you get your name up and get a little bag of M & Ms. You get bragging rights for the month. Everybody has to ask, "How'd you do it in 20 minutes?" And you get to tell. We all want to be there, so we have a little competition going here. You get so good at taking care of heart attacks. You get so good at taking care of pneumonia. But to get to the point of excellent, a shift toward real excellence, you've got to get playful. You've got to have a little spirit of competition in play. You're looking for the opportunity to give somebody a high five.

In our professional pursuit, we're trying to find the solutions to the health care crisis in the inner city. The ER isn't the best place to provide primary care solutions. We're on a Holy Grail hunt here. Every patient we see, we're trying to find a solution that isn't the ER. We'll take care of you in the emergent situation. We're the best place to take care of you when you're acutely sick. But what we're trying to do is find a place so you won't have to get sick again, and have someone to provide you an ongoing {medical} relationship for all your routine problems.

The traditional way that emergency medicine has been working here in America doesn't make sense to me. But the house of emergency medicine has been resistant to looking at itself. What are we doing wrong?

In a good natured attempt, we have taken the position that we're society's safety net for medical crises. We'll take anybody and we'll help anybody. But that's reinforcing the behavior by saying that it's okay not to go to doctors' appointments.

There's something passive and reactive to a safety net, as opposed to being proactive and directed. Safety of our patients is our number one concern. That's exactly what we should be concerned about, but our patients don't really know what's best for them. That's why they're coming to a doctor. But the doctor has an obligation larger than just the problem at hand. We should be thinking about the whole scope of the person's life, medical problems and risks.

We've had a collapse of the social safety net in the health care systems. There aren't alternatives for some people, but there are more than you think there are. Some safety net patients, such as Medicaid patients, use emergency departments just because they can. There's no cost to them.

Can't you refuse to treat somebody like that?

Ah, actually, you can't. There's federal law that says everybody in America has a right to be evaluated at a hospital's emergency department to see if an emergency exists. If one doesn't exist, the law no longer applies. So what's an emergency? Nobody's ever answered that question. We've tried. The house of emergency medicine has said an emergency is what a prudent layperson would define as an emergency. So if I get 12 prudent and reasonable people, and ask them, what's an emergency? They will give you answers. We did that when we came here. We did focus groups and we found out from folks that you shouldn't use an emergency room for a cold. You shouldn't use it for a work excuse or a little backache or headache. You should never come here in place of a doctor's appointment. It's really criminal if you use an ER to get drugs. Yet, 50% of the people in many urban ERs are using it for those reasons.

A lady came and she had a rash. I asked her how long she had the rash. She said, "All my life."

"So why did you come to see me?"

"My dermatologist is out of town."

"When did you see him last?"

"Two weeks ago."

'So when are you going to see him next?'

"Oh, next week."

I said, "Explain to me why you think I would know what's going on with your rash, if your dermatologist who's followed you for how many years can't tell you?"

My assumption is that when {a patient} is having an asthma attack, he's really having a catastrophe going on because he {should have} access to an allergy doctor, or pulmonology doctor, or an internist who's been following him. His coming to the ER means something bad happened. He got pneumonia, at which point I'm the best place in town.

But that's not what's happening in many of our ERs. Thousands of people come to the ER every six to eight weeks to have their asthma cared for because they take their medication until the first prescription runs out. Then, they wait until they get in trouble. They call the ambulance to come to the hospital again and go through another asthma attack.

Now, the literature says that if you study that population, they will have as much as an 800% increased chance of being admitted {to the hospital} and possibly dying, compared to folks who regularly see their primary care doctor and take their medication faithfully.

All the house of emergency medicine has said is we're the best place to take care of asthma attacks. Absolutely, but when people are using it for primary care, it's your responsibility to tell those patients the risk they're taking when they use the ER continuously.

You have to understand the environment we're working in and the human beings we are caring for. How do we teach people to use resources appropriately, when for years they have found their solutions in our ERs without any instruction about alternatives?

It costs a hospital about $800 for an emergency department visit. This includes the equipment, personnel, doctors, nurses, paper, towels, lights and security. Medicaid only pays $125. A hospital loses $675.

Primary care doctors are the right ones to go to for chronic illnesses.

For lots of other care, specialty doctors are the right people to see. America has some of the best medicine in the world, and now we also have some of the worst medicine. We have Third World medicine in America, because there are people who can't get access to anything except in the emergency room.

We have to find solutions here. America needs to put out a national health insurance policy for everybody, but we need to put a decision rule into it. It might mean "everybody gets vanilla." If you want more, you pay for chocolate. But vanilla may mean you don't get dialysis after some age like 65, which I believe is the limit in England. You don't have open heart surgery after age 75. We save lives and tangle ourselves up in all sorts of ethical dilemmas.

Instead of having sensible limits placed on end of life expenditures, we put in gastric feeding tubes. Then, we send people to the ER doctor, so we can work on their fever and replace their blocked feeding tube. We spend thousands of dollars taking care of people who have no meaningful chance of experiencing any happiness or quality of life, and we have no one to advocate for them to terminate medical care.

I would be furious if I was in that position and my family didn't speak on my behalf to protect me from what our medical system will do to you. We've always emphasized the rights of the disabled to be treated. We seem to have never considered the rights of those terminally disabled not to be treated. And then we claim we don't have the resources to give a measles shot to a baby? That's perverse. It's the ER that sees the insanity of those terrible dilemmas.

At some point we have to shift accountability to the individual. If somebody wants to pay for it, they can pay for it. But medicine is on a one way fiscal trip here and our trip has limits to it. None of us can live forever, so we need to make some ethical decisions about what those limits should be. Soon I'm going to be able to say, "I can transplant this into you. I can keep you alive until you're 110. It'll cost us $110,000. Now, if you don't have insurance, we'll just let society pay for it." Society can't keep doing everything.

The public already voted. They've said, "We don't want to pay more taxes." In Milwaukee, we elect a fiscally conservative Republican to be our county exec and he says, "We don't want to pay for mental health anymore." He's trying to close down the mental health unit and downsize that, and get the government out of it. Milwaukee's already succeeded in closing its public county hospital. What the voters are saying is they don't want to pay for medical care for everybody forever.

It's time to start naming what's happening, defining what we're willing to pay for as a society. But we do need to also start recognizing that in each of our families we have mentally ill people. Not paying for basic services ends up costing all of us much more. In each of our neighborhoods, we have friends, neighbors and family members who have needs for disability care. Each of us is only temporarily enabled, but are you willing to pay for another person's disability?

We need to start tying what we vote for to what we can pay for and provide. In society, we want to be more and more generous, but we don't know how to do it. Most cultures clearly define their limits to their social safety net. If you want more, you have to pay for it. Some countries do it openly and blatantly. In India, if you want blood, twenty bucks on the barrelhead and we'll transfuse you. That's the price of blood in a hospital that I know. You don't get the transfusion until you pay it.

You sound pretty familiar with India.

I grew up on a chicken farm in India. My grandparents were missionaries. My mother's dad went out as a GP {general practitioner} and became an eye surgeon, because that's what he found was needed. He was working in the very poorest parts of India. My dad was a chicken farmer.

I didn't come back to live here permanently until I was 18. My roots are on the Minnesota prairie. There were a bunch of farms just west of Byron, Minnesota, close to Rochester that family members used to own. I'm a little bit of a Midwestern guy, but I kind of took a detour far east of here.

Did that missionary experience have anything to do with your choice of professions?

I have no idea. I wasn't one of those kids who had a clear view of what I was going to do. I remember my guidance counselor in high school saying, "Oh, you'd make a good doctor. You ought to go to college and be premed."

I thought about that. A missionary surgeon in India, I remember, about seventh or eighth grade, he took all of us and made us scrub in and put on masks and gowns. We stood in the operating room while he took out an appendix. You couldn't do that in America today, but in India, that was sort of okay in the 1950s. It was thrilling, and then six or seven years later, he came back to America. He went to Madison and got an advanced degree in plastic surgery, and he was India's first plastic surgeon. He was working with leprosy and burns and all sorts of things. He was a strong influence on me.

Those are childhood influences, but I remember showing up at Johns Hopkins, where I went for college. I showed up 10 days before the term started. The guidance counselor said, "Where've you been?"

I said, "Well, traveling back from India."

"We thought you weren't coming."

What I didn't realize is that they had given away my spot.

He says, "Well, what do you want to be?" He looked mad, and I wasn't about to confront him, so I remember saying, "I don't know."

He said, "Premed or something?"

"Oh, sure." I was a premed student.

So at that point, you hadn't even decided if you wanted to become a doctor?

Heck no. A kid who grows up overseas undergoes an awful lot of culture shock. We feel like world citizens. We don't necessarily believe we're American citizens, because my childhood was growing up in India, which was extremely critical of the United States during Vietnam. I grew up with a very healthy dose of skepticism about some of our foreign policy, which continues to this day.

I knew how to study. British discipline in a British boarding school—by golly, I could study. I don't think I'm the brightest bulb on the tree, but I knew how to work. For me, it was an easy decision. Friday night, you went to study hall. The only kids there were my fellow Asian students at Johns Hopkins. I went to this big old, heavy-duty school, and I didn't have the best SAT scores. But after a year, I was one of only a few kids in the class who had straight A's, because I was willing to study. Well, that's what gets you into medical school—A's in chemistry and organic chemistry.

It wasn't hard, partially, I think, because I'd grown up in the world of possibilities. We traveled all around the world, three or four times, back and forth to America on furlough. I'd been given the gift of being taught how to work. I'd seen examples of parents who'd spent their childhood working against incredible barriers and finding solutions to them.

You see that same optimism in America, with people who grow up in Iowa, Kansas or South Dakota. Part of the optimism of America is that we have this "can do" attitude, and the Midwest is the best of it. We have lots of common sense folks in Wisconsin. We solve a lot of problems. Little ideas that you stick with, that make common sense, can change the world. You don't know when to cast your fate to the winds, or when that's going to connect, but somebody has to say, "Let's take this idea and do something with it."

When I went to Yale, we all had to work on a research project. I was running out of time and couldn't afford to spend six weeks in a clinic seeing patients. That clinic had a hideous reputation because you never had any relationship with patients. I was the student who said, "Why don't we hold clinic once a week? Then, we can see the same patients for two years and follow some patients, and everybody would have relationships."

Well, Yale was the first school to design an evening clinic. Now, there are many medical schools that do that. Yale has now had the 30th anniversary of its primary care clinic run by students—I was integral to starting that.

We had so many faculty members who were Nobel laureates. They'd done all these fantastic things, and you'd just have to say that you were in the midst of an awful lot of creative genius. But I really didn't have a good East

Coast experience. The optimism, friendliness, openness and willingness of anybody in the Midwest, to give you the time of day just doesn't happen on the East Coast. When you put human beings in a stressed environment, the East Coast is more congested and busier, and more dense—that's what happens when human beings get put in those environments. We have open spaces here. Whatever it is, we just have more possibilities.

What led you to the ER?

You marry a clergywoman and she follows you off to some little town in Iowa. When you finish your residency, she looks at you and says, "I followed you here. Don't you think you should stick with me, now?" She'd found a church in Iowa City, but the Public Health Service assigned me to an Indian Reservation in North Dakota. Holly said, "See ya. I can't go there. I don't have a career there."

I borrowed all the money and paid off the Public Health Service. I had a huge debt and there were only 100 million doctors in Iowa City, so I went to a town 90 miles away and offered to start an ER group for them. They said, great.

I drove to Ottumwa, Iowa. If you're in emergency medicine, Ottumwa is a special place because it's the home of "Radar" O'Reilly[†]—the ultimate triage officer. I discovered the thrill of taking care of sick folks. Emergency medicine sees all the sickest. You see a lot of others, too. I got adrenaline addicted.

Ottumwa had a John Deere factory for raking equipment. It was just a Midwestern agricultural county seat sort of place.

Emergency medicine's kind of fun because you got to know everybody. You knew every doctor in town. They knew you like the back of their hand. The nurses knew everybody in town, so you'd hear the EMS going to an address and the nurses would say, "Oh, that's Uncle Joe. He must be getting short of breath again because his emphysema's kicking up." We knew all the scandal, all the dirty stuff, and all the funny stories. In a small town like that, you realize that there's an intimacy that on one side is wonderful and on the other, kind of stifling. I fell asleep one day coming back from work. When you fall asleep while driving and find yourself in a corn field, you say, *This is a wake up call of the worst kind. I'll get killed if that happens again.* All I hit was a bunch of corn stalks. I fall asleep at about the 20 minute mark after night shift. I've got to live within 20 minutes of work.

We uprooted both of ourselves and moved to Milwaukee. Milwaukee had 25 UCC {United Church of Christ} churches, so that seemed like a good mix for Holly. We've been in Milwaukee now for 25 years. That's how we got to Milwaukee—cornfields and falling asleep.

[†] "Radar" was a character from the hit sitcom "M*A*S*H.

You went from a very small town to a rather large metropolitan area. That must have been a night and day experience.

Well, it was, because I came here on the faculty of the medical college. I came here to teach emergency medicine. I used to send people to the trauma center. Now, I'm suddenly at the trauma center.

I was only here two-thirds of the time and one-third of the time at the Medical College. The problem is, the Medical College in those days, you had to fly in the helicopter. It sounds like a lot of fun, until you find out that you're deadly airsick. Airplanes have a certain kind of motion to them, in two dimensions. Helicopters do it in all three dimensions because they go tipping, backing, rolling, yawing, and I couldn't do it.

The day the helicopter started was January first and all the big chiefs in the department signed up because they want to be the first people on the helicopter. Well, that year, 1983, we had a blizzard that lasted for about three days and the helicopter couldn't fly. And the first day it was clear, I'm the guy on. I got to be the first doctor in Milwaukee to fly on the helicopter. We had to fly to northern Wisconsin to pick up somebody who had broken her back and didn't want to come down in an ambulance across rough roads.

Every news channel in Milwaukee is there and I'm carrying a barf bag getting off the helicopter. That was a moment of discernment. Life was telling me something. I can't do helicopters. I flew on the helicopter about ten times and each time it was confirming. It was just humiliating, being so nauseated. I had to get back to work and I couldn't. It would take me a half day to get my middle ear back.

It was about nine months before I could find something else. Okay, so much for that false lead. But at that point, St. Luke's was thinking about going to a full-time emergency medicine, so I approached the administration there and they were very eager to have us come. I developed that program and started the first practice there. We expanded St. Luke's practice. The ER doubled in size in the 18 years that I was there.

Then, when you've done something for a while, you say, that's run its course. We did some research on what was happening elsewhere in America. Medicine in America needs a revolution. You have to keep saying what's right, and how to innovate. What's the proper way through? Let's sit back and examine what we're doing and be honest with ourselves.

With asthma, that single patient can be multiplied a million-fold. I've done that repeatedly with patients at this hospital. This hospital was losing $32 million per year three years ago, when I came here. I made a gamble and came to a hospital that's losing $32 million. Two years ago, we lost $16 million. Last year, we're slated to have lost 12, but we had a variance and we only lost 9. Okay, so this hospital's going to make it, which means we're still going to be in this community, still serving the folks who need access to care, as opposed to simply saying, we're out of business.

But you're still losing millions of dollars?

Nine million dollars, in bookkeeping. We're actually $10 million in depreciation, so we're really $1 million cash flow positive. Now, our hospital says we have a mission to be in the community, we're going to be here. The graph is now going down. Our good lines of business are now going up.

We saved something in the order of $16 million a year in this emergency department, in this single hospital. But that's not all we saved. We saved ten million a year for the Medicaid folks in Madison. So Madison says, "Can you do this in every ER in Wisconsin?" We said, "Of course, we can." Unfortunately, you have to convince the other hospitals that they want to do it, and they have to see it as a benefit.

Medicine changes very slowly, so we've got some slow leadership. We've got three or four other hospitals in the Milwaukee area starting to do it. Many of the emergency room doctors at other hospitals feel very threatened by what I'm doing, because they're saying, "Oh, they're just turning away poor people and making it harder for access to care."

Come talk to me. I'll tell you what we're doing. When I see somebody from Medicaid, I have many patients who come to me and say, "My doctor told me to come here." I go through the work of calling their doctor and saying, "I have your patient here. Would you like to see them in your office?" And you know what I find 90% of the time? The doctor says, "Send them right over. They never called here."

There are a lot of things doctors can handle in their offices. I wouldn't ask that question if it wasn't looking like a trivial situation. But it puts me in the position of, am I challenging the honesty and integrity of my customers? Yes, I am and I'm recognizing that one of the most horrible things about our entitlement programs are that with the best of intentions, when we want to save people from poverty and illness, when we give away something that's free, what we do is reinforce attitudes and behaviors that are destructive to the dignity of the human spirit.

What do human beings need who are using emergency departments? They need access to health care. There are lots of people willing to see them. If you just go on face value and say, "Oh, your doctor told you to come to the ER," you'll miss the entire story. You have to go through the time and the effort of checking and finding alternatives.

There are some people who are perfectly honest with you. "My doctor told me to come in because they were busy." Sometimes that's true. Or the doctor's front desk was really the barrier and the doctor didn't even know their patient was turned away. In that case, you have to create access points where they can go to for common problems like colds.

But you also need to have doctors in ERs say to patients, politely and appropriately, "The good news is that you aren't sick with an emergency. The bad news is we don't treat non-emergencies. There's nothing to treat. It'll get better on its own. If you want some medicine written for you, only your family doctor can write that. We want to teach you the right way to get your health care, where it's also cheaper for society and has a better outcome for you." We want to find those solutions, so people start bringing fiscal sanity back to our health care, so we don't lose our hospitals.

Here's a small idea. We're going to say if you don't have an emergency, we aren't going to treat you. We'll say, "We want to be here when your mother has a heart attack. We want our doors to be open and ready for when true emergencies arise."

When you walked in, did you realize there were only two or three people in the lobby? That lobby used to be jam packed. What's interesting is our patient satisfaction went from 20% to 46%. Forty-six percent of patients say, "This is the best experience I've had in an ER."

So the people who really need the care are getting in.

{He nods} If you fall off your bike and get a nasty cut on your leg, we get you in right away. We have a room waiting for you, and there's a doctor to care for you. With respect to the crisis in emergency rooms across the country, some of it is of our own making.

What about all those people who were coming here. Where are they going now?

Well, they aren't just going to other hospitals. They're not a single kind of person. There are different categories of patients who use the ER for a whole raft of reasons. The way we categorized them is by how many visits they make per year.

For example, if you categorize by frequency of use, you can say there are those who come more than 20 visits a year. There are some who come up as many as 109 times a year. Those who come more than 20 times per year are typically mentally ill, drug addicted, or alcoholic.

One example would be as follows: A 17-year old came in and the EMTs who were with her, were just steaming mad. Why? It was the fifth ambulance call she made that day, four different hospitals. {Sighs} This young lady is mentally ill. We don't have an information system in our hospitals to share her mental health issues and an effective plan of care with each other. I was the first person to put it on our internal system for her.

How come nobody's done this before? I went to the effort to find the phone number for her caseworker. When I got a hold of her, the case worker told me exactly what was going on in the patient's life. The second I identified that to the young girl that we were aware of her issues, she said, "Well, she can come pick me up. I'll go home." But basically she'd been flying around to hospitals all day long. Nobody else would pick her up. Our information system now picks her up every time and she comes here—about once per week.

That's one strategy for those folks who come to ERs very frequently. There's a similar one for those who come 10 to 20 times a year, who typically have chronic diseases—asthmas, high blood pressure, diabetes, the big heavies. Many of these folks are usually amenable to logic and resources. Many of them have doctors. Many of them simply haven't realized how risky it is to allow them to let their chronic illness get so out of control that they need to use an ER. So, the treadmill of coming to an ER has never been broken.

The third category is those who come here five to 10 times per year. Those folks are usually primary care patients. They come by when they have a rash or when they have an ache in a joint.

We've categorized our patients by different kinds of strategies. We have different strategies, in a sense, for all of them. Much of it comes down to information, teaching, directing to the right places, and taking care of people when they are sick. We're still an emergency department. We still see folks who are sick, but we're also spending the time to teach each and every customer with a dignified answer.

It doesn't seem that complicated when you look at it. It's just a bit of common sense, but we were the first private hospital in America to do it. The State of Missouri wants to start what we have. Missouri tells me that if they succeed, the whole country will do this.

The population you didn't mention is the uninsured who have nowhere else to go. What do you tell them?

Folks who come to me with no insurance, who have no other option, there *are* places to go. There are federally funded clinics that get paid to see people. There are private doctors willing to see people for reduced fees. The clinics actually get cost, plus reimbursement from the federal government, to see people with Medicaid insurance.

There are also a variety of charitable institutions around town. I personally work at a free clinic. We offer healthcare for about 400 folks. There's also one thing you say to folks without insurance, "When you come here for a cold, you're going to get almost three hundred dollars in debt. Next time, here's an urgent care place that's much cheaper."

I'm the medical director for Quick Care. There are 13 of these clinics. There are six in the Milwaukee metro area, and we've got them all over the place.

You're medical director for all 13 of them?

That's why I carry a cell phone. It may be a nurse asking a question, so I carry my cell phone everywhere until seven o'clock at night and they're all closed. But imagine, a simple problem, sore throat, sore ear, a little cough, or a cold. You go to Quick Care, and for $30 you can have a skilled nurse practitioner see you and write a prescription and you're done in 10 minutes. Thirty bucks, 10 minutes. We don't care whether you have insurance or not. Actually, half of our customers in Quick Care don't have insurance.

For middle-class folks who got thrown out of healthcare. My health system has innovated and has done a dramatic shift and said it's time for us to make another layer of resources. We don't claim to do long term care. The Quick Care nurse's job is solely to take care of simple tests and simple diagnoses. Then, if somebody comes who has a chronic illness, they have lots of people to refer them to.

You have to innovate. Americans are crafty people. Let's find a solution. It won't be long before every Wal-Mart and Target in America is going to have a Quick Care type "retail" clinic in it.

The world runs on competition. Medicine is going to face that pretty soon. Just like other white collar industries. Look at all the brokers who got put off by on-line stock trading. How many industries do you want me to go through? The fact is, the privilege that any of us thinks we have is at risk if we don't innovate and be part of a solution. If you're part of a solution, the world is always going to be coming to you.

We're doing the right thing and we're doing it for good reasons. Medicine has had sort of a privileged run that we, to a large degree, earned. Medicine earned a wonderfully esteemed place in American culture. But we can't own it forever, unless we continue to take care of America. Any doctor who says, "You don't have insurance, I can't see you," is being part of the problem; not part of the solution.

We can make a national vanilla policy work for everybody for half the price we're currently doing and have pretty close to what we have now as a national level of health care. Everybody deserves vanilla. We don't have to be as restrictive as the Canadians. For people who can afford it and want more, they can get it.

Is that fair?
Life isn't fair. I wish it were.

So, rationing and getting rid of the waste are the two key ways to make the system work?
Right. The promise of care management has not been provided by many in the health insurance industry. That whole HMO industry was meant to be the gift that was going to save American medicine, make us more efficient. Instead, it has ended up being an expensive, extremely complicated set of procedures that so confuses people that they give up.

You pay more for your insurance, and I pay more for mine, and hospitals get paid less and doctors get paid less. We haven't managed our own house. It's time hospitals start providing their own care management for their vulnerable populations and say, "We'll take on that risk. We'll do the care management."

Hospitals would do a much better job if they were given a population, given the resources to do it, and took the HMOs and insurance companies out of the middle because I don't see them as adding any value, except for brokering a policy and paying bills.

How did we get to be such a complex, convoluted health care system?

Money. It's not really that complicated. It's just lots and lots of money. There's lots of demand, because you insist on getting health care for everyone.

We've discovered that if you have a heart attack, you are better served if you have cardiac rehab. Right? So everybody who's had a heart attack is put on cardiac rehab. It's suddenly striking us that if cardiac rehab is good for you after you have a heart attack, why isn't it good for you before you have the heart attack?

Medicine of the past is what's gotten us to where we are today. It's episodic care for single conditions. You have appendicitis. I take it out. You're fixed. Episodic.

Medicine of the present, which is currently very expensive medicine, is spectacularly successful. We're now living into our 70s and 80s. We've discovered all these degenerative diseases—we call them Alzheimer's, arthritis, cancer, vascular disease. But they're all degenerative diseases, and they all have common underlying themes. Where does that come from? What we're trying to do now is patch all these degenerative diseases we discover. We're frantically trying to fix them.

Medicine of the future is going to be, how do we prevent those degenerative diseases and apply what we're learning today towards the future? How do I live longer well? How do I prevent Alzheimer's?

If you go to India—the middle class, slender people in India—who have all the health resources they need, they only have 20% of the Alzheimer's we have in America?

In America, if you're 85 years old, you have a 30% to 50% chance of developing Alzheimer's. Oh, I don't want to live to be 100 in America. I'll be living here, dribbling, babbling, and striking people. What a nightmare. But you can reduce your risk of Alzheimer's by 80%. That's interesting to me.

The trend in America to get industrial, healthy food that is produced in an industrial fashion has dramatically changed the nature of the way our bodies deal with it. Our bodies evolved in a very different environment than we're in today.

There are a whole lot of things that are subtle that have long term trends attached to them. Look at the nerve tissue of different cultures around the world. Look at the omega fatty acids—fish have a lot of omega fatty acids. Most primitive cultures have omega fatty acids in their nerve tissue and their membranes of 40% Omega 6 and 60% Omega 3s. In America, the ratio is 80 to 20—very dramatic shifts.

Omega 3s are the part of vegetable oils that make vegetable oils go bad, so we industrially purify rapeseed oil. If you purify it and take much of the omega 3s out of it, what's left is a higher concentrate of omega 6s and we call it canola oil. We say, "This is good." Whoops.

But, over 30 years, all our food from Omega 6 makes our nerve tissue and our brains different. You can't change a membrane without having a change in chemical reactions. We don't know the implications of that.

What are the systems that adapt to learning the lessons of how to prevent diseases? How do we start presenting that to the public? The Internet makes the world very flat with information coming at us from lots of places. How do you start integrating that information into your life? So, Steve Busalacchi, you need to personally start taking fish oil tablets every day. I have done that. Have you?

How do we find places where we work well and live well? That's where I believe the future of medicine is going, because the house that Washington built isn't going to pay for my health care, because I don't believe we're going to pay for everything coming down the road. Society can't.

The best thing for me to do, personally, is to take control of my own health care. I believe there are 100 million other discerning customers in America who are just as smart as me, who know the same thing and are also doing the same thing.

In this hospital, we're considering putting up signs on our stairs that say, "employee gym." Can we paint the stairwell to make it interesting to walk up? If you walk up four flights of stairs, on the fourth floor it says you just burned one percent of a pound. Congratulations, because you burned 40 calories. Do this a hundred times and you burned a pound, four flights. My wife loves to walk, so we're taking many more walks together. Alzheimer's and walking—there's a 40% reduction in risk by walking three times per week. A half hour of walking three times per week, your risk of Alzheimer's drops 40%. Is that enough to motivate you?

In India, they eat a lot of turmeric. Turmeric is one of the most potent antioxidants. If you don't eat lentils or curry very often, there is no way of getting turmeric. Turmeric is this yellow that makes curry powder yellow. It's got its own flavor, but it's a very strong antioxidant. Anybody who lives in India, eats it twice a day—lunch and supper.

In America, you have to go to a health food store and buy curcumin—that's the active ingredient in turmeric. We know that Alzheimer's is related to antioxidant effect. For example, we know that there's a mouse model that gets Alzheimer's. They get plaques in their brain. They get confused. They can't learn new mazes. When you feed them 10% of their food in blueberries they don't get their Alzheimer's. Blueberries are one of the most potent antioxidants, so if you can't eat turmeric, eat blueberries.

I don't want to take a supplement that often. So last summer, I bought eight trays of blueberries and froze them all and every morning I have a handful of blueberries in my cereal. Is health care adapting to that environment?

Thirty years from now, I'd love to be playing bridge with you in my retirement community. But 50 years from now, we won't be here—at least for me, pretty unlikely. You're going to die from something. I just want to hold it off as long as possible. I don't know how to transition from this world to the next one, but I hope it's not through an agonizing nursing home.

When do we prolong life? That's something we need to keep looking at. As a society, we all say, don't do that to me. And yet, when the moment of indecision comes, when you're having a sudden crisis, people give in and say, oh well, for right now until we get a decision, do this. In the emergency department, I'm the guy making that decision.

We haven't figured that out and taught our consuming, grieving public how to deal with that. We haven't made a science of teaching that. We'd better, because 90% of the cost of our healthcare is the last six weeks of your life.

I don't want to be on dialysis at age 30, so I'm going to treat my hypertension. That's another strategy for how we make our healthcare costs dramatically less. Each one of us can only change it for ourselves and our very immediate friends.

You keep talking about continuity of care. Even as a young man, you prized that. And here you are in an ER, where you have no continuity of care with patients. Do you ever think about that?

Yes, especially in my 50s, when I realized that emergency medicine is very hard to do. But I have a public health bent about me, so I've kind of got interested in these bigger pictures, and how you affect larger populations of people. That's why I'm interested in the ER reform, and the wellness stuff goes to the public health ideas. I'm really looking at the world from a different plane. If I were to go back now, I'd get a public health degree. I went into medicine to do good things, and I see the world as changing, so how do we change to fit or adapt to it? That's the life stages you go through.

Emergency medicine is thrilling. When you get to be 50 years old, you find it's kind of hard to work until two in the morning and the thrill of taking care of sick folks gets supplanted by the anxiety of, am I going to be able to keep my attention? Am I going to be able to stay alert? Am I really going to be able to provide optimal care?

CHAPTER TWENTY-FOUR

HOMOPHOBIA AND HEALTH

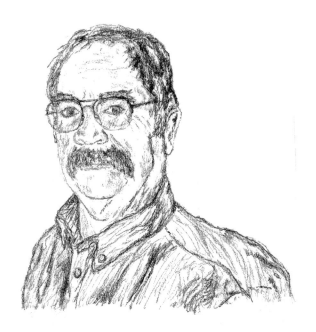

"Why in the world, even if you don't believe in gay marriage, would you want to penalize kids? Hardly anybody wants to do that."

Paul Wertsch, MD
Family Medicine, Madison

Republicans across the country are on a quest to outlaw gay marriage through constitutional amendments. What they don't realize, don't believe or just don't care about, is that changing the law may create tremendous health care hurdles by invalidating insurance coverage for gay partners and children.

That's the message Paul Wertsch, MD, is trying to get out to the public in Wisconsin, and across the country. In his early 60s, he's chair of an advisory committee to the American Medical Association's Board of Directors regarding gay, lesbian and transgender issues.

Being a big Sherlock Holmes fan, Wertsch loves assembling facts to fig-

ure out a solution. Doing that with respect to the gay marriage issue may be the biggest challenge he'll ever face, but he is undaunted.

He pulled off an impressive and unlikely political victory by spearheading a controversial resolution at the Wisconsin Medical Society, putting the organization on record against any attempt to ban gay marriage, out of concern for health care implications.

Doctor Wertsch's interest in this area stems from the fact that he has a gay son. His own childhood memories of discrimination figure prominently, as well, as he recounts how black people down South were treated unfairly by the health care system. I heard the story after he had just put in a very long day.

~~~~~~~~~~~~~~~~~~~~~

We were down in Florida, and my cousin and I went out at night. I felt guilty because I shouldn't have been doing that. My mother was out looking for us and she tripped and broke her leg. She went to the Palm Beach Hospital. They had a white entrance and a black entrance, and she, of course, was taken in. But there was a big gate in front of the black entrance. While they were taking care of her, a husband came up with a sick, black wife and was trying to get in. She was really sick and needed help, and they just sort of ignored them because they were at the black entrance. They were taking care of white people. Hearing mom's story of that and how it bothered her, it stuck with me from that time.

That really wasn't so long ago.

There used to be the white and colored watered fountains and I thought the colored was chocolate milk, so I wanted to drink out of there. So yeah, a lot's changed in my lifetime.

I grew up in Oshkosh. My mother was a teacher and retired to raise the kids. After my sister was in school, she went back and got a degree in special education. She got a Master's later on, and taught school.

My dad ran an auto agency at the same place that his grandparents had a carriage manufacturing place. There's a long family history of the automobile and truck industry and carriage making.

I have a younger sister by three and half years, who's also a physician now. There were some influential doctors in the family and my mother always had high respect for medicine.

When did you seriously start considering medicine as a career?

In high school. I remember reading some of the college catalogues and looking at what the requirements were to be a doc. I also was very interested in zoology, animal behavior. That was my major in college. I could have gone into PhD zoology also. I loved science.

One of the reasons I really became interested was my family had all sorts of medical problems. My mother was a diabetic who had trouble way back before you checked blood sugars and tried to manage diabetes by just checking your urine.

My father had health problems, including a cancer of the intestine that they missed up at the Mayo Clinic. The local doctor, in Oshkosh, picked it up because he sat around and waited for the small bowel follow through that they had kind of rushed elsewhere. You didn't need to be in the big, famous places to do good medicine.

My sister had some medical problems, so I figured somebody had to go into medicine to figure out what's happening in the family. I went to undergraduate here and really loved Madison. Medical school was just a continuation, of course. The courses were very hard, very intense, but fulfilling, and intellectually satisfying. Once I got in, I really enjoyed it.

I get bored with stuff pretty easily. With medical school rotations, I really liked surgery, but I didn't like the long cases where you just stand around all day doing one thing. I just liked the variety of general practice and sort of the challenge of doing a lot more things than strictly doing one specialty.

I'm just a generalist doc who delivers babies and sews up lacerations and treats pneumonias. It's what I thought would be the ideal, and I love it. I have trouble thinking what I would do if I retired. Gee, I'd miss all of this. It's very rewarding. It's great. It's fun to build up your practice and see the kids you delivered grow up and start having their own babies. As you age, your practice ages, too, so I have a lot of geriatrics, which I enjoy. But they're so much harder. They're much more work, so I love to be on call and see some of the younger kids and some of the easy problems once in a while.

You've been a leader in the profession. Why did you choose to get so involved?

I always want to know what's happening all over the place, so I'm interested in politics. I'm interested in how things work. I'm interested in how to get things done. I've seen others do it, so you can pick up a lot of tricks and get better. I'm also very interested in the health care system and how it's not working too well, and how it's not covering the 44 million people without insurance.

When I started, racism was really a problem, before the civil rights acts. It was just appalling to see how people were treated differently and not treated well. If you don't have the finances, there's still some of that. Not on a racial basis, but on an economic basis. There certainly is a fair amount of discrimination and some of it is just ignorance from people not understanding the issue. I'm interested in that because of my gay son. You see the world differently when your family members are affected by it.

As a doctor, I don't think society even understands the causes of homosexuality and discriminates on the basis of that, specifically, with money to pass a constitutional amendment that would disallow gay marriage. It wouldn't allow civil unions and would discriminate against people who love each other and want to have a relationship.*

Do you believe homosexuality has a genetic origin?

There are definitely genetic factors. If you have an identical twin, there's a 50% chance that you're going to be gay. If you have a non-identical brother, there's a 20% chance that you're going to be gay; the same with lesbians. It runs in families. Some will display it. Some won't.

How it actually comes about that some people have a sexual orientation to gay or lesbian, we're not exactly sure. It's widespread in nature. In animals, we actually know some biochemical basis for it. Is that the same in humans? We don't know, but I suspect it is.

Does being gay or lesbian affect the kind of health care they receive?

One of the big issues is that we in medicine have difficulty in taking a history because a lot of doctors are uncomfortable with people being gay or lesbian, and so we ask if you have a husband or a wife. We don't ask if you have a partner. A lot of our forms make it apparent that we don't even want to know, so we don't have people being honest with us with their answers.

We don't understand illnesses as well as we should that affect gay and lesbian people. That's not a small thing. It's a significant thing how to take an adequate sexual history, which a lot of doctors feel uncomfortable taking, anyway. And when you're dealing with something that you don't understand as well, it's tougher.

The big thing is health insurance. If you have a partner who maybe has a good job and you have a job and get fired, there's no way to get health insurance. In a married relationship, one person can have health insurance and cover everybody.

If you have some dependent children and they're your children from a previous marriage and you are in a gay or lesbian relationship, the other person has the health insurance, your kids are not going to be covered. There's a lot of discrimination, in terms of coverage by insurance, just because of sexual orientation. It wouldn't occur if you were heterosexual and were married.

What reaction have you noticed from your colleagues, since you took on this national leadership role?

There are a lot of people who thank me for doing this and they tell me about their gay brothers or gay children or their gay everything, but they're

---

* In November, 2006, Wisconsin voters overwhelmingly approved the constitutional amendment to ban gay marriage and civil unions.

very quiet and they don't say anything to anybody else. They come and tell me about it, but they're kind of quiet little mice, all the rest of the time.

Some people have taken a stand against it. I've heard some say the medical society shouldn't be dealing with this issue. It's a social issue or it's a political issue and we shouldn't be dealing with it. A lot of people, because of their religion, feel that this is wrong. But I've heard four positives for every negative.

What do you say to people when they have these concerns?

I talk about the fact that 33% of lesbian couples have dependent children in their relationships and that insurance is a very important thing, or taking sick leave or benefits that married couples take for granted. Twenty-two percent of gay couples have children who are dependent and that these are indeed, families. They are real people that get sick and need medical care. It is a medical issue.

I purposely didn't ask {the Wisconsin Medical Society} to endorse gay marriage because that would be a step too far, but to at least oppose a law against gay marriage or any other relationship that could be interpreted that way. Companies have good partnership benefits because they want to hire gay people and they have to offer benefits to do it. But the State Constitutional Amendment, theoretically, may eliminate all those benefits and the tax deductibility of businesses, so we got the Medical Society to say we're going to oppose anything that negatively affects the health of dependent children.

Spouses have visitation rights that another person doesn't. Being able to speak for people if they're ill, being able to accompany them to visits, to be able to take off for sick leave. The insurance part is an important part, but a small part. Can you take off from work and help your partner, like if you had a heterosexual partner?

There are a lot of things that go with marriage, such as survivorship benefits. You name it. Social security benefits for somebody who's disabled, but insurance would be a good place to start.

People who are against gay marriage or relationships are against them because they've been told this is against their religious beliefs. All the people I met are not bad people. People are doing things they think are right.

When I sit down and try to analyze the biblical basis for where they derive this from, you can find a lot of flaws in their argument. There are other things in the Old Testament where people eat pork and other things that are clearly prohibited in the Old Testament and don't think anything of it. They interpret some of these biblical passages, not understanding when they were written.

If you sit down and have a really good religious discussion, there's a lot of possibility that this is misinterpreted. But even so, most of the people are good and you sit down and really show them that people are truly affected, that you're dealing with lives. Bringing up the dependent children—why in the world, even if you don't believe in gay marriage, why would you want to penalize these kids? Hardly anybody wants to do that. There are a few. Just letting people know what can happen with these actions is helpful.

The AMA is very interested because they have a lot of gay doctors and certainly a lot of gay patients with dependent children, so they're very far sighted to look at this issue and deal with it.

I think of myself before I had my gay son. He really helped me understand a lot of these issues. I certainly wasn't as educated. I certainly had more prejudices than I do now and I thought I was being good and sanctimonious when I had those prejudices. I really didn't realize how they hurt people. I've been interested in homosexuality for quite a while and I was reading a book before my son came out, so he was kind of wondering whether I knew ahead of time.

I remember exactly when he told me because it was a surprise, even though I had no problems with it, on a theoretical basis. When it's your own child, you wonder what this really means or how is this going to affect things. Of course, you're interested in your kids and worry about your kids and want the best. When it hits home, it makes you do some soul searching and thinking.

He's been with his partner for about four years and he's a great guy. They tell me a lot of things and I've learned a lot from them. But part of it is he's a very talented fellow and he doesn't want to be known as the gay son. He's not ashamed of it, but he's got plenty of other things in his life that are important and that he likes to talk about, too.

When my son moved out to Colorado, one of the questions was, Gee, I need a new doctor. How do you find somebody who is gay friendly, who is not prejudiced against you? The answer is there's no good solution. If you're gay friendly, certainly the word gets out. You have to just wait and make appointments and see how they react.

I'm really hoping that our American Medical Association can actually develop a national list of doctors, at least those who self-register, that they are interested in working with gay and lesbian patients. People may not be telling the truth, but it would be a start.

How was homosexuality dealt with in medical school?

There was very little discussion of sexuality at all when I went to medical school. Masters and Johnson had just come out, but very little mention of homosexuality. There was some discussion about infections that are more common in gays and lesbians, mostly sexually transmitted.

That's a problem, because a lot of doctors don't have homosexual friends, or they have them, but they just don't know that they're gay and lesbian. Their only contact is though illness and disease and just dealing with gays who are sick or diseased or depressed or whatever, which is one of the problems with medical school because you're dealing with illness, mostly.

Do you treat many gay patients?

I have a fair number of gay and lesbian patients. They not only go to doctors they feel comfortable with, they tend to migrate to areas that are more gay friendly. In metropolitan areas, up to 16% of the males are gay just because people are drawn to those areas. I realize how patients feel, and I'm better at my communication. I use words a little better. Just by the way you ask questions you show you are open to the possibility that their answer may be a little different than other people give.

We have a little sticker on our mirror that says feel free to discus sexuality and any issue is safe for discussion here. We try to be open and honest during physicals and ask the kids whether they're attracted to the same sex or the opposite sex—at least let them answer the question, however they will. We let them know that that's a legitimate thing to discuss, if they want to.

Are they different as patients?

Not a whole lot different. HIV AIDS is more common in the gay populations, although that's changing. That was sort of thought of as a gay disease, but now it's spreading in the heterosexual population more. Otherwise, issues are pretty much the same.

VII

Physicians who Listen

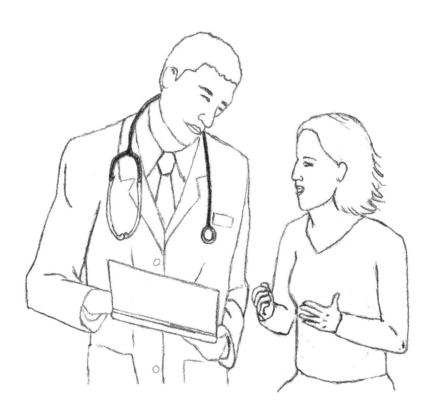

"Most of the successful people I've known are the ones who do more listening than talking."

—Bernard Baruch

Chapter Twenty-Five

Strong, Silent Types

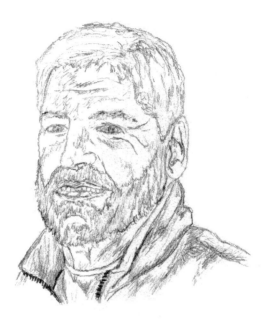

"For people who say on a survey that my doctor understands me, cares about me and listens to me…they also have better blood sugar control, if they have diabetes, they have much better blood pressure control, if they have hypertension, and they take their medicines more reliably."

Norman Jensen, MD
Internal Medicine, Madison

Doctor Norman Jensen is the kind of physician who keeps lawyers up at night. Jensen tells it like it is, and believes it's critical to the patient/doctor relationship to admit to a patient when and if the physician screws up. Jensen, who's in his late 60s, has taken his own advice in that regard and doesn't regret it. Now, he's trying to convince his colleagues to do the same because he says such honesty leads to a better relationship, as well as healthier patients and more satisfied physicians.

Doctor Jensen explains how he handled a mistake he made long ago.

Early in my practice, I made an error. My residents had gone home, so I decided to write a prescription for a blood-thinning drug that I knew really well, but I hadn't written an order for it in a few years. I ordered 10 times the recommended dose. I came in the next morning and found the patient bleeding in her urine, obviously from too much anticoagulant. I looked and indeed, I had made an error and had written it. A pharmacist and nurse were there and I asked them if they knew that I had written this wrongly. They said, "Oh yeah."

I said, "Why didn't you say something?"

They said, "We thought you knew something we didn't know."

That was in the days before pharmacists and nurses were really willing to challenge physician orders. That wouldn't happen today, very likely.

The patient didn't have a permanent injury. She was going to be in the hospital a day or two longer than she would have. I had to decide whether to tell the patient or not. She knows that she's got blood in her urine. She's an experienced health professional. Or, should I just not say anything about it, knowing the patient will probably recover without injury? I decided to do the right thing, which I always believed was the right thing to do, and so I told her. "You're bleeding in your urine."

She said, "Yes, I can see that."

"Do you know why?"

She said, "No."

I said, "Because I gave you too much medicine last night. But it looks like there's not going to be any permanent injury. We're going to watch to be sure you're not harmed at all by this."

She looked at me and was kind of stern, and said, "I could sue you for that."

I said, "I know you could. But I hope you won't."

And she didn't.

That was before I knew much about the science of doctor/patient communication. But I always thought that she didn't sue me, in part, because we'd had a good relationship, and in part because she'd gotten good care, except for this error. I didn't wait for her to discover it, while I tried to keep a secret.

We're now trying to accumulate quite a bit of evidence that people who believe that their doctors care about them, and are working hard to help them, even if that doctor makes a mistake, the person is much more likely to forgive them and not file a lawsuit.

I learned this very strongly when I was a medical expert witness against another doctor, on behalf of another patient, the only time I've ever done that before. It was a painful thing to do because we all say, "There, but for the grace of God go I."

But this patient, I thought, had been mistreated and it was my duty to help the patient. He was suing his doctor for malpractice for about

$25,000—this was a few years ago—because the doctor had failed to diagnose a fractured hip. The symptoms were atypical, but the doctor behaved himself in a way that the patient thought the doctor didn't respect the patient, and didn't take him seriously when he kept telling the doctor that the pain in his knee was so bad that he couldn't stand on it. He couldn't do physical therapy. The nurses and the therapist kept talking about how the leg was dysfunctional and wouldn't work. Yet it was 13 days before a consulting surgeon got an x-ray of the hip, which showed a fracture. The man had a surgical repair, recovered nicely, but sued his doctor.

The patient was awarded $18,000 for economic damages. After the trial was over, the patient came up to me as I was on my way out of the court room and said, "Doctor, may I talk with you?"

We sat in the courtroom and talked for about a half an hour. What this man wanted me to know was why he sued his doctor. "I would have changed doctors for sure, because I don't want a doctor who makes mistakes like that, but I wouldn't have sued him if he had just come and talked to me."

After the diagnosis of the hip fracture, his primary care doctor never, ever, came back to talk with him and the patient felt insulted and humiliated by that. That is what made him mad and want to sue the doctor.

We're accumulating all kinds of cases now that show us that people who are angry at their doctors, feel humiliated, and feel disrespected are much more likely to sue if they get a bad outcome, whether or not the doctor made a mistake.

Now, something like 80% of lawsuits are called frivolous. The doctor didn't make a mistake. There was just a bad outcome. Why do those people sue? Well, certainly, a lot of them sue because they're mad at the doctor. They believe the doctor didn't listen, didn't respect them. The difference between doctoring that allows people to feel understood and cared for is really very small. It results from communication skills. Virtually all doctors aspire to the ideal and their skills just don't allow them to show it.

Is it harder for physicians to admit error, because they're put up on a pedestal as these figures who are all-knowing?

Probably not any harder than an airline pilot who crashes an airliner. But, I think probably just about as hard. I have a friend who flies large airplanes who says, "You kill your patients one at a time. We kill our clients hundreds at a time."

Any time you're dealing in a life and death situation, where an error can result in a death, it becomes very hard to admit to yourself, let alone anybody else, that you made an error. But that comes with the territory. That's been reinforced by attorneys who practice defensive law. That's decreasing now, but our tradition has been, and our attorneys tell us, if we're in an auto accident, you never admit you made a mistake. Never admit it was your fault, because "fault" is a legal concept, and it's complicated and has to be worked out in court in order to decide who's at fault and what percent they're at fault.

Our attorneys in health care have been telling us that it's not so clear you made a mistake. If something goes wrong, it might have been the system that was at fault. If a doctor says, "I'm sorry. It was all my fault," that may unnecessarily prejudice the case against the doctor.

We're told, don't admit any fault. Express regret over it. Doctors make mistakes. We're beginning to see evidence that when people do apologize, admit an error, they are less likely to be sued.

Back when you made the medication error, you didn't consult a lawyer, did you?

I'm not even sure we had a lawyer on staff back then. Malpractice suits were pretty rare in those days. They were just beginning to become more common in the 1970s, so I really wasn't very concerned about a lawsuit. No, I didn't consult a lawyer or anybody else. I just did what I knew to be the right thing.

But we live in a litigious society and attorneys consult on everything. Could you do the same thing today?

Yes, I could make that choice. But our attorneys now would advise I not tell the patient that it was my fault alone. They would advise now that I tell the patient that she had gotten an overdose of blood thinning medicine and tell the patient everything else about the event. But not tell the patient whose fault it was.

How do you feel about that?

Fault is complicated, and we're beginning to understand that. A lot of errors that appear to be caused by an individual are really due to a system that sets up people to make errors. We're now beginning to understand that systems are as responsible for errors as individuals. People shouldn't be so quick, just because they feel bad about it, and they feel guilty about it, to say, "It was all my fault. I'm sorry."

Now, in this particular case, it was all my fault. My colleagues in nursing and pharmacy probably would have had to share the fault a little bit because they knew it was too much medicine. Now, if the pharmacy had called me within five minutes and said, "Did you really mean for this dose to be given?" I would have immediately recognized the problem and said, "No, no, no, this is an error. Please don't give that." We would have corrected it. That's the benefit of teams, and about people in different professions jointly caring for patients and reducing the kind of errors that humans are all subject to. I don't see any reason not to own up to an error, when it clearly is my fault, and it was.

If I were the patient, I would want the doctor to tell me, "It was my fault. I wrote the wrong order." Doctors need to be that trustworthy. If we're transparent, I'm convinced that we could reduce malpractice suits. It will increase the forgiveness factor. Humans have an enormous amount of forgiveness in them.

When did your interest in this develop?

I trace the roots of it way back to my first interest in medicine. What interested me most about medicine was the care of people. My other interest was in teaching, which is just another way of caring for people. My brief interest in clergy is another way of caring for people. What won out, ultimately, was my interest in biology, and human biology and health and illness. The chemistry, physiology, pathology and all that also very much interested me, so medicine really allowed me to combine my interest in people and my interest in biology and human medicine.

It was very clear when I got into my internship. I feel very lucky to have gotten to be an intern at Harvard Medical School in the Boston City Hospital, where they had a tradition started by Francis Peabody, who has been quoted frequently in modern times, talking about the secret of patient care being to care for the patient.

During my internship and residency there, I really had the distinct privilege of participating in an environment that was extremely compassionate and concerned about people, and also intellectually very rigorous and curious, cognitively, operating at a very high level. The exposure to both of those environments in the same place really showed me that you didn't have to choose sides over the care of humans or one or the other. They were best combined.

During my residency, early in my career as a teacher, I began to realize that I was most intrigued from an academic point of view, by the care of humans, which really comes down to communication. Except for people in a coma, doctors can only work through their powers to communicate with people, to understand people's needs and to persuade and instruct and motivate people to change whatever they're doing to be healthier.

It was realizing that communication is the main medium of medical care that made me become interested in it. That was after I was on the faculty for about five years. Since I got a job in an academic environment, it seemed important to focus on something. I looked around for mentors in medical school in this area, in communication, and didn't find any, so I went to University graduate school and found mentors in the Department of Sociology. So in the middle of my career I focused on social psychology, which is small group sociology. I learned research methods, and studied communication. I finished all my PhD coursework and got a Master's degree, and as they say, ABD—all but dissertation, for my PhD. I followed this with a two-year distance fellowship within the American Academy on Communication in Healthcare. These experiences really gave me substance and confidence to work with in my interest, and provided me with some credibility among my colleagues in medical school. This has really allowed me to specialize in my teaching work and in communication.

What is the status of doctor-patient communication today? How are we doing?

Well, we're doing better, but we've got quite a ways to go yet. Public opinion polls still rate us rather poorly. There's still a tendency for people in the public opinion poll to comment generally on doctors that we appear not to care about them as much as they wish we would. We don't listen to them like they wish. We don't spend enough time with them and we don't teach them as much as they would like about their illness, the treatments, and their prognosis.

When they talk about us, generally as a profession, they express disappointment in the human relations part of our work, in terms of listening and teaching and caring. That grieves me, because in my teaching work I've gotten to know the hearts and souls of a large number of medical students and residents and, to some extent, physicians in practice, and so I'm convinced that that's not the case. I'm convinced that most physicians care very deeply about their patients, but that there's a failure somehow in people understanding that.

It has to do with a tradition that our mentors, William Osler* in medicine, and even in nursing, Florence Nightingale taught us, at the beginning of the 20th Century, that doctors and nurses need equanimity—that patients were in the midst of great emotional turmoil, and they didn't need doctors and nurses who were also emotional. They needed doctors and nurses who were strong, affectively neutral, who could be sort of rocks in the storm-tossed sea.

For a long time, we interpreted that to mean we should be strong and silent, and we learned to be silent, really, really well. Nursing is getting over this more quickly than we are in medicine. But now, because doctors are so silent, their patients don't understand that they care. They don't understand that the doctors care very deeply and agonize about their patients and suffer along with their patients. If they don't hear or see we care, they assume we don't.

In just an everyday example in my clinic, I hear a story of suffering from my patients, that they're experiencing a lot of pain. Like yesterday, a man was telling me how much pain he had, how it was disturbing his sleep, and that kept him from doing his work. He's had to retire on disability. It keeps him from doing his hobbies. He has to depend on his grown children to do tasks that he used to do by himself with a great deal of pride.

I could have just simply listened to that story, remained affectively

* Canadian physician who was hired in 1888 as one of the first four doctors at Johns Hopkins Hospital. He revolutionized the medical curriculum in both the US and Canada.

neutral and not even responded verbally to that story, but simply focus on his pain and how to relieve his pain, not express any appreciation or understanding of that problem and suffering.

But what I've learned that's important to do, and what I did, was to let him know, by paraphrasing his story, that I was hearing about how much pain he was having, that he was unable to work, that he was unable to do his hobbies, his life has changed enormously, and furthermore, he had to put up with a lot of pain, which is also difficult. It took me maybe 30 or 40 seconds to let him know that I heard all that by reflecting it back, and then assessing it, saying that, in modern vernacular, it sounds like your life really sucks now, compared to what it used to.

He very much agreed, and brightened up a little bit just on hearing me say that. So a minute or less of empathy and reflecting back verbally, communicated to him that I not only understood his suffering, but that I cared about it. It's the kind of stuff that really good friends do. Women do this better than men, in our culture. But we've learned that men can learn how to do it, and once they appreciate how important it is to the mission of healing, they can do it really well.

What do you think of these "I'm sorry laws?" They seemed to be designed to let doctors do what you suggest they do.

What that's going to do is encourage doctors to be less frightened of saying I'm sorry, to inform patients. Right now, doctors are allergic to the word, sorry, because we've learned so strongly that saying, "I'm sorry," might well cause a lawsuit rather than prevent one. It's not an implausible idea. But the empiric evidence suggests that it doesn't work that way.

Now, if you're a doctor who doesn't have good relationships with patients, whose patients don't feel heard, understood, and cared for, then saying, "I'm sorry," might be risky. But what the law's going to do, just like the Good Samaritan laws did, it made doctors less fearful of stopping on the road and helping somebody who's had an accident. As long as they don't commit malpractice, they are really immune from any lawsuit.

This apology law would help doctors feel less fearful about honest communication after something goes wrong. I don't think the "I'm sorry" laws are going to change anything in the legal system. There might be a rare case when a patient says the doctor said he was sorry, and that's why I sued him, because that's tantamount to an admission of guilt. In those rare cases, where a lawsuit comes mainly from those words, "I'm sorry," that will, under these laws, make that inadmissible into court. But lawsuits that come only from the words, "I'm sorry," have to be extremely rare. I've never heard of one.

We've spoken only about the physician. But there's another person in this conversation. What is the patient's responsibility in good communication?

For a variety of reasons, patients have learned to cooperate with doctors in this interrogational style of communicating. People don't know how, maybe, and don't know there's an opportunity to really enrich the conversation, so many of my patients are really minimalists. They don't speak very much at all, unless I really encourage them and invite them to tell more of the story and pay attention to it, so they know I'm interested in it. But yeah, citizens and patients also have a lot to learn, because it's two-way communication.

How much is honesty an issue in these patient doctor relationships?

When people go to the doctor for the first time it's a meeting of strangers, because people don't know whether the doctor can be trusted. The doctor doesn't know that the patient can be trusted, so there's sort of this dance that goes on any time strangers meet and begin to work together.

But, over a short time, two or three meetings, trust should easily be established and the patient, at that point, should feel confident that the doctor not only will keep things confidential, but the doctor will be respectful about things that the patient talks about. Many people are embarrassed by the facts of their lives and are afraid of being humiliated and judged. For example, people are still embarrassed to tell me that they consulted a chiropractor for an illness, because they expect that we doctors are going to judge them and humiliate them about doing something foolish.

I know a doctor who prefers that patients call him by his first name and lose the formality.

I don't feel like I have a judgment about that. It's important for the patient and the doctor to have some degree of distance and I'm going to call it affective distance—that's social distance. I don't think we need doctors to be in a social class, superior to their patients. In fact, many of my patients are socially superior to me, and that can be a challenge in itself. At least they think they're superior to me. If you wonder, they'll tell you.

Doctors are among the most highly educated people in most communities, not necessarily just Madison. That means something to people. People expect something special from a highly educated person. People expect something special from their doctor. Most people don't want their doctor to be their best friend. They want their doctor to respect them, to listen to them, and to be their advocates when they need it.

They need their doctor to hold confidential the stories of their life. And, they want doctors to be special, in the sense that doctors know about illness, they know how to diagnose illness, they know how to treat illness, and they know how to help the patient get to specialists and specialist services when they need them. They expect the doctors to have a fair amount of expertise and be well trained, be reliable.

Now, that's going to make it very hard to also have the doctor be a best friend and buddy. Out of that belief comes my style of doctoring, which is to be fairly formal. I resist referring to patients by their first name, for example. Mr. or Mrs. or professor or doctor or whatever to anybody over age 18. And in general, people like that level of respect.

But it's a social distance, and the distance comes from both the patient and the doctor. Patients are most comfortable when there is that bit of social distance, because if your doctor's your best friend, you've got to worry a little bit about what the doctor is also telling about you.

Just like your lawyer, your clergy person, your doctor, your professor, or your social worker, you want to have a little bit of social distance. Not status distance, not class difference, but social distance. When you're in the room with the doctor and the door's closed, there is intimacy. Apart from that, there is not. My style of practice is to keep it formal, but intimate. Sometimes people think you can't be both formal and intimate. I think you can. But I do have some patients who very much want to call me by my first name. I'm usually uncomfortable with that, unless we have had a strong friendship before I became their doctor.

So tell me how your practice works. You see patients and teach?

My plan B was to become a physics teacher after high school and college. Teaching always interested me. Never, ever thought I would be a medical school teacher. That was far beyond what I thought I would ever be able to do. But I was really pleased to be invited back to start what really amounted to a new program in primary care for internal medicine.

In those days, we were just beginning to see that internists were going to have to become primary care doctors, whether they wanted to or not. There weren't enough family doctors or general practitioners to take care of all the adults and there weren't enough hospital patients for physicians to support all the internists. By necessity, if nothing else, internists became generalists for adults.

My work for about 35 years has been about half-time practicing. I have about 800 people who think of me as their doctor, and then the other half of my time I get to teach, and prepare for teaching and learning, and participating in an academic environment.

Sounds like the best of both worlds.

It is for me. Overall, I'd say it's about as perfect a job as I could ever have gotten. I'm very pleased with my job here at the University of Wisconsin.

Was there any question that family medicine was going to be the specialty for you?

When I graduated, family medicine hadn't been born yet. It was an idea in the minds of some people, but I didn't know about it. I really wanted to be an old fashioned general practitioner, just like my doctor, who cared for me when I was a child. But by the time I got through and I maintained that idea, by the time I was preparing to apply for residency and internship, my mentors all told me that that was not a very good idea. It was what they called impractical. What they meant was that the ethic in the profession in those days was that general practice was not a competent way to be a doctor. You had to specialize in something.

I chose internal medicine, which seemed the most general of all the specialties. Then, in internal medicine, my mentors told me that I had to sub-specialize in internal medicine. Infectious disease seemed to be the most general of all the specialties, so I thought, all right, I'll do infectious disease.

My family doctor, who was a general practitioner, was really my ideal of a doctor. He worked long days every day of the week, 11 months out of the year. Then, took a month off. I remember very vividly that he treated me when I had rheumatic fever as a child. He treated me for appendicitis, and took out my appendix as a surgeon. My parents couldn't come and get me when I was ready to come home, so he drove me home in his own car. He encouraged me to go to medical school and came to my basketball games when I was in high school. He was like my favorite uncle, as well as my primary doctor.

Was he around to see you develop into a physician?
Yes, he was. He was retired at the time.

Had it not been for this doc, might you have pursued something else? Was he that important to your decision?
Oh yeah, very much. I never expected I would get into medical school. I probably would have been a teacher. I had a brief interest in seminary, which would have very much pleased my mother, but my wife-to-be informed me that that wasn't her idea of a good life, so I changed my mind.

I grew up really in northwest Wisconsin, Burnett County, a rural area, a town of about 600 people in an area of poverty, and kids up there really didn't believe they could go to college or make it through college, let alone professional school. I was very much influenced by that idea, that I probably wouldn't be able to do it. My high school teachers, unfortunately, had a similar attitude. They didn't really think kids from that area and that school could go to college and professional school. It was my family doctor who encouraged me to go for it.

I later found out from my college roommate that my principal had told him that he didn't think I would make it through college and medical school. It was less a personal assessment than a general attitude.

Tell me about your family.
My dad worked most of his life on construction, operating heavy equipment. My mother is a retired school teacher.

What did they think of your interest in medicine?
My father was a man of few words and never really said he was pleased,

but I think he was. My mother thought being a doctor was almost as good as being a clergyman.

By the time I graduated high school, I was pretty serious, and maintained that all the way through college. Of course, every time I got a B in one of my courses, rather than an A, I assumed that meant I wasn't going to get into medical school. But I did manage to get enough A's to get in.

During the first year of medical school, I kept having this nightmare where the Dean of my medical school said he was very sorry to tell me that there were two Norm Jensens that applied to medical school, and I was the wrong one. I'd have to leave medical school.

What was that first year like?

I had to support myself during college so I worked 32 hours in a hospital, which served two purposes. It confirmed my interest in health care in a real life environment, and I also got several more people, physicians, on my side, who encouraged me to continue to pursue medical school. But it also exhausted me and took me away from being a full-time student. One disadvantage was that I didn't get to play basketball in college.

My main worry was whether I could succeed and get through medical school; whether I had the talent to do it. By the end of my first year in medical school, I was able to see that I was as well prepared as anybody, and could survive, and even thrive, in medical school. The thing that really cemented it was my original inspiration from childhood. My second family doctor, who I also much admired, hired me to work with him after my second year of medical school.

It was during that summer that his partner left him to go into a psychiatry residency, so he was all alone in a large practice. I got to work quite independently, actually, having completed just two years of medical school. That was at a time when hospital regulations were not what they are now. One could never get away with that now. He was always available by phone, to come in if he needed to.

It was in the area that I grew up, so I saw several people who came in for treatment. The father of one of my best friends came in with migraine headaches. He came in to see me to get relief. I was able to look it up in a book and get some guidance from one of the nurses, and it was very gratifying to be able to relieve his very severe migraine headache.

I also got to treat a baby who had meningitis. I knew enough after even two years of medical school to do a spinal tap and sample the fluid. The laboratory technicians helped me to do the gram stain necessary to identify the meningococcal bacteria. I was doing all this, of course, in cooperation with my preceptor who was on the phone from home, approving of what I was doing. I actually saved the baby's life by treating the infant.

Whether lives are on the line or not, today's doctors are under even greater pres-

sure to see more patients. How likely is it that they will take the time to treat them in the respectful manner you recommend?

Doctors are learning to appreciate the value of communication with their patients. The opportunity's changing, and their skills also will have to be upgraded. People too, have a ways to go before they can get the most value out of their minutes with the doctor.

For example, the minutes are limited, so people have to think ahead of time what they want to tell the doctor, what they want to get out of the 15 or 20 minutes they have with the doctor. They may have to appreciate that their agenda exceeds what can be done in 15 or 20 minutes. They may have to schedule a longer visit, or maybe two visits, in order to complete the work that they're interested in. People have to be clear about their agenda and prioritize their agenda.

Now, my colleagues, like the culture in America, generally don't appreciate how much skill is involved in communication. There's a deep cultural bias in America, and perhaps all over the world, that communication is something sort of natural, that by the time you're 18-years old, it's grounded in your personality, and your personality is relatively fixed by the time you're 18 or 21. You're already a good communicator or you're not, and therefore communication skills training is rather pointless. At worst, it's a waste of time. It's even insulting to some doctors to think that anybody would recommend that they get skills training in communication. The same thing applies to teaching. There's a cultural bias that teachers are born, not made.

But now we're beginning to understand how wrong that is, and now it looks to many of us like utter nonsense. You wonder where it came from, but it's deeply embedded in the culture, to the point where doctors will say, "Communication is very important for our work, but you know, there isn't really much you can learn about that. You either have it or you don't."

We're at the point, now, where our profession is just beginning to understand that good communication is very skills-dependent.

The story that illustrates that, a few years ago, involves an intern who brought in his videotape to my office because we were scheduled to review his training. On arrival, he looked pretty unhappy about the whole thing. Being the empathic person I am, I said to him, "You're not very excited about being here today."

He said, "No, frankly, I'm not."

"Tell me what's going on."

He said, "I have a lot of patients to take care of. You're a good guy. I don't mind spending time with you. But I don't think there's anything for me to learn about this communication stuff. I'm 24 years old. If I haven't learned to communicate by now, it's pretty hopeless."

I said, "A lot of people think like you do. I appreciate your being candid about it. But, since we have an hour assigned to us, we've got to do something with this hour. Why don't we just watch your videotape for a while and see what happens? Maybe there will be something to talk about, maybe not. If not, we can quit early."

So we watched his videotape and he was talking to a patient who had pain. He was conducting a very standard history of the present illness.

"I have pain."

"Where's the pain?"

"It's in my head."

"How long have you had it?"

"About three months."

"What's the pain like?"

"Well, it's sharp."

"How strong is it?"

All those are questions doctors know to ask to try to understand pain really well. Those questions are important, because they help us make up a differential diagnosis to figure out what's causing the pain. They're very important questions, and I don't mean to depreciate them.

But, after we listened for about seven or eight minutes, I stopped the tape and said, "Well, let's talk a little about your style of interviewing here." We pretty quickly agreed that it was an interrogational style. That is, the doctor asks the questions and the patient gives minimally sufficient answers. It's kind of like the old TV program, *Dragnet.* "Just the facts, ma'am."

When I was a medical school student, they talked about extracting the medical history. It tells us a little about how doctors have traditionally thought about doctor-patient communication. It's almost as though you have to extract this truth from this patient.

I said, "Since you believe that communication is really grounded in personality, I presume that this is also the way that you talk to your mother. This is the way you talk to your girlfriend, to your pastor, to your teachers. You talk to everybody pretty much this way as an interrogator. Would that be true?"

He smiled and said, "Okay, I get your point."

The point is that we have lots of different ways of talking to people. When it involves the important people in our lives, we talk a whole lot differently, so doctors are not bound to interrogate their patients. They can learn to talk to their patients in a variety of ways. We all have a huge repertoire of ways of talking and communicating. Doctors can learn. We can change.

My experience in teaching doctor-patient communication to students, residents, and practicing doctors, tells me that doctors not only can change, but once they figure out that they can change, they quickly become quite enthusiastic about it.

Chapter Twenty-Six

War Rapport

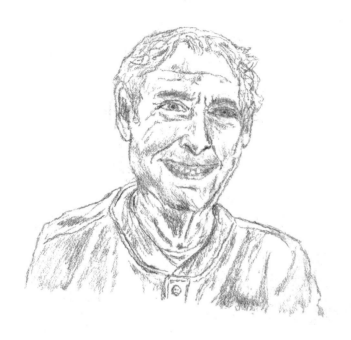

"My practice was kind of a private health club."

Paul Vastola, Jr., MD
Internal Medicine, Madison

I introduced Doctor Paul Vastola to my family a few years ago over dinner. While Paul was talking to somebody else, my dad whispered, "He's a doctor, right?

"Yeah, he's a doctor" I replied.

"So why are you calling him, Paul?"

"What do you mean? That's his name. Paul."

"Why aren't you calling him, doctor?"

"He's not my doctor. He's my friend," I explained.

My dad just shrugged, worried that I wasn't paying proper respect.

The irony is that even if I were Paul's patient, I wouldn't call him Dr. Vastola. Hardly any of his patients ever did, and that's the way he prefers it. Vastola's philosophy on this goes back to his World War II days, when his *very life depended on getting along with a bunch of soldiers who came from a completely different station in life than he.*

Paul, who's in his early 80s, explained it to me during a wonderful three hour conversation in his den at home, where he spends a lot of time on his computer. He's continually keeping up with medical advances, even though he's been retired for all of the 12 years that I've known him. We've biked and played tennis together many times over the years. In fact, he's the only guy I've ever known who actually built a full-size tennis court in his backyard! Paul is a remarkable guy in many ways, especially with respect to his gift for developing rapport with people.

You had an especially close relationship with your patients. How did that develop?

I certainly never had any pre-formed conceptions about how I should act with a patient, but part of my Army experience very definitely played a role in how I related to people. My unit was an armored infantry regiment {from the South}. I came there as a replacement in England, before D-Day, in June of '44. As an Italian, who they called a Yankee, I was constantly badgered and beat up. It was a very traumatic experience.

The regimental colonel called me in one day and said I was out of place and if I wanted to get out of there, he would certainly consider transferring me to another unit. That's how bad it was. These guys were really Southerners. Believe it or not, some of them had used the Sears and Roebuck catalogue as the only kind of toilet paper they ever knew.

I was so intent on succeeding at where I was that I said, "Absolutely not. I'm staying where I am."

You can look up there and see a picture of myself with my buddies. {Points to a photo} Those are the guys I related to for two years. These fellas would not accept me as I was, but I became one of them.

How did you win them over?

The first thing I did was play my harmonica. We would sing along over wine. It developed a sense of camaraderie. The song they loved the most was *"Take Me Back to the Red River Valley."* It was a song I could play endlessly, and they loved it.

The second thing is I was a good soldier. I worked hard, I stayed with my unit, and was on night patrol just like everybody else. During the war, I was promoted to corporal, and eventually to staff sergeant. But think of the journey I made. I came from a doctor's family to a bunch of fellows who were typical GI Joes. I was entrenched in that society for a long time.

Why was this experience important in terms of rapport with your patients?

I developed what I saw as a working relationship, the same way as I did in the service when I joined that unit in the Second Armored Division. I used the same techniques. My practice was kind of a private health club.

When I worked my way into a Tennessee society in the Army, I knew that the first thing you had to do was look at a guy. You could always read their eyes. Eye contact with a patient was the most important thing I could do, especially in the first two or three moments. They had to connect with me, and I had to connect with them. Once that happened, we were one.

I never sat at the desk. I had a chair on wheels. We're talking 1958. No austere conference room with padded chairs and pictures on a paneled wall, so it was easy for me to take my chair around and look somebody right in the eye and say, "What's going on?"

Was it a conscious decision to have patients call you by your first name?

It just happened. The fact is, I felt we were all equal. You've met people around town who think they're doing you a favor by making eye contact with you. Those people I avoid.

You worked hard to become a physician. Isn't the title, "doctor," appropriate as a sign of respect?

I definitely don't like it. For me, it doesn't work because I have always gotten my pleasure out of pure contact, one on one, without worrying about who you are or where you came from. It's the experience that you and I are having.

But wasn't it a kick to get out of medical school and be called Doctor Vastola? Didn't that mean something to you?

You know what happened the first time I got out of medical school? I graduated in Boston, and I went down to New York City to see a friend. I had come by train down to Grand Central Station. Integrated within Grand Central is the Biltmore Hotel. I went there for old time sake. In prep school, we used to go to New York for parties. We usually ended up having a drink at the Biltmore bar.

I sat down and had a beer. Who comes up to me but one of my old prep school buddies, who said, "You're a doctor, hanging out in a bar like this?" He was serious. "You don't do that. Don't ever do that again. People won't respect you. That is wrong."

That was eight or nine years after we had even seen each other. I couldn't understand his position at all. I was just being myself. He was disappointed that he saw me. He was telling me I would amount to nothing as a physician if I'm going to hang out in a bar and have a beer. That reinforced my feeling that I should not, in any way, ever have to change my basic behavior to become someone other than just myself. First, I'm myself—and not a doctor.

You seem to have just the right attitude for being a doctor, because the nature of the work involves dealing with people from every station in life.

A lot of doctors don't want that. They want their own sphere, to be on their own pedestal, and they are not going to move sideways or anywhere else. That's one of the real flaws in a large institution, or a medical school, where people are professorial and academic, but who do have obligations to work in a clinic and see patients, which they do, and I respect them for their total dedication. They see patients. They write. They do research, and a lot of administration, so they wear four hats.

I wear the hat of the world and that's where I want to be. You see one of those people and you see how often they make eye contact with you, and you listen to their inflection. It's hauteur. Now, there are some marvelous people who relate exactly the same way I do, but I'm talking about institutions I've been to and know well, all over the country. But the people who have developed the humanistic approach are not necessarily the doctors. The paramedical personnel play this role, too. You have to relate to the person, or else the consumer is not going to feel totally fulfilled. There's a great deal of emotionalism involved in the patient's illness. "You're not listening to me. How can I tell you how I feel, if you're not listening?"

An academician may be talented, but is he smiling? Is his voice changing in intonation, responding to the kind of emotional stream that you're trying to give him? It doesn't happen. You might say the academician, successful in the national arena is trying to tell you, "Look, I'm here and I'll do my best to help you, but I've got a lot of other things to do."

My experience with the upper levels of society, during my early childhood and my primary school childhood, was that these people would be doing you a favor by just looking you in the eye. I grew up in Waterbury, Connecticut. Waterbury, at that time, had made canons ever since the Civil War. It was primarily a heavy manufacturing city. The social levels at that time included the very rich industrialists, who were mostly Yankees. Then there was the mixed culture of the more recent immigrant groups. The Yankees, of course, had been in that area for four or five generations, so they had a certain level of acceptance that other people never really penetrated.

I was part of, what you might call the upper professional families from outside the Yankee {sphere}. As part of an Italian family, I was accepted on the edge. The three of us, as boys, got most of our pleasure not from social boy-to-boy contact, but through sports. I was big into baseball. We didn't have any social outlets for much pleasure.

The school system was geared for vocational training. We had to go to a private school to get a college preparatory education. We were very comfortable with where we were as children, and when we got to private school, we met abruptly with the upper levels of society and wealthy children from all over the country. This was a real strain, primarily, for me. My other two brothers, who also went there, were more comfortable, but I was more a rough and ready kid who would be quick to challenge anybody in conversation, primarily because I was so competitive in sports.

My brothers enjoyed their four years in private school with these people, but I never did. I never felt that I belonged to them. I grudgingly accepted my role, but I was glad to get out of there.

Your dad was a doctor. Tell me about him.

Our father was a very kindly, gentle person. The three of us accepted him as our role model, which contributed a great deal to what all of us went on to do ourselves. Dad, in our house, was a person of some reverence. He had the European tradition of the man of the house. Whenever he would get calls at home that my mother would answer, she would begin the conversation by saying, "Just a moment, I'll get the doctor." The doctor was either in or the doctor was out, and this was extremely formal. She was a lot more formal with his patients than he was.

We knew he was a completely dedicated surgeon. At home, he had periods of silence when he would do his own reading and we, by unwritten mandate, were careful not to bother him. He used to sit in the living room with big blocks of gum arabic. These are huge pieces of erasers that you could buy at that time. It was used primarily for packing. With his scalpels, he would sit in his chair in the living room and carve out abdominal organs to fix in his own mind the architecture and the relationship of organs to each other.

He would bring us down to his office frequently, and show us his new x-ray machine. If he ever turned it on, you'd die of radiation. His nurse, who was with him for over 40 years, was a certified technician. Nobody got radiation sickness, so it must have been a lot safer than it looked.

He would talk to us about his patients and how interesting they were. He had a marvelous practice with people all up and down the social scale. I can tell you a lot about some of his patients, whose children remained in contact with us for years.

My father went to Yale. He came to this country when he was eight, with his family. They became moderately well provided for, and dad went to Yale.

In 1941, after Pearl Harbor, we were at war. Just a few days before, my father was at a ceremonial dinner in New Haven, with the Italian Ambassador. He came home and related to us what the problems were. He was very concerned that bad things were going to happen. Within a week, federal agents came to our house and took out all the radios because we were felt to be a security risk to the country. They came out of the car with long coats, wide black rim hats. It looked like we were all going to be hauled off to a concentration camp. We used to go next door to hear the news.

Dad was also a community leader. He was heavily involved in the

Italian-American community. He was the founder of the UNICO* Club, which most Italians of my generation knew. He formed UNICO to get academically qualified Italian children out of the Italian ghettos and into mainstream American Society. He always felt that he rescued these people.

My mother was a school teacher. They were married in Waterbury, so there was this Anglo-Italian mix, which at that time was not always a friendly one, socially. We identified ourselves primarily through our father, because he was a successful surgeon who trained at the Mayo Clinic, when the two Mayo brothers were there. I trained there myself, and we hoped that our son, who is a surgeon, would have trained there, also. He chose not to, and went to New York City.

Was it your father's influence that led you to medicine?

I don't think I became a physician because my father was my role model. I made the circle and came back and discovered it for myself. I was in the Army for almost three years. I signed up early. I volunteered when I was 17, and was out of education for that time. I was in a tank division. This is a long way from the academic life. Truly, most days were a life and death experience, and you weren't thinking of anything like coming home. You even forgot your family.

When I got back, Connecticut was extremely generous to their returning veterans with their mustering out pay. It was five hundred dollars, which was a lot of money at in 1945. In addition to that, they gave me a scholarship to Wesleyan University.

After the end of the war, in May of '45, I went to the Sorbonne {University} in Paris for four months to study French. Then, I was transferred to George Patton's headquarters in Germany, where he was compiling a history of the war. After that, I went back to a communication company, which was part of International Telephone & Telegraph, and was at Nuremberg for about a month before I came home. I could've accepted a position there at twelve thousand dollars a year, running local communications. I notified my family that I intended to stay in Europe for a while, and they almost disintegrated. They pleaded and they called, "Can we talk?" I agreed to come home.

When I got home, the first thing I did was decide whether I should get a job in this country related to what I was doing, or should I go to college? At that point, I made my own decision to go into medicine. I've got to make a living. So what am I going to do? And that's what I did. I was very good in science. I got a prize for the most significant work in science when I graduated.

But it's very difficult to figure out why I became a doctor. One reason

* UNICO is the largest Italian American service group, whose members support charitable, educational, scientific and literary projects while promoting Italian heritage.

is that it's a feeling of empowerment, with no one to answer to but yourself. It's an independent vocation that allows you to be your own person. When I came to Madison in 1959, I picked the office where I spent my whole career because they were called not associated physicians, but assorted physicians. We were all our own individuals and we respected that.

Why are there three brothers who are doctors, whose father is a doctor? There may well be programming that I'm not aware of: that children are imbued with a sense of tradition, no matter what it might be, no matter what your decision. That may be so, but it would have been subliminal, in my case.

You have a son who's a physician. How does that make you feel?

Very proud that he continued the family tradition. I never pressured him. That would have created a terrible gulf between us. I always said, "You follow your own stream and do what is fulfilling for you." He always said he wanted to be what his father was.

How was medical school for you?

From my childhood and in my college career, I would not have considered myself very intelligent, so I had to work. I did graduate in the upper third of my class. I had excellent training appointments. But my God, during medical school, I don't think I ever saw the outside. I spent my evenings working as a librarian in the medical school to supplement my GI Bill check. I was always determined to get to where I wanted to go, and I excelled during the last two years because this was the doctor/patient relationship in hospital and clinic training. The last two years of medical school were pure joy.

How did you decide on your specialty?

It was my interest in coronary artery disease and the electrocardiogram. From there, I wrote an honors thesis on the role of cholesterol, arteriosclerosis, coronary artery disease and myocardial infarction. After my internship, I accepted a fellowship in cardiology at the Mayo Clinic, where I did all my work.

You became a jack of all trades, didn't you?

Well, yes. I took extra time training in rheumatology, cardiology, and pathology, primarily relating to coronary artery disease. I expanded in that area, and had a broad education in internal medicine. As an internist, about two thirds of the people you meet in the office are either well or worried well, and one third of your patients are sick or in the hospital.

Tell me about your approach. How did that all develop? You have such a nice rapport.

At that time, nobody had any training in medical school on relating to patients, or on developing a patient-doctor relationship. I can't believe

403

there was such a gap. I don't think I had any standards that I was prompted by, either from my father or anybody else.

Have you ever had trouble relating to certain patients?

The general perception when I was practicing was that the new patients who came to see you for one reason or another would stay with you. Those who left probably didn't like doctors in the first place. Two, people who really didn't like that kind of familiarity and preferred to be on a more formal basis. Number three, a person who did not like me personally for how I might look, how I might be on that day, circumstances that I might have no control over.

Early on, I would develop my practice from doctors in the office who wanted me to see patients sooner rather than later because of their own appointments, and then who I might keep under my care. People who might find me in the phone book, or who were referred by someone I took care of.

I saw a lady who came to see me because she thought I was Finnish. A suffix in Finish is—ola. Another one is—i, which is also Italian. A lot of Finish and Italian names end with vowels. We had a very good relationship, until this patient talked to one of her friends. This story came to me from a doctor who asked, "Do you remember Mrs. So and so?"

I said, "Yes. I've seen her quite a few times."

"She's not coming to you anymore. Do you know why?

She was talking to another lady and said, 'I am seeing Dr. Paul Vastola, and he really is a fine doctor. He's Finnish, which I think is wonderful, because I've never been able to find a Finnish doctor.'"

"He isn't Finnish. He's Italian."

'He's a what? {Laughs} An Italian?'

I never saw her again! She thought I was working a conspiracy on her. I was masquerading as a Finnish doctor.

Another doctor called me up one afternoon and said that he had one of his patients who was sick out of town, under the care of an internist there. He had been in the hospital, wasn't doing well and thought he better come back home. The doctor said he would arrange for me to see him. He arrived with this wife. He obviously was developing fluid retention from taking a new medication, which was on the market for several years and was withdrawn, not by edict, but because it wasn't a very good drug. On exam, you could hear fluid in his chest. This was a time when we'd hospitalize a person for a situation like that, instead of treating them at home, which I would today, because we have better medications.

I hospitalized him. After a few days, I advised he go home, stay around; I would see him once a week for two weeks, make sure he's stable and he could go back home.

The first week he came for his appointment, I had a beat up station wagon, which I parked behind the building, full of all the athletic gear that my kids and I used—soccer mainly, a couple of jock straps, tennis balls, and whatever else. What do you know, I'm getting out of my car and he's coming in for his first appointment. He parks next to me.

I said, "Come on in and we'll get going, so you can get out of here and go back home."

I could tell that he wasn't receiving me very well. I should have just taken him in the back door, which is where the physicians went. I didn't because he would have had to climb two flights of stairs. So, he walked around to the front and into the office, but I never saw him.

A half hour goes by and he doesn't show up. The first thing I'm thinking of, *Did he collapse somewhere?* I went out, looked and saw nothing. I told my nurse to check with the fire station across the street. They had no calls. We called three emergency rooms—didn't show up. In the meantime, I had to see my other patients. Every time a patient would leave, I'd say, "What's the news?"

My nurse finally said, "You don't want to know." I said, "Let's have it."

Well, he looked in the back of my wagon and said, "If the inside of his head is anything like the back of his station wagon, I don't want him. I am out of here." And he never did come back.

He actually admitted that to the nurse?

His wife did. She said, "I hate to tell you. I couldn't convince him that this was just his wagon and it doesn't have anything to do with how he practices."

He said, "He practices the same way he lives, and I don't want anything to do with him."

I cleaned up the wagon and got all that stuff out of there.

Were you insulted?

Oh, I thought it was a riot. {Laughs}

You were never one of these doctors who would drive around in a Mercedes or Porsche.

Oh, no. I would never want that status. That's just repugnant to me. It's awful.

You weren't one of these 100-hour a week guys, either. How did you decide to manage your professional life with your personal life?

Jackie was a big part of it in this way. The two of us are East Coasters. We developed the relationship that led to our marriage when we both found out the most important thing we wanted to do in our lives was get out of New York City. Our life was somewhere else.

I felt that I had given enough for my country, so that we ought to get a piece of the capitalization in the country. We got married and left.

I would not be the kind of a doctor who got up at six o'clock in the morning, be at hospital meetings at seven, and work all day, and get home late because it was our schedule to see hospital patients in the afternoon. We had a morning hospital meeting, morning hospital rounds, evening hospital rounds and then home. That meant I would miss all three meals with the family. I felt a big responsibility toward helping to raise our children. Medicine was going to have to be part of a bigger picture.

I refused to attend seven o'clock meetings. The meetings that I had were always at noon. I was responsible enough to my wife. We've always had a fine relationship together. I knew the kind of doctor who left his family for his practice to be the usual egomaniac, with a great sense of empowerment as to what he did, without any real concerns about his wife and children. That was terrible. I knew many of them.

Given your concern about having a reasonable schedule, did you ever have to do house calls?

Once or twice a week. It began as a gesture of convenience for the patient. Most patients could have come to the office, but I made house calls at their request.

Early on, one of the doctors in the office said, at the end of the day, "On your way home, would you stop and see so and so? She's a retired woman. She really sounded sick and you ought to make sure she doesn't have pneumonia because if she does, she's living alone and she doesn't belong there. She ought to be in the hospital."

She was unmarried, straight as a ramrod and prim to the last measure, and was sick with a bad cough. I examined her. It was my judgment that she had a bad bronchial infection, but she didn't have pneumonia and she didn't have a fever. I told her I would call down to the drug store nearby for a prescription. She was only two or three houses away, and I would go down and get it for her. She said, "No, I can go do this myself. How much is the house call?" Well, believe it or not in 1959, a house call was $8.

I said, "The office will send you a bill."

"Just a minute. I'll pay you right now."

She went to her bedroom and came out with eight crumpled one dollar bills.

"Here you are. May I have a receipt?"

I wrote her a receipt and called in the prescription. Going out the door, I suddenly remember, *It's our wedding anniversary.* I knew this particular pharmacy was the only one in town that had a liquor department, so I went in and bought a bottle of Champagne with her money. I never carried any money. It was six dollars. I'm rushing out to get home with my hand around the bottle in a paper bag, and here she comes. She saw the bottle, and she looked at me, and that was it.

The next morning, she called up the doctor in the office and said, "John, you've got a drinking doctor there. I just thought you ought to know." I never saw her again. {Laughs}

When you made house calls, did you have a little black bag?
Yes.

What was in it?
A stethoscope and a blood pressure cuff. Most house calls would be for respiratory infections. At that time, before emergency transport, they only thing you had was a private ambulance, which were not that plentiful. You would go to the home, make an appraisal and get a person with a serious problem to the hospital.

When you went to the home to examine a patient, the only thing you could lean on was the history and the physical examination, not the laboratory work, because it wouldn't have been available then. The other items in the bag would be a whole mini pharmacy—pain medication, morphine, cold preparations, some bottles of cough syrup.

Do you still have that bag?
I do.
{Within three minutes, he's back with a well worn, black bag that opens lengthwise across the top}.

When was the last time you opened this?
A long time ago! That's a laxative kit. Here is a rubber glove, and a kit to test for blood by rectal exam, which was important. Here's a tuning fork, and this empty box was for an ophthalmoscope, which I gave to our son. Here's an oxygen mask for resuscitation. Here's a thermometer, a book of standard values, a reference for using antibiotics to care for infections at home.

Would you carry this thing around as a matter of course? If you and Jackie went out to dinner, would you have this in the trunk?
Yes, always.

This looks just like what you saw in the movies or on "Marcus Welby,"[†]
Yes. I remember when we got here {Madison}, Jackie and I had $200. That's all I had. The first thing I bought was the bag. That bag cost about $100.

That was essential to being a doctor back then.
Very much so. I went down to the bank to borrow $3,000 and they wouldn't give it to me because I didn't have any credit. Then, I had to wire home for money. I never stepped into that bank again.

---

† Marcus Welby was the doctor character in a hugely popular TV series that ran from 1969-1976.

Are there any memorable experiences in medicine since retirement?

Since then, I've successfully resuscitated four people. I had two at an athletic club. One was an older gentleman who was working out in the exercise room on a slant board doing sit ups, when he collapsed and died right there on the board. The club has a loudspeaker, medical alert code, so they had three people in there who had received Red Cross instruction in CPR.

These three people flew up and started chest and respiratory resuscitation, but the man didn't respond. They knew I was in the building. There was also another doctor, Peter Karofsky, from the medical school. The two of us raced up. We were both in the locker room at that time, and here this man who was by definition, dead. Peter started mouth to mouth breathing and I did chest compression. We placed this gentleman on the floor. We continued resuscitation for about five minutes. And all of a sudden, the man started foaming at the mouth and salivating. You knew that you were purfusing because this was a sign of life and circulation.

We continued CPR until the EMT arrived. They shocked this man, established normal {heart} rhythm and brought him to the hospital. He never did have a coronary. He had diminished flow to the heart and went into fibrillation—an ineffective heart beat—but survived, and went home.

We had all sorts of responses from the family. They wanted to take us out to dinner, etc. Peter and I conferenced on this and said, "Look, we don't want to get involved in any of those public displays of appreciation because they can get very emotional, and the man could collapse again."

It was a very rewarding experience. You feel like God. You can't go around feeling that way for too long.

I recall you telling me about another heart disease case years ago that you managed over the phone.

That gentleman was in a phone booth out of town. He was having terrible chest pain. He was obviously having a heart attack.

I had been taking care of his wife. He was not my patient, but he related to me at a time when he needed some help. He thought he had bad indigestion, but he was feeling very weak and was afraid to go anywhere or doing anything.

But you're in Madison. This guy's in another city on the phone.

Right, but I had a straight-line communication with the hospital. I called the local hospital and it sent a helicopter over to the phone booth. The 911 car was already there with the flashing light and got him out of the booth. They developed a community rescue program. He was brought to the hospital within minutes. It was just a phone call.

You don't sound impressed with that one. Tell me a story you are impressed with.

I saw this man at home. His wife called me and he has terrible abdominal pain. I went in the front door and here's this man upside down on the stairway with his head on the floor and his feet up the stairs. Okay? With abdominal pain, looking badly, death-like, smitten. All you had to do was read the face and you know when somebody's in trouble.

He put himself there purposely. It was the most spectacular demonstration of what was happening that you could ask for, and it was well described. He had ruptured his aorta and his animal instincts said he was more comfortable upside down because the blood was less likely to leak out of the aorta. He was right.

What did you do at this point?

Ambulance and emergency surgery. He made it.

If it hadn't been for going upside down...?

I'm sure he would have died. He saved himself by pooling all his blood in his upper body, so he wouldn't lose it through his ruptured aorta.

You still keep up on medical advancements. Why?

I still continue to be a licensed physician and keep up all my continuing medical education credits. It's all computer-driven. I want to remain licensed. I'm intensely interested in medicine and I continue to write primarily for myself on the current scene. It's really important to be engaged. I also spend about an hour a day, hopefully less, managing my own financial portfolio.

I've had a marvelous life. I couldn't ask for anything better, especially knowing that, at least every other day during the war, I never thought I was going to survive.

Chapter Twenty-Seven

Fill-in Physician

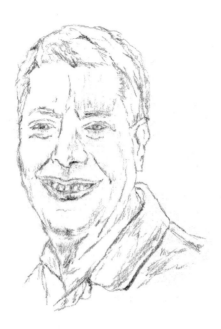

"'Do things your way, and I'll fit into that.' That does separate me a bit from many of my colleagues, who do like to have things their way."

Alan Schwartzstein, MD
Family Medicine, Oregon, Wisconsin

He doesn't make house calls, but Dr. Alan Schwartzstein is on the road every day. He fills in for colleagues who are sick, on vacation, or for whatever personal reason, unable to practice that day. Schwartzstein, in his mid 50s, is a Locum tenens. It's Latin for "holding the place."

Despite the fact that he's always working with somebody else's patient, Dr. Schwartzstein enjoys getting to know patients and developing strong relationships with them, which he considers essential for an effective patient/doctor relationship. The doctor explains how he accomplishes that when his job rarely allows him to see the same patient twice.

I had a mentor in medical school help me before I went into my third year. One of my best experiences was getting out for a summer externship in a rural area. I worked in Andover, New York, with a family doctor, who was just out of residency, named Toby Atkins. There were two other docs there; one internist and one family doctor. I spent eight weeks, mostly with Toby. I lived with them because they didn't have a place for a medical student to live yet. Toby taught me many of the things about family medicine that I continue on today. I lived the life of a family doctor and realized it was something that I enjoyed doing. He had three young kids. I saw how he balanced his family life with his medical life. I saw how he worked with patients who were having problems, and helped them to accept the ones that he couldn't help them with, or that they couldn't deal with.

One of the first weeks I was there, I was talking to him about one of the technical aspects of medicine and he said, "Alan, it's always been my goal to be the best doctor I can be. I don't care if I'm only an average physician, but I want to be a really, really good doctor."

I asked him to explain the difference. He said, "Well, I think of the best physician as being a specialist who knows all the science, reads all of the latest articles, and knows the latest, technically, about how to do something. I think of the doctor more in the way of *"Marcus Welby,"* or a person who can work with a patient. I may not know the latest thing, but I want to be able to work with my patients. That's what they really want, more than the latest science." That struck a chord in me. That's what I try to do when I try to be the best doctor I can be.

You have a rather nice rapport with people. Is that a natural thing or something you've developed?

It's a little bit of both, Steve. It's more the former. Medicine is a very social career. There are branches of medicine where one doesn't need to be as social, where one is using their technical skills, and those are very important parts of medicine. I'm thinking of neurosurgeons, cardiac surgeons, pathologists, and other fields like that.

I really enjoy the interaction with people and enjoy the opportunity to help people, both in the office and outside the office. I see myself as a jack of all trades, which is probably why, when I was a kid, it was hard to decide what I enjoy doing best.

As I went through {various medical rotations}, I found some role models and learned how to interact with patients and how to adapt myself to a family practice mode from them. One particular interaction I had in residency was with a mentor, Jack Cunningham, who was an old-time general practitioner. I was doing an exam on a nine or ten year old girl and wanted to do a complete exam and do a good job. Part of the requirement was to examine the private parts. I had done this with other patients without problem so far. In this situation, it was not very comfortable at all to examine those areas. I worked with her. I worked with her parent about how important it was that I do this examination to make sure things are okay. I got to a point where I stepped out and spoke with Dr. Cunningham. Jack came in the room and he knew the family and he said, "Hi," and did a little bit of an exam and finished and said, "Everything's fine" and left.

I talked to him about how we hadn't done this part of the exam and he said, "Alan, part of being a family doctor is to develop a relationship with the patient. This is the first time you've seen this girl. She wasn't comfortable, and our job is to really develop a relationship, so we can help people. Part of developing a relationship is building confidence. That's often much more important than the actual technical aspects of what we do and how we do things."

I like to learn. I like to be sort of a passive observer, but I had to learn how to adapt that to an interaction with the patients and have them trust me. When I counseled patients, I found it very exhausting. That was part of why I didn't go into psychiatry. I did eventually learn, after many long tours in my career, that there is a certain wall that a person has to put up at times in order to be able to help people. I enjoy people. I want to have an emotional bond with them, and yet as a physician I do have to step back and realize I'm in a therapeutic relationship with them, not a solely personal relationship. They're not coming to me as a friend or a relative. They're coming to me as a physician.

At times, I try to share bits of my life that might be applicable to what's going on, but I do that very carefully, and certainly not on a daily basis.

One of the hardest things, Steve, is hearing from people who are in trouble. A good doctor empathizes with people who are having a tough situation, helps to guide them to understand it, and yet is able to do that in a somewhat objective manner. The best doctors can do that very well.

Did any physicians in your family influence you regarding your decision to pursue medicine?

Coming from a Jewish family, there were influences from my relatives in New York City, toward becoming a doctor or lawyer, but my parents never really pushed me in that direction or any direction.

I really grew up doing fairly well in classes, but I didn't have a specific interest of what I was going to go into. I enjoyed math, history, and a lot of subjects, which is probably why I ended up in family practice.

As I got into college, I got interested in math, but I didn't really see myself being a researcher or a professor. I had too many social interests, and enjoyed being around people, so I started thinking more of social things to do and psychology interested me a lot. I had a couple people suggest that I should perhaps become a psychiatrist.

At the time, I had very little interest in the physician side of it. It was more as an avenue to fully do psychology. In college, I had a couple of experiences that probably led me more towards the physician side of that. I spent a summer in Europe with three friends, rented a car, and drove around Europe. It was the first real independent experience I'd had. I wanted to get away from my friends and do more on my own, to be more independent. That helped my sense of self-confidence and gave me a sense that I could accomplish more.

We picked up a couple of hitchhikers along the way, one of whom was going to medical school. We talked about what his interests were, and why he was going into medicine.

When I got back, I talked to one of my cousins, who was a pediatrician, about medicine itself. And then, based on those interactions, felt I needed to spend some time in the medical field to get a sense of what it's about. I volunteered in the emergency room at Princeton Hospital for the winter session of my junior year of college. I worked there for two summers, paid as a unit clerk and as an orderly, pushing stretchers, cleaning bedpans, giving back rubs, and taking orders from nurses. It was really the key to the decision.

All doctors should have to take orders from nurses because the nurses are the ones who really take care of the patients. We give orders. We make diagnoses. We make recommendations. But in the hospital, anyway, we pass that along to the nurses, who actually care for the patients. Everybody in medicine should have to clean some bedpans before they become a doctor. It's very challenging for doctors, actually, because many doctors don't have experience in the medical field before they go into medicine. We get to medical school and we spend our first two years mostly with the books and then, in the third year, we walk onto the wards and work with interns and residents, and we're instructed that we should be writing orders to nurses and unit clerks, who sometimes have been in the field for many years before us.

It's unlike many other fields, where a person works themselves up from the ground up, and as you work your way up, you're treated by those above you in a way that you can learn respect and humility. You understand how the world operates, and that you're not the greatest thing since sliced bread.

In a way, our medical education puts physicians who've always been successful in their educational career in a setting where they're automatically respected, but we really don't know very much, clinically. It robs us, sometimes, of the opportunity to learn empathy, humility and interaction with other people, so I applaud a medical education that takes them out in their first year and connects them with elderly patients and people without health care.

When I did my volunteer work in the emergency room, I fell in love with medicine. I enjoyed following the doctors, watching what they were doing. I enjoyed their process of trying to figure out what was wrong with

the patient, trying to help a patient, and I especially enjoyed the artful interaction, which I think was the side of psychology that interested me.

Medicine is not a science, as much as we'd like it to be. It's very much
an art. It's a person meeting with another person, talking about what's going on with them and figuring out with them the best thing to do in order
to help them, be that short term, such as giving an antibiotic, or long term,
as encouraging them not to smoke.

Then, as I learned more and talked to some psychiatrists, I realized if I
went into psychiatry I would be working with people in a thoughtful way
all day long with a lot of mental work. That was something that I didn't
think I could handle on a full-time basis. It takes a lot out of person to do
that.

I learned from doctors that I was with, that family medicine has as awful lot of psychiatry in it, so I started leaning more toward family practice.

What's an average day like for you now?

Early in my career, I had a life threatening illness which put me in a
situation where it would be difficult for me to practice the full spectrum of
family medicine, so I made a decision with my wife, as we were just starting
a family, to do a more limited practice. Initially, that led me to do urgent
care medicine. I took a job with a medical center, a large multi-specialty
clinic in south central Wisconsin. At that point in my life, being a little
more insecure with my illness, I thought being involved with a large organization would be easier for me to find the right path in medicine. I practiced
in the urgent care setting for about seven years and that worked well for us
as we were starting a family, but I still missed the family practice setting. I
didn't feel that I could go into traditional call, being up at night. I missed
delivering babies. There were aspects I definitely wanted to get back into.

At Dean Health System,* our department grew large enough that we
needed a full-time person to cover other physicians when they were on
vacation, when they had babies, when they got sick, went to conferences.
That position was created and I immediately applied for it. I was accepted
into it by my partners and have done that for ten years.

I have a scheduler who takes requests from the 22 clinics, and it's es-
sentially a full-time practice. This past week on Monday, I was in Madison.
On Tuesday, I was in Oregon. Wednesday, I was in Stoughton. On Friday,
I was in Milton.

So an average day for me is getting my kids off to school with my
wife, and then heading in to the clinic. I'll spend half an hour to 45 minutes
catching up on any chart work from the day before, checking my e-mails
for any of the community activities I'm involved with, and then start seeing
patients.

---

* Dean Health System is very large, physician-owned clinic with multiple locations in Southern
Wisconsin.

The patients are mostly established at that site. They don't know me as a physician, unless I've been fortunate to have seen them before. But they know their nurse, they know the exam room they're in, hence they're fairly comfortable. It's a challenge to adapt, to use my social skills to gain their confidence, to be able to practice.

You talked about how wonderful it is to develop that doctor patient relationship, and here you're working with other doctors' patients. Every day it's starting over, isn't it?

Yes, it is. I miss the continuing rapport with patients, and miss the satisfaction that a physician otherwise gets from seeing patients they've helped, and being thanked. I've had to accept that as part of where my life has guided me. I've developed my social skills to have the interaction with the patients there. I make sure that I'm very approachable to the patients. I make sure that I'm approachable to the staff at the clinics, so that frequently when I'm at the clinics and someone will come in and say, "Who's this Dr. Schwartzstein?" The staff says, "Oh, he's very nice. You'll like him." Of course, just that simple phrase from a nurse they know will make them much more comfortable and receiving to me when I come in. I get back to the clinics often enough, so I get to see some of the patients I've seen before.

If I wasn't there, that person couldn't be seen. If I wasn't there, the clinic couldn't get the patient in, so they're very appreciative.

Besides the rapport, you have to actually understand what's going on with them. Is the chart crucial in that respect?

It's not crucial, but it is very valuable. When I started in urgent care, we didn't even have charts when we went into see patients, so I had to learn in that setting. That was probably a good experience for me, how to interact without the chart. It was very frustrating at times, not knowing what happened. At times, we had to talk to patients more, do more testing, things they hadn't done before.

Dean is now converting over to an electronic medical record. That's made a world of difference in practice, because no matter what clinic I'm at, no matter what's happened anywhere in the system, I have at my fingertips the laboratory tests, the x-rays, and the thoughts of people who've seen the patient before. I can review that in my office before I even go to see the patient, if I know whether they have a complicated history or recent issues. I can walk in, fairly well armed with the information and background, to help the patient.

Doctors don't always agree with each other. Have you ever had to change course because you simply wouldn't do it that way?

Yes, I have. Most often, I figure my job is to practice in the way that the patient is comfortably treated and in the way my colleague is comfortable practicing medicine. There is no single best way in many situations. I respect my colleagues' approaches to how they do things.

In clinics, often when I work with a nurse I haven't worked with before, she'll say, "How do you like me to do things?"

I'll usually say, "How do you do things with Dr. Smith?"

"Well, this is what I do."

"Well, you do things your way and I'll fit into that." That does separate me a bit from many of my colleagues, who do like to have things their way.

The appreciation of the nurses and the doctors I work with is great. Occasionally, I'll work in a setting where the patient is not doing well, and there's something going on that we have to change, and I go ahead and change course. It takes some diplomacy and some tact to do that in a way that doesn't undermine the patient's relationship with the physician they're seeing. I'm usually successful in guiding the patient to go in that direction.

My colleagues respect my ability and my medical sense, so they'll go ahead and accept what I have done. Of course, it's their patient, and if they don't accept what I've done, they can always come back a week later and switch horses.

I bet there are patients who like you and would just like to make you their regular doctor. What do you do when that happens?

That does happen frequently. They'll often ask where I'm practicing. I explain the sort of practice I do, and that I very much appreciate their confidence in me, and that if I did have a single practice, I'd like to see them. Some have actually traveled to the various clinics I go to, just to see me. I try to limit that because it's not the kind of practice I'm in. I only do it in a situation where I believe it will work right for the patient and will not undermine their treatment or medical care.

What about the other side of that coin? It's almost like you're the substitute teacher. And substitute teachers get no respect at all.

At times I run into patients who are suspicious, and question what I'm doing. That usually just runs off my back. If I notice that this is happening, I just offer the patients options. "Would you prefer to hold off until Dr. Smith is back next week?" It's their life and their health, and I respect any decision they make for themselves.

Outside of the office, you've taken an interest in obesity prevention. How did that develop?

My main interest is in helping people's health in the community. As a family doctor, one of the things I've learned is that a doctor is not just a doctor in their office with patients. Part of family medicine is working not just with the patient in the room, but with their whole family, and in a way, their community—be it the extended family or the actual community.

Four or five years ago, I looked around in my practice and in my community and recognized how big people were becoming, and what effect this was having on people's health. I was a little bit ahead of the curve at that point. Now, of course, this is big news and everybody is following it. I decided it was something I could do for the community as a family physician and try and raise awareness. This is our biggest health hazard after cigarette smoking. If a person is overweight, it puts additional strains on their organ systems, including the musculoskeletal system, their heart, their lungs, and their endocrine system.

Diabetes is a big killer, and a big cause of morbidity. One type of diabetes happens almost exclusively in people who are overweight. Fat kids become fat adults. If you start off fat, there's a good chance you're going to go on in life fat, and stay that way. The best way to deal with this is through prevention, just as with tobacco. If people don't start smoking, they won't have to worry about cancer or heart disease from it.

I gradually started thinking about working more with parents and communities, so kids don't become fat. This is a struggle that has to happen outside the doctor's office. What I can do with a patient in one annual visit or even a few, is really limited in combating what society has done over the last thirty or forty years with making life more convenient, less necessary to have physical activity, and providing less healthy foods.

Today, TV has multiple channels, so it's a lot more seductive for kids. In addition, computers used to be the size of buildings. Now, we all have computers, and they're very easy. Passive entertainment is a lot easier. Kids want to spend screen time and don't want to get outside.

The second thing is the proliferation of junk food. We have so much media exposure, and so much advertising, that kids get unhealthy foods at an earlier age, and in unhealthy quantities.

Another thing that's changed is the amount of physical education in school. I think as we went through the '60s and '70s, and the Vietnam War era, some of society started to see physical education in school and connect it a bit with the military and fighting. There was a bit of a backlash against physical education, that it wasn't as important in school, and could be moved out for more important, cognitive activities.

I now go around and talk to people about physical education. It means educating kids about the importance of physical activity, the importance of the physical body and taking care of it in the same way they take care of their minds. That's just as important an endeavor for our school system to teach our kids as the three R's.

There are so many schools that don't have physical education all through the school year, or they start off with only every third or fourth day. We can tell them to be physically active all we want in health class, but when we bus them to school, provide them with non-nutritious foods, and only have them be physically active once every fourth day, the message is not the same.

Parents are the most important conveyers of that message. With the loss of the extended family, and with some single-parent households, the parents don't always have the skills, the knowledge, or the resilience and strength to be able to pass that message on to their kids. We now have a much higher incidence of single parent families. I struggle with the challenges of raising three, and I'm in a fairly stable situation with a spouse who doesn't need to work. For single parents, who may be away from their families, working as hard as they can to make ends meet, it's hard work to get a kid outside.

The school becomes the second most influential place where society can pass that message along. Our public school system is society's opportunity to demonstrate to kids what societal norms are. If our society is going to be healthy, and not be ravaged by the problems of obesity, then our schools have to show kids, and also have to help parents to educate kids, to take care of their bodies as well as their minds.

People have grown really large. Could genetics be to blame in many of these cases?

Genetics plays a small part in determining whether somebody's going to be fat. But genes don't change in a matter of years or a decade or two, so the fact that this has changed over a few decades, it's been pretty well studied and confirmed that genetics is not the reason why we've gotten bigger.

We're eating too much and not exercising.

Exactly. I'm worried that for people in their 20s and 30s's who have gone through this, it's going to be a gigantic struggle for them to reverse that. The studies show that so far, the medical treatment of obesity is not good. It's not that doctors don't want to help. We do what we can. But when a person develops certain habits in their life, and this happens over 20 or 30 years, they're very hard to change.

That's why I key in on the pediatric population and on prevention, rather than treatment. The best treatment we have now for adults who are fat, the most successful, is surgical treatment. That's a very expensive treatment that involves a lot of risk for people's lives, and I don't want to see that being the answer for our society. It's going to cost so much money and use so many resources that we won't be able to use those resources in better ways in health care and outside of health care. Learning what a community needs is important to a physician, to provide that help to the community, as opposed to what the physician's interest is.

But why the hell am I doing this? I don't have to do this. I've worked through my specialty society, in the schools. It's not something that I need to do to make money, to take care of my family or to practice medicine. It would be satisfying to me to see the changes made and see school systems make changes. I'm giving back to my community and that makes me a complete doctor.

Part of medicine is a calling. It's a calling that we accept and say, we want to do something better for our society. Some of it is probably a reward for ourselves and some of it is the oath that we take. We're going to do things to help our patients. That's more than just prescribing medicine and it's more than making money.

I was raised by parents who said, "It's important to give back to your society. It's important that you do well, and take a certain amount of your income and a certain amount of your ability, and give back without any expectation of a reward for it."

There's a concept in Judaism called Tikkun Olam, which translated from Hebrew means "repairing the world." Jews believe that when God created the Earth, the world, He made a little corner of the world that was not quite perfect and said to the people, "It's your job through your life to try to perfect that part of the world." I grew up seeing my father helping in our Synagogue; helping the community and give what we call Tekamah, or charity.

I grew up in Princeton, New Jersey, going to Sunday school and taking a quarter, a nickel, a dollar bill sometimes, putting it in a little box, and recognizing that there are people who are less fortunate than me. That's part of what I brought into medicine.

My parents were two generations away from moving from Europe, so their parents settled in the New York City area. I was born in Jersey; grew up in Princeton.

What did your parents do for a living?

My dad was an accountant. My mom finished college, which my dad did not, and had bookkeeping skills. She worked when we needed money, but when my sister and I were growing up, she was at home.

My mom died six years ago. She was 85. She had breast cancer twice. She suffered from depression her whole life after delivering her daughter. She was in and out of hospitals the last few years of her life with various ailments and clearly was not enjoying life.

She and my dad moved from our original family home to an assisted living facility about three years before she died. She sat in her chair most of the time. A couple times during that time, she had bouts of depression and said, "I really don't want to live anymore." That scared my dad and my sister a lot. It scared me some, but probably less, because of my knowledge as a physician.

I talked with my dad, my mother, and my sister about some end-of-life decisions. My mom developed a bowel obstruction six years ago, which meant that food could not transfer to her digestive system, and this is usually treated by having a feeding tube put in, taking some of the pressure off of the bowel and seeing if it won't fix itself. That was done in the hospital. The feeding tube was taken out and my mother was fed and she developed the infection problems again.

She'd had abdominal surgery a couple of times, and there was a possibility that she might have adhesions, connections between the bowel that needed to be stripped away, so a surgeon was brought in, gave his opinion and recommended surgery.

My mom said, "No. I don't want any surgery. I'm 85. I'm too old for surgery. I want to die."

My sister called me in a panic from out East and said, "You need to come and convince mom to have surgery." I spoke with her a bit on the phone. I spoke with my dad and my sister and I spoke with the doctor. We did convince my mom to have the surgery, with the idea that this might be a simple problem.

Then, I had a very spiritual experience. I decided I had to fly out East to see what was going on. I was torn myself, because I recognize that surgery at 85 does have problems, especially with somebody who has ailments. It's possible my mom might make it through the surgery without any problem. It's also possible she could have respiratory problems and other situations that come up. She could end up on a respirator. Many families don't recognize this, but when they tell doctors to do everything, they don't necessarily recognize what's going to come up down the road because of the care that they have requested.

While I was on the plane at 10 o'clock at night, I asked God for guidance. For one of the only times in my life, I think I actually heard God, because this was a moment when I heard a voice say, "It's time." It wasn't anything I said, it was just something that came to my consciousness.

I arrived out East about 11:45. My sister picked me up at the airport. I was going to stay at her house, but I asked her to drive me to the hospital. She said, "Mom's asleep."

I said, "That's okay. I just want to be with her for a few minutes."

So I stayed with her for about 15 or 20 minutes, just to get a feeling and then went back to my sister's house. I needed to be there to kind of confirm what I heard on the plane.

Surgery was scheduled for the next morning. Went to the hospital, met my dad and my sister and we sat down. And I said, "You know, I don't think surgery's the right thing."

And they said, "But the doctor said there's a good chance this could work."

"Yeah, I know. But there's also a chance it could go this way."

My mother had said a long time before in our discussions, "I don't want to have my chest pounded on." But in medicine, when you go into surgery and you go through anesthesia, those kinds of requirements are taken off. So I said, "We need to talk to the surgeon about this. During surgery, they're going to put a tube in her. If she has problems later, are they going to take it out?"

In fact, he confirmed that if her heart stopped while she was on the surgical table, they would pound on her chest. They would try to resuscitate her.

I asked, "If she gets through surgery and her lungs don't seem to be working right, will you take the tube out?"

He said, "No, we're not going to take it out right away. It may take a week or ten days to get out."

My mom clearly said before this that she never wanted to live on tubes. She didn't want to be resuscitated.

Even temporarily?

Even temporarily, yeah. At that point, I thanked the surgeon and told him I wanted to talk to my sister and dad a little bit. He essentially refused to leave the room. He continued to try to convince us that this was the right way to proceed. I don't know if I hadn't been a physician, if I could have diplomatically insisted that he leave the room, so I could talk to my sister and dad.

I told them, "I love mom dearly and there's nothing more I want than for her to get through this, but I have to tell you my experience as a doctor in these situations. We all want the best, but many of the situations we hear about people who are in the hospital on respirators for a long time because a decision was made like this early on, which might work, that hopefully would be simple. Mom's lived 85 years. She's said several times she'd lived her life and has had enough. I don't think we should let the surgery go through."

They had lots of questions. They wanted to believe what the surgeon told them, that this might be easy. I made the decision based on my medical experience of things going wrong, based on the voice I heard on the plane, that this was the right decision.

My sister finally said, "We can't make this decision without asking mom."

I agreed. So we went into the preparatory room where they were getting ready for the surgery and I explained to my mom as best I could what was going on. I said, "If you decide not to have the surgery at this point, you are going to die. The only other option is to give you some morphine to help control the pain and send you back to the nursing home where, within three or four days, without nutrition, without food, you will die. It's no longer a theoretical. It's a definite. If that happens, no more me, no more Rhoda, no more dad."

She looked up and said, "Mom and dad."

I didn't quite understand. My sister said, "She'll be with her mother and father."

So we went to the surgeon and said we're canceling the surgery. He was not happy. At that point, the chief anesthesiologist had heard what was going on, showed up and said, "You can always change your mind. At this point, there's no surgery."

We arranged for my mom to go back to the nursing home. That was Wednesday. She was on a morphine drip. She was comfortable the whole time.

My nephews came from across the country to say goodbye to her. I spent a couple of days saying goodbye to her, knowing I would never see her again. My dad spent time with her over the next four or five days, whenever he could, and went back to his apartment. He got a call Sunday morning that she had passed away.

In reflection, my sister, my dad, and me all believe it was the death my mother wanted. It was the perfect way for her to go. The whole family knew she was going. We could all say our goodbyes.

There have been times, Steve, when I've thought back wondered, should we have done the surgery? Maybe it would have been simple. Maybe mom would still be around. But I'm convinced as a doctor and as a son, that we did the right thing. I'm sorry that every family doesn't have a physician or a nurse to provide that knowledge to their family at that point in life, to give advice to avoid some of the situations that people get into.

I feel for your family, but I also feel for that surgeon. He wants to help your mom. He's dying to try. Do you feel for him, too?

I absolutely do. I actually sent him a letter afterwards, telling him how much I appreciated his efforts and how much I regretted that we had gotten into a confrontational situation. In a way, he was doing the same sort of thing that I try to do with patients, which is to provide them with the best information that I can. Then, let them make the choice or decision.

In this situation, we made the choice. He'd seen many successful situations and believed he could be successful in helping her. Whether he crossed the boundary of trying to force that decision on to the patient, I don't know.

At times I look at my surgical colleagues and realize that they believe very strongly in their abilities, and their technical abilities to get people through. If I'm in a critical situation, and I'm on a surgical table in the operating room and something tough comes in, I want somebody who's a little cocky, a little confident in their ability to do what they need to do and keep me alive. So perhaps it's good, in a way, that this fellow was very confident in his ability to protect my mom.

My role as a physician is much more as an educator and an advisor. When a patient comes in, they bring me a problem, or they come in and tell me, "I want to know if I have a problem." I'll talk to them, do whatever test is necessary, and then I tell them my assessment of the situation and what I think they should do. Sometimes that's as simple as saying, "I think you have an ear infection and I want to prescribe an antibiotic for you." At other times, it's a very different situation. One is end-of-life situations. We've become technically excellent in our society at keeping people alive at the end of life, even when their body may not be functioning well. We have many more decisions now than we did before I was born. People bring their own feelings about life into that situation at the end of life. Some value life very strongly and want to live regardless of the situation in which they're living and the conditions in which they're living.

Some feel just as strongly that if they can't be capable in certain aspects of their life, that life is not worthwhile. Those are situations where I see my task as a physician, to assess the situation, tell people the options and explain to them not just how this will affect their life, but also what, from my experience, I've seen happen to people when they go down this road. I allow them, and their families, to make the decision.

As I've conducted these interviews with several dozen physicians, spirituality and education come through almost every time. What do you make of that?

You've obviously hit a thread here about what perhaps happens to us as we're in the field. We can't always heal people. We can't always cure people's problems. We can always care about them as they're working through those problems. We can always provide them the best help we can and the best advice we can. In that role, we're educators.

If a person didn't have a certain spirituality, it would be very hard to accept the cycle of life and the fact that some people who get sick don't get better. Some people we treat don't respond to our treatment. And some people die too early.

When I was in practice my second or third year, I vividly remember having a man come into the hospital at about four or five o'clock who was having an acute heart attack. He was about 55 or 60. It was a very severe heart attack and I was in the coronary care unit of the hospital for five or six hours.

In between, I had a young woman come in who was in labor, who I was following. I went in between the labor unit and the coronary care unit, taking care of these two patients, which became three patients. This was the first baby I delivered in my own practice. I got about four or five hours of sleep that night, between giving orders for the fellow who was suffering the heart attack and examining the woman in labor.

At about three o'clock, the fellow with the heart attack passed away. About 5:30, the woman delivered a healthy, newborn baby. I left the hospital tired, but educated about the cycle of life and found that to be something that really reinforced for me one of the joys of medicine. A life passes away, and new life comes into the world. One of the most exciting parts of medicine is to be involved in the birth of a child.

We're privileged as doctors to be involved in people's lives. Our job is really to respect them and to understand that we do our best to make each of those processes to go as well as they can for the people we're working with.

That night when I delivered a baby and the gentlemen with the heart attack passed away, reinforced for me that practicing medicine was not a success or failure sort of endeavor. There's a circle of life. People are born. People die. Some people are healthier; some people are not. How I do is not whether the patient is healthy or lives or dies, but how I adapt to the situation. That is where the art of medicine comes in.

VIII

Medicine on Trial

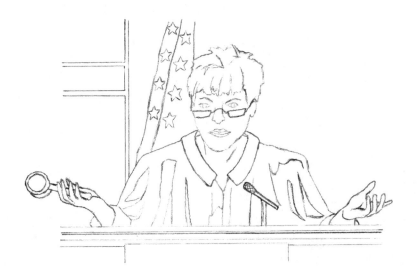

"Law and justice are not always the same."

—Gloria Steinem

Chapter Twenty-Eight

Courting Medicine

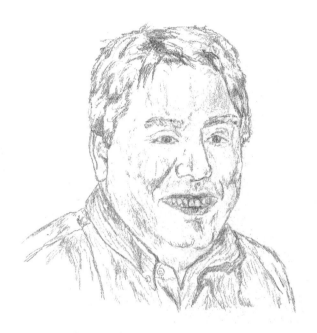

"There are lousy doctors who never get sued and there are great doctors who get sued all the time."

Richard Roberts, MD, JD
Family Medicine, Belleville

Lawyers and doctors go together like oil and water, unless of course, they're one and the same. At age 41, Richard Roberts, MD, JD was sworn in as one of the youngest presidents in the Wisconsin Medical Society's long history. He also served as president of his national medical specialty society. By virtue of his many activities, the guy seems to know just about everybody.

He's a mover and a shaker alright, but mostly the former. To call Roberts, now in his early 50s, a frequent flier is an understatement. He has been traveling the globe regularly for the past couple of decades, often because his dual training as a doctor of both medicine and jurisprudence has become increasingly relevant in medicine today. That's why, as a reporter, I so frequently called him for comment.

Doctor Roberts says he doesn't require a lot of sleep and it's a good thing, because he claims to regularly work 100-hour weeks. So it should come as no surprise that he's in his office on a Saturday morning, where Dr. Roberts explains to me why it was important for him to practice medicine with a law degree.

~~~~~~~~~~~~~~~~~~~~

I wasn't one of those guys, who wanted to be a doctor from age five. But when I finished high school, I wanted to do something where I was help-ing make a difference in the world, and could do that in a way that you could touch and experience fairly immediately. I was also conflicted by wanting to paint on a larger canvas, in terms of policy, of making systems better. The way that the tension between those two aspirations played out was really to go both paths, the law and policy route, as well as take care of patients through medicine.

Part of the law interest came from a guy named Fred Kriss, whom I got to know as a college student. Fred was an inspiration to me. I painted hous-es in the summer. One of the guys I was painting with—his best friend's dad—was a doc in town, so we were getting all kinds of doc jobs, and one of the physicians was Dr. Kriss.

Fred and I really hit it off. He would allow me, as a college student, to accompany him on hospital rounds and scrub in on neurosurgical cases. It really solidified my vague interest in medicine. Fred was one of the most compassionate physicians I had ever met.

One morning, we were looking in on a guy who had been in a persis-tent vegetative state for many years. You couldn't really communicate with him. Fred came down and sat next to him on the bed, told him about the Packer game that day and what the weather was like outside. There was a young nurse who was standing there listening to this, too. Fred asked me to go out to the nurses' station and get something. As I walked out there, she walked with me.

She said, "What's wrong with him?"

Well, I said, "He's in a persistent vegetative state."

She said, "No, no. I mean the doctor."

I said, "What do you mean?"

"He's talking to that patient like he's with us, and he's not."

"Well, you have to understand Dr. Kriss. He thinks that everybody's very important, and that you just don't know what's going on inside, so you always assume the best."

He had a big effect on me in that way, and he was the guy, in the end, who really encouraged me to pursue a law degree because he was pretty much involved with the legislature. This was in the early, mid '70s, and we were just beginning to have the first malpractice crisis, so Fred was doing a lot of testimony before the Legislature. He used to complain incessantly about these idiotic lawyers who were making health policy that had nothing to do with taking care of patients. Wouldn't it be nice if we had a doc who could actually understand that stuff and help make things better?

I was a philosophy major in college, and so I was already interested in chewing on a lot of ethical issues, like Roe v. Wade, euthanasia, eugenics, and the law was a big part of that. The law was seen as an instrument of social change in the '70s. It was the Watergate era.

When I wrote my law school application at 19, I said I do not intend to practice law. I want to practice medicine. I said I wanted to practice primary care medicine in an underserved area for a while, and then do patient care and change the health care system.

Before we get into that, tell me about your upbringing.

I lived a comfortable middle income life as a kid. I was born in Beaver Dam, Wisconsin. I moved to Madison, two years later and spent the rest of my formative years in Madison. I was the oldest of five kids—two sisters and two brothers.

We had one car, no garage. Five kids in a three bedroom house. My dad worked for the Singer sewing machine company. By the time we came to Madison, he was like a store manager. As I was growing up, he became a regional manager and quite often traveled across the Midwest to oversee different stores.

My mom was a homemaker all of her life, until my sister was probably ten. Then, she started working. That was fortuitous, because a couple years later, when I was just starting my second year of med school, my dad dropped dead with a heart attack, out jogging one morning. He didn't have any health problems. He was 51. That's why I said it was fortuitous that she had this job. It was helpful, obviously, financially, but emotionally, just to have an outside thing that she could do.

How did your parents feel about your interest in medicine?

They were very proud that I chose that path. We had never really had anybody in our family go to college, much less to medical school, so they weren't quite sure what that meant. My parents weren't really in a position to fund school for me, so I was working two jobs, and played football for a while at the University. I was juggling so many balls in the air, I thought I'd better get through this pretty quickly, because it's either going to kill me or I'm going to go broke. I accelerated, and got through college in three years.

The way I always started the registration process was that my first visit was always to the Dean's Office. I'd get permission to take an illegal number of credits. They just got used to it at the undergraduate level and in law school. "I'm Rich Roberts. I need 24 credits this semester. Is that okay?"

It was law school, and then medical school?

Absolutely, and some people think that's a little odd. It is. The typical path is you go to medical school, do a residency and then you practice for a while. Then you decide, because you're angry about malpractice, that you're interested in doing other kinds of work. You go to law school. Then, most of those folks end up doing the law, which is less physically taxing. Medicine is very long hours. It's very emotionally draining, if you're dealing with dying people. I never practiced as a lawyer, but I'm sure that being in the middle of conflict and controversy can be pretty emotionally taxing. I just found the medical training much more intense, because you're actually doing it. Law is more about talking about doing it.

But that wasn't what I was about. For one thing, I was a little nervous about coming up with a couple hundred bucks to be admitted to the Bar, because I didn't have it. When I went to law school in DC, we probably spent the first three or four months on a towel at night. We stayed on a mattress all the way through residency six years later, so there wasn't a lot of discretionary income.

I feared being tempted away into the law and leaving medicine. And I did have some interesting plane conversations during my medical school years, with guys offering six figure incomes to go help them sort out med mal cases and things like that, because somebody who has medical training who's a lawyer—that's pretty good. I don't know if it's a big deal anymore, but it was then.

I loved law school. The two professions approach things very differently. How they think about things is different. Under the law, all the rules you operate under are human-made, by judges and legislatures. Those people change, so you live in a bit of a relativistic world.

As a law student, there's not a correct answer, but there's the strong or persuasive answer. In evidence class, you were sitting in a class of 500 people and professor calls on you. "Mr. Roberts, give me the plaintiff's argument in this case." Then, he'd snap his fingers two minutes later and say, "Give me the defense argument." You shift gears and deal with that. It makes for a kind of mental nimbleness that I enjoyed. People who tend to do well in that environment have good written and oral skills; they're people who are pretty good at logic and deductive thinking.

Medicine, on the other hand, tends to, at least philosophically, deal much more in the absolute. If I can just learn these rules and apply them properly, things will turn out well.

What I always tell students and residents is that half of what you learn is going to be out of date, incorrect, or incomplete by the time you finish your training, and you're not going to know which half. The doctor's absolute world isn't as absolute as he or she would like to think. It was interesting for me to live between those two worlds, where knowledge and truth, and how to help society best, are viewed somewhat differently.

Did your legal training pan out as you had hoped, as you progressed through your medical career?

I think so. At one level, in terms of just my own personal growth, it was great because I got to watch *"Star Trek"* reruns and play Sheepshead. But I think it improved my speaking skills, my writing skills, and, most important, I got to understand better how America works.

Whether it's constitutional law or contract law, it makes you think about what's the point of all this? We talk about rules and regs and laws, and conflict in the pursuit of what? Who are we and what are we about? What matters in life? You have to think about that stuff because, in the end, it has to work for some reason. It's about more than just making money. It's about trying to make lives better.

I got through law school in two years, and that saved a couple years of tuition and time. I went to George Washington Medical School in Washington, DC, did the usual four years there, then ended up doing a family medicine residency through UCLA-Santa Monica Hospital for three years, and then returned to Wisconsin, where I did about three and a half years practicing in an underserved community in Darlington, Wisconsin, from '83-'87.

There's enmity between these two professions. I wonder if you see lawyers in a different light than your physician colleagues do?

There's no question that you can find lawyers who do it for all the wrong reasons—for greed or ego. But there are lots of people who are just trying to do a good job. The people who are being pointed at and beat up on are people I used to call classmates a while ago. They didn't cheat at cards and they cared about the world, just like I did, so perhaps I have a somewhat different perspective. Nobody likes a lawyer until you need one, and then you want the toughest, meanest S.O.B. you can possibly find on your side.

The financial motivation appears to be quite high among lawyers who want to get rid of award limits in medical malpractice cases.

Plaintiffs' lawyers remind us that they are not going out there getting folks. Most of the time, it's folks coming to them because they're unhappy because the system hasn't treated them right. But I bet most lawyers think of a cap {on pain and suffering and other intangible losses} as a reasonable balance. There are lots of limits out there in life. I might like to drive without speed limits, but in this country we've decided that that's just not permissible. And so, for the good of all, we've put speed limits on our roads.

The law reflects the culture of the people, and we have an anti-authority mentality, so if I'm a patient and I feel like I've been done wrong, I'm going to want to tackle that. I don't care that a tribunal of doctors said the doctor done right because I don't trust those guys anyway. They're authority figures. Does the law get it all right? Heck no. Making laws and adjudicating them is a pretty complicated process. Most of the time, they probably get it right.

What are the main reasons why we have med mal lawsuits?

It's where medicine's failings are most glaringly illuminated. The thing about medical liability that surprises me is that there aren't more lawsuits filed. We know that there is a two out of 100 chance of getting hurt any time you show up at a hospital, but only one out of ten times will you file suit. Only one of 20 times will you get any money, so there's a lot more malpractice going on than is being recognized, litigated or compensated.

There are many lawsuits filed where it's not negligence, but it's only after you have worked through the entire process, done discovery and have both sides tell their story, that you, as a jury, can decide that. Four out of five times, the jury finds for the doctor.

But doctors find it so unsettling to have to go through that process. The goal of the tort system is to make people who are negligently injured whole again, to punish the person who hurt the individual, and put others on notice regarding the behaviors they should avoid or do, to not have those injuries occur. Our system doesn't work very well in any of those three regards.

In terms of punishing, most docs have insurance, so other than the embarrassment and time out of practice to deal with it, and the aggravation, it doesn't hit them in the immediate pocketbook. In terms of putting physicians on notice, most doctors don't know what they'll get sued for. We're blowing smoke in the wind. Many doctors use malpractice risk as the great boogey man to justify all kinds of other dumb stuff—over-testing, over procedures, because I'm going to get sued. Where is the evidence for the statement? It's actually pretty sparse.

Some of the blame, I lay squarely at the feet of physicians, because we're excessively sensitive to it. Docs have this mental image, and society enforces it in some ways, that we're perfect, and we're not. Every one of us makes mistakes. We're going to make a bunch before we retire, and we hope, in our heart of hearts, that none of them ever comes to the light of day. More important, we hope nobody is ever hurt by them.

The whole culture of medicine is, bury your mistakes. The patient safety movement, which I'm very involved in, is trying to help us get past that because we find in most kind of systems you're just not going to improve your performance unless you get out of the name, blame, and shame game. We practice in very complicated health care environments, and no one doctor is usually going to make or break a patient's outcome.

We have an 18th Century system trying to catch up with 21st Century medicine. In the old days, it was only the doctor. It wasn't the nurse. There wasn't a hospital. It was the doctor.

Today, you have a whole bunch of players, and everybody's got a role, and everybody's got a role in the outcome, so to hold a doctor singularly accountable, which is how the system by and large works, sucks. It's inappropriate. It creates all kinds of strange stresses on doctors and on the system. Part of it's the system, and part of it's the patients. Patients have unrealistic expectations.

I get this all the time from policy wonks: Doctors see themselves as God. That's bull. Most of them don't know what they're talking about, in terms of the hours that I've watched people at the bedside, young doctors and old doctors, trying to explain things to people, approaching them with great respect and great humility.

People, understandably, project their own biases and assumptions onto the doc. Unless you're mature enough to recognize it, you're going to stay stuck in a bad system. My conclusion is a pox on all our houses. We all have more than enough blame to go around.

What's the smarter way to do this?

You'd like to go to a either a scheduled compensation approach, sort of like the Workers Comp approach, or find less fractious settings where people could work through these disputes with much less animosity. I don't think either of those will happen in America, any time soon.

From an affordability standpoint, you probably do have to put a cap on non-economics.* It's the most volatile part of the judgment. It's the most lucrative part for plaintiffs. It's a very complicated issue, and, in some ways, embodies all the dramatic elements and tensions between the law and medicine and insurance.

When somebody has a bad outcome that none of us wanted, it's perfectly appropriate to let them know that you feel bad. But to the extent that you screwed up, it's also appropriate to let them know that and to say to them, "I'm going to do my best to fix it."

When I was on our inpatient hospital service, a woman who came in late one night was admitted with chest pain that was not very typical for heart trouble. She didn't have many risk factors, other than being in her 60s with high blood pressure.

The usual protocol at the hospital was to get three sets of heart muscle enzyme and blood test levels, and do two electrocardiograms. All those were normal. We saw her early the next morning, and she was feeling fine. We thought the pain, based on her exam and history, was due to her chest wall muscle, which is very common. We sent her home. We told her the tests look good, but at some point, she should probably consider getting other testing done, just to be sure this wasn't an unusual presentation of heart disease. And, here are the things to watch for. If any of these things come back, please come in.

---

* Noneconomic damages are the part of the judgment that compensates for intangible losses, such as pain and suffering, loss of companionship, etc.

Unbeknownst to the team, just before she left, had another electrocardiogram done. None of us had ordered it. I didn't see it. Nobody else did, and she goes home. Mistake number one was having a third ECG performed that was not ordered. Mistake number two was allowing my patient to go home without any physician being made aware that she had had a third ECG and that it was abnormal.

The next day, she's back in the emergency room and they do another electrocardiogram. She's got chest pain again. By this time, they had that ECG from the day before and both of them were abnormal, showing evidence of heart muscle damage. The emergency doctor says to her, "Well, why did they send you home with this abnormal electrocardiogram?" She was admitted to the hospital. I saw her the next morning.

I was stunned. Where did this thing come from? So I said to the residents, "Come on, I'm going to teach you something about doing right by people." I took the three electrocardiograms and I sat down and said, "Here's what's been going on. We had these tests done. They were all normal. This other test should not have been done. You didn't have chest pain. I don't know why it was done. None of us saw it. You went home. Thank goodness, you listened to us before leaving and came back when you had the symptoms come back. But now you can see, on this last electrocardiogram, that it looks different than the first two. It's abnormal. And that was also what they saw when they did the new one on Sunday. And by that time, they had the last one that was done on Saturday, just before you left the first time. That shouldn't have happened. That was a screw up. I'm sorry. I don't know why it happened or how it happened. You shouldn't have gone home. But, thank God, you're okay."

And she was. She was very appreciative that I was just straight with her about it. Nobody can design a system that absolutely eliminates all possibilities of error. But you have a responsibility as a human, and as a professional, to step up and take responsibility, and try your best to make it right with people.

What keeps docs from doing that is a lot of things. It's part of the culture of training; partly practice anxieties. You're too busy as it is. This is going to be lots more work to try to make it right. There's also this weird thing. There's this ethic among physicians and health professionals that we're going to treat everybody the same. I don't care if you're the CEO of a company; you wait in line like everybody else. It's the guy who's got the most pressing health need that gets my attention first. Many people feel very strongly about that.

I believe that's wrong, because people's needs go up and down. When you've got somebody who's had a bad thing happen to them because of what you did, you have to go the extra mile because you put them in harm's way.

It's not always so clear that a mistake was made, is it?

What's interesting is that doctors will sometimes conclude that they committed malpractice when they didn't. You have to prove four things: First you have to prove a duty or relationship to the patient. Another thing you have to prove is that there is harm or damage resulting from the care. Very few people sue for frivolous reasons. Most people have pretty horrible outcomes that they wouldn't want for themselves or their families.

It's the other two parts of this that are much harder to prove. Did the doctor commit negligence? Negligence means he did not perform at the level of a similarly situated practitioner. That's pretty hard to prove. Why? Because we don't know what most doctors do. Nobody does that kind of research. We can tell you what we think the doctor should have done, but when you ask doctors what they actually do themselves, they're often wrong.

I do lots of talks, and I'll say to a physician audience, "How many of you in the room have seen a patient with a sore throat?" Every hand goes up. "Can you tell me in the last month, how many did you see?" Not one hand goes up. If you can't tell me how many you saw, can you tell me what percentage of them got a strep screen? And what percentage of the strep screen people got a strep culture? How many got penicillin? Doctors don't know this stuff because we're like battlefield surgeons. We're sitting in the trenches and they just keep throwing bodies at us. We don't have the time or wherewithal to climb out and see how the war is going.

What the expert witness in a lawsuit testifies to is what the average doctor does. He doesn't know. He's making it up. It's a legal fiction that we engage in, as a system.

The other element that you have to prove is that the negligence is the cause of injury. That's probably the hardest of all to prove. The example I use is breast cancer. The doctor will have identified a lump in a woman and advised her to come back in a month, after the next cycle. The woman forgets, the doctor doesn't have a tickler file system, and so the woman comes back 15 months later. By now, the cancer has spread and she has a very low chance of survival. Was there anything he could have done 15 months earlier? You don't know. Sometimes you could have, many times not. We don't know. One of the reasons docs win 80% of the time is it's hard to prove this stuff to the satisfaction of the jury.

Doctors want to help patients get meaning from what happened, and sometimes they'll blame themselves for stuff they shouldn't blame themselves for. You have a child who has cerebral palsy. He has a catastrophic outcome. He has seizures and mental retardation, and you feel terrible. You know that it was a long, pushing, second stage labor, and so you say to yourself, "Maybe we should have done that c-section two hours ago."

You know what? Less than one out of 10 times does the birth process have anything to do with those neurological, handicapping conditions.

Ninety plus percent of the times when you're blaming yourself for that, you're not only going to be scientifically incorrect, you're going to be, 100% of the time, legally inflammatory because a kid who has a handicap is going to be very expensive. There's no mechanism in the U.S. system to cover those costs.

In other countries, their healthcare is already covered and there's some sort of disability coverage in place to cover that. The poor family, they have to turn to somebody to help feed this kid, provide nursing and other care costs, and they use the liability system to do it.

In some ways, what makes the liability system suck is that so many other social support systems in the U.S. suck, in terms of health insurance and other social welfare mechanisms. If we don't want to pay for those other things, as docs, for example, then we shouldn't whine too much because the arena that we live in also isn't very functional. You can't have it both ways.

For the people who are found negligent, do they tend to fall into the same category as other professions? There are lousy cops and lousy journalists, and there are some lousy doctors, too.

There are. If this was more consistent, we'd probably all feel a little better. In other words, if the lousy doctors got sued the most often and the good doctors got sued the least often. Yet, I can also tell you that there are lousy doctors that never get sued and there are great doctors who get sued all the time.

The New York studies on heart surgery have shown us that if you're going to hold my results up to public scrutiny as a surgeon, my tendency is not to take the hard cases because I don't want to look bad. If they know that people are second guessing them, they may not take that risk.

The liability system is a pretty inefficient and ineffective way of sorting out good and bad performing doctors. When you look at the literature, there's not a very good correlation between the two at all. To get a lawsuit filed, to get it through the system, to win the case against the doc, that's a pretty unpredictable crap shoot. Society would be ill advised to ever depend on that as a way of weeding out bad doctors or bad practices.

I do think that the other mechanisms we have are pretty good. We have lots of overlapping review processes. Everything from the group that you're in, the hospital you have privileges at, the health plan where you provide services to, to the Medical Examining Board, to our quality improvement organization. I can promise you that there's no other profession that is reviewed and re-reviewed to the extent that docs are.

You were the first physician I had ever met who was also an attorney. Have you found that throughout your career, your medical colleagues have also been interested in your dual expertise?

It happens nearly on a daily basis. It plays out in a lot of ways. I'll get calls from around the country from physicians who've just been named in a suit or are about to be, or had some other sort of a legal problem come up and they want some help with that. I still sit down with our residents and I help them with their contracts and their negotiations, and their first employment group that they join.

The thing that's been kind of fun for me with the experiences that I've had, is there almost isn't a town in America where I could go, where I wouldn't know somebody now. I've been to every state—I can't even count how many times—at least a half dozen times. And I've been to 85 countries. The traveling started in a big way when I started getting involved with the American Academy of Family Physicians. I've served on national commissions for them since I was a second year resident, so that goes back 21 years now. In the late '90s, I became president of the American Academy of Family Physicians. I had to travel so much for those duties that I went to part-time in my University job.

When I first entered practice in Darlington, Wisconsin in 1983, I was also volunteering half a day at the University of Wisconsin, teaching through the family medicine program. I really liked that. They kept working on me to join the University full-time and I finally did, in early '87. I'd come to very much enjoy taking care of rural folks, farmers. I started in Belleville, Wisconsin, which was then 1,500 people and is now 1,900. I've been there for the last 20 years.

I've also had the chance, because of the University position, to do all kinds of other interesting and fun things. I've been the department chair; headed up our Madison campus. The University of Wisconsin Family Medicine Department is a very large, complex department. We have campuses in Milwaukee, Eau Claire, Wausau, and Madison. We cover about 110,000 square miles of the state. We have 150 faculty, 150 residents and fellows.

When I got into academe, it got lots more intense. I was giving talks around the country; around the world. I conducted exchange programs, where you'd have students from Nigeria, Ghana, Barcelona, and elsewhere come spend time with me and I sent students to them. I did the Kellogg fellowship. That was four years of traveling all over the world.

It's an unusual month that I'm not in airplanes a dozen times. I'm still doing 120 days on the road, also on weekends. When I'm not traveling, I'm on call. It's kind of what my life is like. I'm a professed workaholic. The last time I worked under 100 hours a week, I was 18 years old, starting into college. You just figure out how to crank it up and keep the tread mill running on high speed. People always ask me, "When are you going to slow down?" I always say, "After I'm dead. I'll have all eternity to rest. I'm having too much fun."

One of the problems many of us are having as docs is that we work long hours and often do not avail ourselves of the opportunity to engage in the community because we feel like we're so busy and we deserve the time away with family. And frankly, it's the income. When you live in the big house on the hill, it means you're not seeing everybody else that's not on the top of the hill.

But my medical school preceptor, Ed Richards, was not like that. He was part of the community, and I loved that. That's why I became a family doc. Ed had just stopped delivering babies. He was a community icon. He saw patients out of his own home. He'd taken care of generations, been there about 30 years. It turned out that when I looked at the list of preceptors, {Richards} lived only a mile from my apartment. I thought, great, I could have two months were I could walk and not have to drive 14 miles to downtown DC in this choking, sputtering, barley alive car. It was a dying car that drove my specialty choice.

How do you maintain a pace like that and have a family?

It's a challenge, but you need to be creative, too. I'll deal with family first, because it's the most important, and it has to be that way. I've developed some strategies for managing all this. I've tried as much as I can to have them involved in stuff, so my kids have been all around the world. A standing rule in our house is that any trip that dad is going on, as long as it works out okay with school, you can go.

When I led a U.S. trip to Vietnam and the Philippines, my two middle kids went with us for two weeks. They saw leper colonies in Vietnam. They visited with the health minister in Hanoi. When I represented the U.S. to the world meeting in South Africa, my youngest went along, with my father-in-law.

My other kids have been to Costa Rica and France. Sometimes it's one of them. Sometimes it's all four. Sometimes it's all six of us as a family. It's kind of what works for people and what the budget can afford. Those kinds of experiences are worth investing in, partly because they're special family experiences, but they're also for the kids—it's opened their eyes to a bigger world.

When I'm on the road, I'm on a regimen that I stick to that has been helpful. I usually try to call the kids twice. I still have three teenagers at home. The oldest is 23, and in college. Once after school is done, and I usually ask about their homework assignments. Then, later that night, I get back to them and say, "Now, what about this English thing?" I probably bird-dog their homework closer than their mom does, even if I'm half a continent away. I would really be in hog heaven if I had a two line with broadband access, because I could use a little web cam I could put up. They could see me and I could see them. I could do on-line editing. I'm working on that.

I won't kid you. It's been stressful. It's hard. For me, on a personal level, it's lonely when you're traveling that much. But it's also one way that

I feel that I've been able to, in my own small way, try to make the world better, because a lot of what I do when I'm at these other places is learning a lot of stuff. I'm trying to change stuff. That's what drives me.

For the practice, as a family doc, people need you when they need you. But they also usually manage to wait until you're there. Here's a story about staying connected in the 21st Century.

In the year I was getting ready to be Academy president—that's a 300-day travel year—I knew that was going to be a crazy year, so I was giving people a business card that had my cell phone number and paging number that worked all across North America. I said, "Look, my partners are great here. If you need help, they'll be happy to help. But if you need me, just give me a call, or send me an e-mail or page me and I'll be happy to try to help you from wherever I am."

Well, people rarely contacted me. One of the lessons that that taught me was that if a patient has a sense that they can get to the doctor, they don't bother them. Part of what's gotten so dysfunctional in American health care with people covering for each other, from the patient's standpoint, it's just another stranger in the night I'm going to be talking to, so I don't mind keeping him up at night.

From the doc's standpoint, it makes call hell. But when the patient and doctor truly have a relationship, where I've said to you, "I'm going to make a leap of faith, Steve: I'm your doctor. You need me. You get me. You don't bother me, because you know I've got a life, unless you need me, in which case I want to know, anyway."

I've been trying to develop this franchise model for how to do this. Patients trust doctors. You have to, if you're going to reveal the most intimate aspects of your life; you're going to take your clothes off in front of me, I'm going to stick my fingers in places nobody else should stick their fingers, do obnoxious things to you and, in a sense, put your life in my hands. You have to trust me to do that.

What doctors haven't done very well is trust the patients not to abuse them. Sometimes it's for good reason, but sometimes not. We have to find a way to get back to that mutual trust.

One of the ways I've managed to make the practice work is to take down the barriers between us. I've explained to patients what I do. I was in Europe a few years back and I got this e-mail. "I've been having all kinds of bruising and I am tired. What do you think?"

I read this and I immediately wrote a response. "This may be just a simple virus infection … But you better get to the clinic tomorrow for a blood count."

Now, she was a very bright patient. She ended up having a very unusual form of cancer. We happened to have one of the world experts right here at the University. Unfortunately, between her travel commitments and this physician's travel commitments, the two weren't even going to be back in the same area for about a month, so I called the cancer specialist, and said, "I've got this patient…."

"Oh yeah, your nurse already sent over the slides. I already looked at them."

"I'm kind of worried because she can't come to see you for about a month."

"Well, the blood count's okay. She's not in a crisis right now. If she watches out for fever and other worrisome signs, she'll probably be okay."

Well, every day for the next month, with the patient, the specialist or me traveling, the patient and I would send at least one and sometimes two or three, e-mail messages. "Rich, what do you think about this study?"

"I don't think it's relevant to you, not the same type of cancer and the sample size is too small."

Finally, we come to the end of this thing. The month is up. She goes to see this specialist and about 20 minutes after she leaves the specialist's office, I get a call from the specialist and the first thing he says, is "What the hell did you tell that gal?"

"What are you talking about?"

"I sat down with her for 45 minutes. We had a lovely conversation. I explained what she had and what our protocol was. At the end of it, I turned to her and said, 'Do you have any questions?' She lifted a briefcase onto my desk and pulled out about a five-inch stack of reprints."

"She said, 'Well doctor, if I understand it right, using the protocol you use here, I'll improve my five year survival by 30 or 40%. Is that right?'"

"'Yes, that's right.'"

"'If I go down to another university in Texas, I'll improve it to about 50%. Is that right?'"

"Yes, that's right."

"'If I go to Paris, I can improve my odds about 60%.'"

The specialist said, "Really?"

She says, "Yeah. Doctor Roberts just sent me this abstract," which the specialist hadn't been able to get to, so the specialist says, "Can I make a copy of that?"

The patient went on, "I did a post doc in France, and still have a number of friends there. They already have a deal worked out with Air France. They'll fly me out one weekend a month for eight cycles of chemotherapy and I can walk the halls of the Louvre during the weekend, get my chemo and look at artwork."

The specialist says to me, "What the hell could I tell the gal at that point?"

I said, "How about the truth? Is she right?"

"Well, yeah. It looks like she is."

"Here's what I advise that we do. We're going to write a letter to her

HMO and I want you to sign it with me, saying we'll let her go to Paris, for treatment."

We did, and the patient did.

Two lessons out of that: In the 21st Century world, you're going to stay connected to people in ways you never imagined. The second is that the way the technology is going to change is going to make the relationship we have with people even more important. I didn't know anywhere near what the specialist knew about the chemo, but I knew the patient. I knew how she thought about things. A key role for a doctor is helping make sense of things for people, to make relevant for them the technologic options that are available out there.

The other story about relationships was, I was getting ready to leave for a meeting one year and had this guy who was dying of very aggressive cancer. He was in misery—terrible spasms, a lot of pain. He was a farmer, and despite all the ups and downs of the dairy industry, he managed to put his children through college. He was the sort of guy who just never quit, even when his blood count was very low and he was pale and exhausted. He would still, as he'd always done, walk the fence lines at the end of the day just to make sure there were no strays out there, that the fence hadn't broken down. He did this, even when he was deathly ill.

Now he's in the hospital, and he's pretty close to dying. I'm getting ready for {an out of town} meeting. I said to him, "What is it we can do for you, anything?" By now, the specialists had stepped away because that's what happens when there's no new treatment left to try. You know, when people get to the end, good luck finding some of these other experts. He said, "I want to go home to die."

I said, "All set up. We've got hospice waiting for you—home health nursing."

"You don't understand, doc. I can't do that. If I go home without trying something again, something new, my kids will remember me as a quitter."

I thought, Geez. Nobody's going to think that. He had experimental treatments. Nothing's worked.

I introduced him to my partner. But before leaving the room, I turned to his wife, and I said, "I wrote on the bottom of my business card the number of the hotel. If you need me, call me. I'll be happy to help you, if I can."

In my room, late that night, I'm checking my e-mail and there's a message. This was kind of weird, because this was back when e-mail was still kind of new.

"Dear Doc, Your partner's very nice, but she doesn't know my husband like you know him. Would you mind if I kind of keep you posted with how things are going with e-mail?"

"Sure, I'll try to be helpful to you." Again, each day, once, twice a day, there were e-mails going back and forth during the week I was gone. She would report that he was struggling with this issue of wanting to go home, but not wanting his kids to think that he quit. And I was struggling with how to help them from afar.

On Tuesday, I woke up at two in the morning from deep sleep—I just sat straight up and I went right over to my computer and typed in, "Please tell your husband to tell the kids that he's been climbing a very steep path of a very high hill and there's no evidence that this path is going to get him down the hill." And I went back to bed.

The next morning, she told him that. He was home Wednesday afternoon, after telling the kids that. I got back Thursday night from the meeting. The first thing I did when I landed was call to see how things were going. He had just died.

Two nights later, his wake was going on. They were going to shut it down at nine, and I got there at five to nine. Driving up to it, there's this lattice work outside the funeral home, like a porch around it. There's this five year old kid climbing on it. It was his grandson, who was my patient too, which is one of the joys of being a small town, family doctor. I had given this kid his school immunizations about two weeks earlier, so when I got out of the car and started walking toward him, he kind of eyed me with suspicion. He asked, "What are you doing here?"

"I'm here to see your grandpa."

"You're late. He's dead."

I said, "Well, I know. But your grandma would probably appreciate my coming in and visiting with him, if that's okay with you."

By then, pretty much most of the town was gone, but there were still maybe a dozen relatives there. His wife and the kids were there, and she was just delighted to see me and she introduced me to all the family.

They had four easels, with these four big poster board placards on each of them, and each one of them represented a different stage of his life. The fourth easel was right next to the foot of the coffin and the widow was standing right in front of this thing, and we were talking. I was apologizing for about the 50th time that I couldn't have been there as he was going through his last hours and days.

She stopped me and stepped aside from the easel and said, "Doc, you were here all the time." The only thing on that easel was that e-mail printout from the hotel. That still chokes me up, even today. So here I have this farm wife teaching me what it means to be connected, as a doc in an Internet world. That, to me, is the essence of what I do as a doc. That to me is the challenge, the struggle, but also the joy of doctoring.

This had to be percolating in your head, to get up in the middle of the night to type that e-mail. What led to that?

I don't know. It's happened often in my life. As a scientist, I was probably processing a lot of stuff and trying to do pattern analysis, and all the things human brains try to do when we're struggling with a decision or trying to develop a solution. It just popped into my head. Perhaps, it was just an awareness at that moment that the metaphor of climbing the hill would be one that would make sense to him because he had found how hard it had been in those last months to climb his hills and that he couldn't always take the same path he was taking, even though he was determined to make it to the top of that hill. He was going to have to take a different path, and in this case, it was home. It wouldn't be that you would quit.

It was never about the kids, in my mind. It was about him coming to terms with all of this and then communicating that back to the kids. It was a defense mechanism to help him cope with the hard reality of his death. For whatever reason, I'd like to think that that metaphor helped him. It's not like a cure for cancer or anything. It's not that profound an insight. But in its own small way, I think it was enormously helpful and important to this man and his family. It doesn't get much better than that. We don't have many opportunities as humans when we feel we really had an impact on people.

You've tried to have an impact in other ways, too. Let's talk about your interest in preventing gun violence. That was one of the issues you championed at the Wisconsin Medical Society.

As I was about to become Society president, there were a whole lot of experiences swirling around in my head. When I was moonlighting in Los Angeles, I was working the ER on a Monday Night Football night. There was a 15-year old who was doing homework right after school at her house in her bedroom, when a car drove by and a guy shot and killed her. A bullet went through her window and hit her right in the head. It's me and this little itty bitty nurse from Guatemala, and a couple of other people in the ER. It was a pretty quiet night, otherwise. We wheel this young woman in, and start the resuscitation.

Within ten minutes, this gang comes rolling in and it's her brother and his buddies—like a dozen of them, and they're waving Uzi machine guns and hand guns. I'm trying to explain to them in my fractured Spanish, what's going on. They're getting more and more upset. Then, Maria, who's no more than four foot ten, 50ish, steps right into the middle of this semi-circle of these angry guys and starts talking to them, very quiet Spanish, like she was talking to a child, trying to soothe them, so quiet, that they had to sort of lean in to hear her. After three minutes of talking to her, they turned on their heels and walked out. I almost collapsed with relief and said to Maria, "What did you tell them?"

"I just told them that she's hurt very badly, that we don't think she's going to make it. She's going to be joining God soon, and the best thing that they can do to respect the memory of his sister is to not hurt anybody here and just to go."

So I've had a couple of life experiences that make you feel angry and sad about the harm that can be done with guns. When you live in stressful society and you give people lethal means that are easy to get at, and ever more lethal, that is not appropriate.

I'm not a hunter. But I'm not an anti-gun person at all. I was not a guy who was on a crusade against gun violence—not at all. I wanted physicians to view themselves, and communities to view their physicians, as instruments of social change in their communities. We knew from polling data that people were concerned about violence; violence among kids.

I didn't want to do this in a way that would get me sucked into all the politics of the Second Amendment. This was about making things safer for kids. The focus was primarily on education and safety. We worked with a number of hunter safety programs and things like that.

As this went on, we went in several directions: bicycle safety, water safety, things like that.

People are more uptight about everything today, and that worries me. What used to be minor disagreements between neighbors that you somehow managed to work out, now you end up with somebody getting shot and killed. Maybe it's a sign of the increasing stress in the times in which we live.

I was trying to poke the docs and say, if you think you can do this by just sitting in your office, you can't. The thing about physicians is that we occupy a rather unique position in society. It becomes a very powerful thing. For people to quit smoking, the one thing we know that works best is to have your doctor look you in the eye and say, "I'm concerned about your smoking. I really want you to quit. I'd like to help you do that."

I want to take that idea and translate it into a community-wide effort, so you have docs at the individual patient level say, "I'm concerned about violence at the community level, and I want to help everybody be safer." You couldn't do this at a state or federal level, because it would become so diffuse, it almost sounds like political sloganeering. The key is that you have to take it by the individual, but that's very slow and inefficient.

The first thing that many docs do, when they have the opportunity, is to talk about the issue. Awareness is always the first step. As a big part of my annual assessment for a child or an adult, I ask whether there are any guns in the house. Are they locked? Are they secured? Do you feel safe at home? That, alone, is a bit of an eye-opener for people.

I approach it in a way that's very non-judgmental. I'm not out to investigate anybody or put anybody down. Trigger locks may be helpful, too. For the impetuous teen or the quarreling couple in the middle of a hot moment, it might slow them down, just enough to give them a second thought.

I had intended to do something to give focus to my presidential year and it did that. I never expected it to go on for 10 years. It was fun. Did we save any kids' lives? I don't know. The point was to open the dialogue, to get docs to think of themselves in kind of a broader role in the community.

What would your dad think of this life you've led?

My dad was a very bright man who went from high school right into World War II. He wanted to go to school to become a lawyer, but he ended up getting married and having kids, so in a sense, that career dream never came true for him. He would view what I've been able to do as this tremendously exciting opportunity. He'd be pretty amazed by all of this and I am, too. It's been quite an amazing journey, but I'm nowhere near done. Looking back, it wasn't a grand plan, and it didn't always feel like work. Most of the time, it felt like exciting, interesting, satisfying stuff.

Chapter Twenty-Nine

Sick—of Lawyers

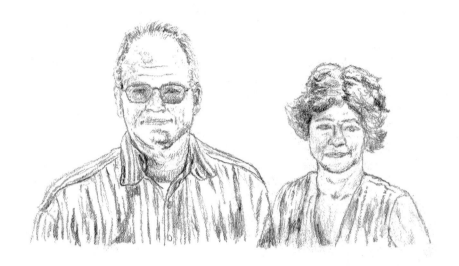

"The check for the two of us to leave Ohio was $250,000 cash. Yeah, that was the ransom to get out of the banana republic of Ohio."

Christopher Magiera, MD
Gastroenterologist, Wausau

Pamela Galloway, MD
General Surgery, Wausau

"Why would a doctor just pick up and leave?" my cousin Mike wondered. In 2002, his wife Lenette discovered her Nevada OB/GYN suddenly had left the state without notice. Since she was over 35 and pregnant with twins, doctors considered Lenette a high-risk patient. They were unable to find another specialist in Nevada to care for her, so she went home to Baltimore for obstetric care, and to deliver their babies. For six months, Mike flew back and forth from Las Vegas, where he still worked, to be with her. Not exactly an ideal way to start a family.

What happened to my cousin is not all that extraordinary. Many families across the country have suffered because numerous states have failed to pass limits on jury awards in medical malpractice cases. Good, responsible physicians, especially those who practice in high-risk specialties, have seen their medical liability premiums soar because the states in which they practice have no limits on these awards. Whatever dollar amount the jury decides is what is awarded. I've met two physicians, a brain surgeon and an obstetrician, who came to Wisconsin because their insurance premiums to practice in Illinois exceeded their income!

For many years, Wisconsin was a safe haven for doctors, attracting them from problem states, including Illinois, Pennsylvania, Ohio, and Nevada. Physicians Christopher Magiera and Pamela Galloway, both in their early 50s, are among those who now call Wisconsin home. They are "medical refugees" from Ohio, a state that was once rife with negligence lawsuits.

I "met" them via e-mail, shortly after they arrived in Wausau in 2002, at which time they became politically involved to help make sure Wisconsin's stable healthcare system wouldn't contract the insurance disease spreading across the country. The married couple explain how exasperating it was to practice medicine under the constant fear of lawsuits.

Magiera:
One friend of mine, a general surgeon, came to work one day in his shorts, sandals and t-shirt. I said, "You got a paperwork day?"

And he said, "Yeah, because I have no insurance. I'm out of business."

He said the company that was insuring him just announced that they were not renewing his coverage. They did that with just a week to go. Just cut him off. No reason. They said we're just not going to insure any surgeons any more.

Galloway:
It was the end of 2001, and you started hearing things from your insurance company that there was this looming liability crisis, but you didn't believe it. The chicken hadn't come home to roost. I was one of those people, who like all other doctors, thought that this wasn't going to apply to me, so I never really listened to them.

But then in December of 2001, the surgeon that I worked with, a very good general surgeon, got a bill for his malpractice insurance premium that was $100,000. He couldn't afford to stay open, so within four weeks, he was gone. Then there were more people getting slapped with these tremendously high premiums, mostly people in the high-risk specialties like OB and surgery.

Magiera:

When I was first sued in 1996, it was something you talked about quietly in the back of the doctors' lounge. By 1999, that's all doctors talked about in their offices in front of patients. That was issue number one. People were just losing their insurance. At that point, my office staff thought I had contracted pancreatic cancer. I was losing so much weight and looking so worried. As a gastroenterologist, we love to eat, so looking sickly was not a usual sight.

That made me personally investigate what was happening with the insurance industry. I began to get a view of the magnitude of the problem, talking to other doctors and finding that this lawsuit business was rampant in Ohio.

I started investigating the politics of this. We found out there was this big movement around the country. During that lawsuit, the malpractice insurance industry was going into crisis. My malpractice carrier filed for bankruptcy as I was about to go to trial. Talk about needing a diaper.

Then I got hooked up with the political end of this with the national picture, and figured out that this was a state-by-state issue. Some states were better and it got to the point where you say, okay, my premium dollars are like, $10,000. Your premiums go up to $20,000. Okay, it's no big deal. Then $30,000, I can afford that. $40,000. I can afford that, but I'm not happy. And you keep going until at some point, it's economically unfeasible. With my costs going up and my revenue going down, the two lines cross and you're out.

I rapidly became knowledgeable about just how out of control the system was. Before, I thought it was just the cost of doing business. I would just drive up my rates and do good medicine, and I won't get sued. But I got sued, trying to be the best physician I could be. It was totally nonsense, a frivolous action.

We did a little plotting of these graphs and figured out when the hammer was going to fall. We needed to get out of Dodge. This is not a sustainable operation.

Galloway:

In May of 2002, we went to a rally in Cleveland, trying to call attention to the crisis. But by then, I had become more knowledgeable about the whole situation. What we had found out is that Ohio had passed tort reform twice in the preceding 10 years, as recently as something like '96. It was overturned by the Supreme Court in '99. The whole package—not just one item—everything in the tort reform package was deemed unconstitutional.

We also found out through our own research that Cuyahoga County, where we were practicing, was one of the worst counties in the country, in terms of jury awards, and had been nominated by the American Tort Reform Association for what's called a "judicial hellhole," where the jury trials are heavily slanted in favor of the plaintiff.

Other states had enacted tort reform and it was still in place. To find out more, I contacted the lawyer who had defended me, successfully, in a malpractice suit. He was born and raised in Cuyahoga County and worked there for years and years.

I said, "We found out that other states have successfully passed tort reform. What do you think about moving?"

Much to my surprise, he thought that would be a good idea, because he didn't think things were going to change much in Ohio very soon, that there was a very bad track record, the trial bar was very strong, and things like that. And, he mentioned that he had just seen USA Today, which listed the states where the medical liability climate was stable. Ohio was one of the ones in crisis. The "safe" states were Wisconsin, Indiana, Iowa, New Mexico and Louisiana. As two Midwesterners, we thought it over. Moving was the right solution.

It isn't just the malpractice insurance rates—it's the threat of getting sued. In my practice, I had many patients who came in with breast problems. The number one cause of lawsuits among surgeons is delay of diagnosis of appendicitis, and the other is delay of diagnosis of breast cancer. The likelihood of getting a suit with my practice was extremely high, because I was seeing all these patients with breast problems and saying, "Yes, you need a biopsy or no you don't need a biopsy." That's when we decided to look into Wisconsin.

In order to leave the state, you had to pay what is called tail coverage, which is two and a half times your annual premium. We thought it would be better to leave sooner, rather than sticking around to see what would happen.

Magiera:

We moved in March of 2003, so we hatched this plot for about a year.

Galloway:

We knew that rates would go up astronomically the next year. Especially mine, being a surgeon—there's no way that they would not. So the longer we waited, it would just be more expensive to move. As it was, I had to pay something like $75,000.

Magiera:

The check, for the two of us to leave Ohio, was $250,000 cash. Yeah, that was the ransom to get out of the banana republic of Ohio.

What's driving this?

Galloway:

It's patients looking for perfection. Somehow, they've developed unrealistic expectations. There was a gal I removed a hemorrhoid on. She came back in the office, and I could tell by the way she was looking at me, that she was really mad. I asked her what was wrong.

She said, "I don't like the way my anus looks."

I kept the shock off my face and said, "What don't you like about it?"

"There's a scar there where you took the hemorrhoid off."

I thought, *God, is she an exotic dancer or what?* It was probably the most shocking thing that anybody ever said to me.

How difficult is it to determine a bad outcome from negligence?

Galloway:

It should be the kind of thing where only a specialist in that area is looking at it, not a family practitioner evaluating a surgeon. And, it has to be something extreme, because physicians are humans. They're not perfect. They're going to make mistakes.

Magiera:

There are eight on a civil jury and they're certainly not my peers. There are alternative, unexpected outcomes, and there's malpractice. Like, if you walk into a room and replace the wrong knee and you did it because you're such a busy surgeon that you didn't bother looking at their record or something, now that's malpractice. Okay, get out your checkbook. You owe that patient some recompense. But the gray areas can't be evaluated by the public.

But, if you replace the knee and the patient doesn't have full function, and they weren't following your post op order correctly, that's not malpractice. You have to have a definition of what went wrong, malice or forethought.

It's politicizing justice. The legislature passes a law and then it can be interpreted differently every five to 10 years, depending on the political and philosophical makeup of the Supreme Court. That's not what the justices are there to do.

Doctors in Wisconsin are complacent. People here think that the lawyers—and the population in general—are not going to get too bad. But it's gonna be just holy hell here once the trial lawyers get the upper hand.

That's the biggest denial part for physicians, thinking that it only affects somebody else. I almost don't know a doctor who hadn't been sued. And Pam and I, by virtue of being on various quality assurance and medical staff committees, we had adequate access to people's records. We knew when they had been sued, so we knew the record on everybody. Everybody had been sued—very good people.

The frightening thing was that the mindset of the population of Cleveland, Ohio, was simply to sue your doctor. I had one guy come into my office with a tape recorder running in his pocket. He was coming there expressly for the purpose of trying to initiate litigation. I told him that he could just leave.

If you have a $10 million insurance policy, the lawyers know they're only going to get $10 million. They can garnish your wages successfully and make you work for them the rest of your life, but they want fast money.

Galloway:

We need caps. The other thing we should do is turn a negative into a positive and look at all of the tort reform we've enacted and see if there are other reforms that can be done while working on the project. Some states have "I'm Sorry" laws, where if you apologize to a patient it can't be held against you.

Most malpractice suits are out there for the patient to find out information. They're the exception. Generally, the suit is an issue of fixing blame and getting money. I've always thought of myself as a good communicator and Chris is a good communicator.

Many states have now enacted tort reform. Ohio actually did enact tort reform right before we moved.

Magiera:

All this talk about the plight of physicians—it's not about us. It's about patient access to quality care. It's about the economy of the state of Wisconsin. If you were a widget manufacturer and there were no good doctors in Wisconsin, would you want to locate your plant in Wisconsin and pay high healthcare costs? No. It just drags the whole state down.

The year we left Cleveland, 14 other doctors we knew from the three hospitals we had privileges at, left. You multiply that by all of the hospitals in Ohio, you have an idea of things to come.

Galloway:

The first field I think that will be hit negatively will be OB, because family practitioners and general surgeons may become reluctant to do cesareans. The rural areas will get hit more quickly. OB will be harder to recruit.

Magiera:

What happened in Ohio is that people who deliver babies are obstetrician/gynecologists, family practitioners, some general specialists, and some rural surgeons. When we left, we knew of no family practitioners who delivered babies, for the fact that if they wanted to do obstetrics, their premiums were so high they couldn't afford them. The hospitals wouldn't give them privileges because the hospital is also liable.

Now you've got family practitioners, who are the backbone of our healthcare system, and if you exclude them from their fully-trained realm of their repertoire, you're truncating the health care system. You'll have people from thousands of square miles with nobody to deliver babies.

Galloway:

In Ohio, 2002, there was a Supreme Court race and there were two positions available. Doctors were able to educate their patients about the importance of having a Supreme Court justice who would be in favor of medical liability stability, and they did elect those two judges. It is possible to educate the public.

The biggest thing driving it is the trial lawyers. In Ohio, where there are no restrictions on attorneys' fees, and for a while, there weren't any caps, there was nothing deterring them from taking a case. Any case could turn into a humungous reward.

Magiera:
My overall opinion is that people expect perfection and doctors do try. Doctors aren't out there hacking off the wrong limbs because they come to work drunk. We're all very thoughtful to our patients. Yeah, there are a couple bad apples. There are bad apples in all professions, but by and large, we're very good and honest people trying to help people.

I entered private practice out of training in 1987, and I think things went fairly well. I always knew that people got sued, and malpractice lawyers always had their pictures on the back of every phone book in every city in the country, and we knew they were vicious. You always heard of multi-million dollar jury awards, which just sounded stupid. This lottery mentality has been driven by plaintiffs' attorneys, not just malpractice attorneys. I go so far as to say that it's all due to the fact that plaintiffs' lawyers are all greedy crooks. They drag out case after case because a baby got hurt. All right, stuff like that happens.

But they're driving the industry just to get the rewards. I know this because I had an acquaintance who I sat next to at the symphony for many years. He had tickets next to me and we shared a lot of stuff. He was the greediest malpractice attorney, and would tell me he's just after this money, because it's easy money.

Galloway:
The other thing is that a lot of physicians will settle to make the whole thing go away rather than fight a lawsuit. That encourages lawsuits because they know they can get 25 or $50,000, which is a lot of money to some people. But there are a lot of doctors out there who won't make the effort to contest a case. They just want to settle to make it go away. And that's like agreeing with the terrorists. They just come back.

It's like nothing bad is ever supposed to happen to you, and that if you decide to have a child, there's some risk to it. The child may not be perfect. But instead of accepting that risk, people are shifting the risk to their physician, saying, well, it's your fault there's a birth defect or a complicated labor. After a while, physicians may not be willing to accept that risk.

Magiera:
One part of me says that if I had a child, I would never recommend this field. I would say go to business school, engineering, anything, but medicine. Then part of me feels that this is unique, noble, and it's a good feeling to be a doctor. My parents were just thrilled that I was going on {to medical school}. Of course, they felt that doctors and dentists were the epitome of the community.

Where did you grow up, Dr. Magiera?

I was born in South Bend, Indiana. My father works as a photo engraver. My mother's a homemaker. I'm an only child. I was the first person in my family to ever go past high school. Well, I always wanted to be in the sciences. I was in school in a rural community in Northern Illinois, where the majority of my buddies were farmers. I wanted to do something different than that, and science looked like the way to go.

Then, my father—he was a labor leader—was involved in a series of strikes and strikes mean unemployment. I said to myself, I've never known a doctor or dentist who's unemployed. That sort of selfish, economic motivation, combined with the sciences, came together, so in high school I decided that was medicine.

I started off at the Medical College of Virginia in Richmond, and Pam was two years ahead of me. Midway through medical school when she graduated and got her residency, I had to transfer medical school. She had a job in Cleveland, so I transferred to Case Western University School of Medicine, so it was not one, but two med schools I went to, which was a little bit more difficult.

The material was hard to grasp, but I was used to that. It became a self-sustaining reaction, just like almost obsessive, compulsive behavior. You couldn't put it down.

Galloway:

I would have been disappointed in myself had I gone into anything other than medicine. I can still recommend medicine as a career, but with the advice that you'd have to be very selective about where you practice. You can't go into medicine thinking you could just hang out a shingle anywhere. You have to look at where you're going to practice, from a liability point of view, as well as from other things. You can't just go work in Florida because you like to go lie on the beach.

When did you start thinking about becoming a physician, Doctor Galloway?

When I was 12. I decided that becoming a doctor was the most challenging, interesting thing I could do. I was born in Alabama. But when I was two years old, we moved. We lived in Berlin, Germany, because my dad was a college professor. My dad passed away when I was 14, so we moved to Virginia, to the suburbs of Washington, D.C., where my mom got a job.

The first couple years of medical school were not that difficult, because there was just more book work, like in college. But I remember having a hard time making the transition from the classrooms to the wards. I wasn't really prepared for the hours I had to put in, being up for 36 hours in a row.

My first rotation was surgery. We were up all night, and were expected to do whatever the residents did, and keep on going. We weren't given any breaks or anything like that, because we were medical students. In retrospect, it was very valuable experience. My educational experience at the Medical College of Virginia was probably the best overall experience I've had in my career, because they set the standards high and expected us to perform. Having experienced those standards and succeeded, served me well. There weren't a lot of women in the class, but enough that we weren't that unusual. The student in our class who graduated at the top of our class was a woman.

At the time, at the Medical College of Virginia, there had never been a woman graduate from their surgery program, so there weren't a lot of female mentors in that field.

Magiera:

In the first two years of medical school, we're just in the classroom. You're lectured to by all the different specialties, and the gastroenterologists, to me, just seemed the most interesting. They asked for volunteers and everybody else took a step backwards. They were the most down to earth. They smiled. Surgeons never smiled. They had an interesting specialty and they were very, very good teachers.

One thing I remember about the gastroenterologists is that they love to eat and drink. Food being very near and dear to my heart, well, I thought this specialty was okay, because you'd always find these people talking about the restaurants they were going to, and what convention cities they are hanging out at together. It was just a convivial group. They were nice to be around.

Actually, I wanted to be a pathologist. When I first got into med school, I thought that was just the coolest thing around because you got to do the autopsies. You knew the answers to everything. Everybody else was just guessing. Somewhere towards the end of the second year, when I was exposed to these gastroenterologists, it just clicked that no, this was the way to go.

We were called digestive disease specialists, so we deal with everything that has to do with the intake of nutrients, the mixing of them, the digesting and the excretion thereof, and it takes into consideration what we call the hollow organs, like colon, esophagus, and stomach, and then the solid organs of digestion, such as the liver and pancreas.

There are endoscopies, surgical procedures that you can do as a gastroenterologist, on the hollow organs, and there are also what we call the intellectual aspects of liver disease because there's not much you can do about it. A gastroenterologist can't do anything to the liver except think about it. We have our surgical side and our intellectual side, so to me it was a good combination.

Galloway:

You almost have to be kind of an egomaniac to be a surgeon. You can't be a surgeon and be afraid. It was something I developed.

Do you recall your first surgery?

My first night on call, a guy came in with a gunshot wound to the back. It just nicked his aorta and he was bleeding profusely through a pinhole injury in his aorta. We took him to the operating room, thinking he was bleeding. It was obvious that he was bleeding internally when he came in, and we took him into the operating room, thinking it was into his abdomen, based on where the entrance wound was. It turned out he was actually bleeding into his chest. We had to call in one of the thoracic surgeons. I was up all night, but it was very exciting.

In my case, since I was a little bit older than the other residents, and had already been through another residency, my age actually really helped me in terms of being able to keep things in perspective.

Magiera:

I trained at a county hospital in Cleveland. It was truly like a MASH unit or the fabled Cook County General. It was—you are on your own. The attending physician would show up in the morning and teach, but in the middle of the night, you were it. And it was a fantastic learning experience because there was nobody to turn around to and say, "Hey, what do you think about this?" You were just talking to the wall. It's just you and the patient.

In medicine, as opposed to surgery, we thrive on what's called the differential diagnosis. We're always sitting on the fence saying, "Well, it could be this or it could be this." But since we can't cut the patient up, we really don't know, so we always have a list of probabilities.

Surgeons are like the captains of the ship. They say full speed ahead. We say, a little bit to the left, maybe a little bit to the right and see how things go before we put the pedal to the metal. It's a little bit more tentative, although at some point, like in an intensive care unit and somebody's heart is failing, you have to make a decision and do something.

Gastroenterology was a more leisurely specialty because you basically dealt with elective things, although there were some critical endoscopic surgery interventions where people were bleeding to death, so that was a little bit exciting.

Back when we were residents, they didn't have this candy pants 80-hour workweek that the residents do now. We were, as they say, men of men. It was like the Marine Corps training. You would be on call all day, all night and then work until the work was done, which was a 36 or more hour shift. You had to ask yourself at times, am I crazy? But it became its own reward. It's like what the marathon runners get—the endorphins.

There were plenty of nights riding home after being on call, and I would fall asleep at stoplights in downtown Cleveland. You'd be riding with the windows down in sub-zero air in your face to stay awake, music blaring and sometimes, you'd wake up to horns honking because you're stopped at a green light. {laughs}

The best learning takes place on the fly and under stress, and if you just punch in eight to five and go home, you're not getting the complete experience.

Galloway:

I agree. You only learn a certain amount from a textbook. You've got to actually see things. See the way people present their symptoms—the physicals signs, the x-rays and you have to see it as it changes. That's especially true in surgery, where somebody may come in the early stages of disease and you're not sure.

For example, like appendicitis, the early presentation isn't always classic, so you have to watch them. After about eight or 12 hours, you're more sure they have appendicitis, and then you operate on the patient. You really have to see things evolve. It doesn't just fit into 80 hours.

If I came to you as a patient, and said, "I work 90, 100 hours a week," you probably wouldn't tell me that's a good idea.

Galloway:

No, I wouldn't, but I never thought about it that way. We don't do that all the time. It's a limited time. Plus, it's not always 36 hours in a row. When I was on call, if I got two hours of sleep, I actually felt pretty good the next day. You aren't always working these uninterrupted 36-hour shifts. You get say, a couple of hours.

The higher up in the program, the less likely you were to be up all night, because the interns and the lower level residents would be in the emergency room admitting people, and they would call you for advice. It did get better within the program, as time went by.

What's it like to have a relationship when you have two really demanding professions?

Galloway:

It puts stress on the marriage. The way you are living at that time is not the way you're always going to be living. If you're married, that may help you just in terms of the stability in your life. The key thing is having an understanding spouse, because if you go home to a spouse, you have somebody who's important to you and who can listen to you if you're having a bad time, as opposed to just going home to an empty apartment. I never thought of it as a negative. I was halfway through medical school, and Chris, you were about to start, weren't you?

Magiera:

Right. I started that summer we were married. If we go back to the old days, like back in the '40s and '50s, they would say that doctors weren't supposed to get married during their training. They could get married once they were out in the community. It was almost like the priesthood, or a religious vocation, because you had to dedicate yourself to that vocation. I saw many of my colleagues in med school with spouses who couldn't understand the dedication needed to do this. There were divorces, break ups, separations, and constants fights, because unless you're in the profession, you have no idea what dedication it takes.

I often thought that physicians should only marry people in the field because no one else understands. Or, the spouse has to be very understanding. As physicians, you don't get on each other's nerves because you're never together that much.

There's one particular event I remember that really showed me just how nasty this is on the home life. I said to Pam that I was on call and that she could fix the Thanksgiving dinner and I'll be home. I then come home at 11 o'clock at night, candles are burned down, the leftovers are there and just feeling like a total worthless individual. It was at that point, that we figured out that if you're on duty, there's no commitment. You just can't do a thing, personally.

Galloway:

We learned that Thanksgiving isn't the third Thursday in November. It's whenever we eat the turkey. You have to be flexible. It's much better for me, because I only work part-time now. When I was in practice in Cleveland, in solo practice and on call all the time, we basically had no social life. Every now and then, I would have someone cover for me so we could go to a baseball game, so my pager wouldn't go off. I made sure I got time off for vacations and stuff like that. But now, it's great. I only work three days a week and I assume more of the household chores, which is much, much better than it was before.

A few years ago, when I was working all those hours and practicing on call all the time, there was no attention going to the home. It's amazing how little things will disrupt your schedule. It's better that Chris can focus all his time on working.

Magiera:

It is good. And it was very hectic when we both had full-time careers, especially her career as a solo, independent, general surgeon, with no back-up. I would say, "Hey, let's go to an Indians game or the New York Yankees. I'm not on call his weekend."

And she goes, "Well, that's swell for you."

I'm an independent practitioner in a small group, and that's a full-time occupation. You have to crank the practice. Pam works for a large multi-specialty clinic, where there's more backup, and they have a job description for part-time. It's a more flexible situation.

Our patients primarily come by referrals from a family doctor. Very few people pick up a phone book and say I need a gastroenterologist. It would be like, "Hey, I need a colonoscopy. Where can I have this?"

Our patients tend to be longer-lasting. Digestive illnesses are more chronic. Something called irritable bowel syndrome, which is also a chronic condition, you pick up one of these patients and you're with them forever, like a family doctor.

But there was a gentleman in my practice who was a vet. He was an incorrigible alcoholic. Started out, one of my partners had met him when she was a resident. Then he eventually moved out to where I was in practice and I started encountering him and his alcoholic, bleeding, cirrhotic binge episodes. He would always be in the hospital, just episode after episode of complications of cirrhosis—GI bleeding, bacterial sepsis. I mean this guy was a survivor. You just couldn't kill him. Not with bullets, uranium, or kryptonite, so it was always the joke.

I was taking care of him one night in the ICU. He had just finished almost bleeding out from esophageal varices* and we patched him together. He was telling me about this nursing home he was in. He was really upset with the nursing home. And I said, "What's wrong?"

He goes, "Well, hypocrites. The world is full of hypocrites."

I said, "Why is that?"

"Well, I'm a boozer. Yeah, all these people who work at this nursing home—they're doing crack. They're smoking weed. They're shooting smack. Hypocrites. All I want is a blankety blank beer and they say, 'No, you gonna be addicted.'"

He was such a con artist, too. They wheeled him into the emergency room in a coma and I said to the driver, "Was he in a coma on the way in?"

"No, but he had us go to Subway."

He got a thing that was a one-pounder Subway sandwich. So here he was, this guy in a coma with a half eaten sub in his hand, and in a liver coma because he'd eaten too much protein from the salami. Well, he finally went to the big veteran's reunion in the sky.

There are very few people who just bounce in and bounce out of your practice, except maybe these screening colonoscopies. They come in once every 10 years

Galloway:

If you're lucky, you'll never see me again. That's kind of the parting line I use with my patients, because that's how it is with a focused specialty. You see one problem once or twice and they go back to their primary care physician. It's much more interventional. I prefer it that way. You don't really develop a long-term relationship with a patient. What may arise is that you do an operation for something like a breast biopsy and then you need to have a gall bladder removed and they come back to you. About the only patients in my practice I see over the long term are patients who had breast cancer, because after you operate on them, you monitor them for reoccurrence, basically forever.

* Veins in the lower walls of the esophagus that are bloated due to high blood pressure, which may burst, causing life-threatening complications.

It's just quick gratification, like removing the appendix and then they're done and they're fine. That's it. Problem solved.

Magiera:

Surgeons—they can't get involved in relationships. {Grins}

Galloway:

Most of the stereotypes are true. If you see gory things in the emergency room, you have to be very cool and almost detached. Sometimes, I feel very bad for the women who are diagnosed with breast cancer, especially if they have a hard time handling it. I try to empathize with them and try to get them to think of things long-term and eventually, they'll recover and get back to a normal lifestyle. I try to emphasize it as something that's treatable, something that's manageable. It's not a death sentence. It's more believable coming from a woman, if maybe the person delivering the news is someone they can relate to.

How do you deliver that bad news?

Magiera:

We diagnose a fair amount of cancer—colon cancer, stomach cancer, liver cancer, pancreas cancers, many cancers. That's the least favorable part of the job. I'll try to establish a good physical atmosphere in the room, so we're not standing in the middle of a noisy hallway or something.

What I like to do is to sit down with them and physically get on their level, not hovering above them like some God, you know. I mean, these are things my professor taught me how to do. You can get really good at it. You have a little bit of conversation. The patients know as soon as you come in the room what you're going to say. I don't want to just blurt it out. I tell them that we found a big lump of tissue and I'm really suspicious there might be some tumor cells.

They say, "You mean cancer?"

I'll say, "It could be. We took biopsies."

I try to go about it a little gently, and then you can see the wheels start to turn and see they're coming to grips with it. Then, you have to talk to them about decisions about treatment, wait for the biopsies, introduce them to surgeons, read things about options. So it's mainly trying to be very calm and reassuring. I've seen some people trying to train residents, and they'll just walk over and go, "Your cousin Smitty has colon cancer. We'll talk to you in a few minutes."

Oh, come on guys. Use a little more finesse here. It's almost a little like being like a priest. You've got to have interpersonal skills, do it diplomatically. That's the most difficult part.

When I'm with medical students or with any kind of person in training that's following me around, I'll say here's the fun part of the job, very sarcastically. The patients and their families are crying and carrying on and you've got to make them feel better.

I've always thought that myself and doctors in general—have to be attached to your patients and give them bad news, but I don't think you can get emotionally caught up with them. You have to give the impression of emotion. I've always thought a good doctor would make an excellent hit man. Go up to some terrorist, pop him and go have a yogurt—just ice water in your veins; no emotion. You can't sit there and let yourself go into an emotional crisis because you're crying with somebody who has cancer—not that you can't do that, if they're a lifelong patient. But you've got to be able to pull yourself up, be objective and move on. In the end, I have to tell hundreds of people they have cancer. I can't let it devastate my life.

The medical liability crisis in Ohio almost devastated your careers. Since Ohio enacted new laws, are you considering moving back home?

Galloway:

No. There are too many other good things about Wisconsin, and things aren't going to change over night into Cuyahoga County. That mindset won't change for maybe a generation.

Magiera:

The insurance agents told us they didn't expect the premiums in Ohio to go down for maybe 20 years. No, there's just no reason to go back—not at this late point in my career. I'll stick it out here in Wisconsin.

IX

World Class

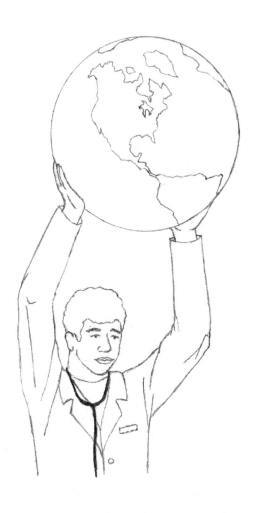

"Do what you love, and you will find the way to get it out to the world."

—Judy Collins

CHAPTER THIRTY

TRANSPLANT FROM TURKEY

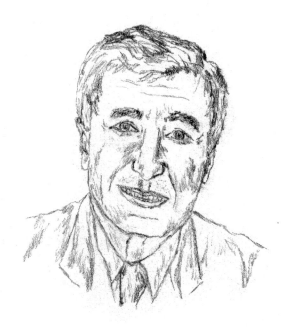

"This kid going to die, definitely. And next day, the patient was awake. In two weeks, he went home. Then, I told my wife, 'Look, I saw some miracle.'"

Munci Kalayoglu, MD {MOON-jee} kuh-LIE-uh-loo}
Liver Transplant Surgeon, Madison

"So what's the grim reality here? Are you waiting for a car accident victim?" I asked my sick friend, Erin Davisson, who needed a liver transplant.

"Yeah, pretty much," Erin said, matter of factly.

"Who's doing the transplant, Kalayoglu?" I asked.

She nodded, and then did her Kalayoglu impression, with a Turkish accent.

'When I have liver in hands, you will be saved,' she mimicked, smiling and with such panache, it was obvious that the doctor's confidence had reassured her. And he made good on his promise! Erin did get a new liver and Dr. Kalayoglu did save her.

I interviewed him once in person in the 1980s, and what I remember most clearly about that discussion in his office, was marveling at a framed copy of "Life Magazine." He and his surgical team were on the cover, draped in gowns and masks, hovering over a patient in the midst of transplant surgery. I'd never met anybody who'd attained such fame, and the image stayed with me.

When I arrived at his office at University of Wisconsin Hospital for this interview, the first thing I looked for was that magazine cover. And sure enough, it was still hanging there, in addition to a wall packed with awards and other framed photos of him posing with presidents.

Doctor Kalayoglu, in his mid 60s, graciously welcomed me, and eagerly recounted how he became the life saver he is.

Tell me about the first liver transplant you did on your own.

I was 43 years old. Trust me, if they ask me to do that operation right now, I will never do that. I come here in '83. Nine months, I couldn't find any patient. After nine months, I find some patient in VA hospital—Vietnam War hero. He was dying from end stage liver disease and coma. That patient was in terrible shape. He was so risky. There was no hope, actually.

I went to Canada. We got in twin engine propeller Cessna. And on the way to Salzburg, tornado hit our plane and we had to land it to Rhinelander.* We had to wait until tornado pass and then the plane was moving up and down, and I was not so feeling well. Then, I go to Canada and we got liver. I have to take a cold shower to wake up. Otherwise, I was shaking and scared.

Anyway, we take out liver and bring it back. We have to stop in Milwaukee. We cannot fly directly because we're coming from another country. We have to have custom check us and we lost some time. I was worried the clock was ticking, and we come to the airport by the ambulance and then come to UW Hospital operating room. I did 12 hours of surgery. I fix it and follow the patient.

Were you confident that this went well?

Yes. After you put the liver in, you can get idea if patient is going to live or die. If the liver is pink and soft and making bile, and if the liver works, the blood starts clotting right away. Kidney does improve right away. Patient starts peeing. You can see it. Blood pressure turns to normal. You can see a lot of changes, dynamic changes. Anesthesia changes, blood pressure, pulse, everything turn normal.

That is one of the magical operations, unbelievable. Everything was bad. Suddenly, you take out the sick liver and replace with new one, and everything may change easily. I knew that patient was going to make it. The

---

* Rhinelander is a small city in northern Wisconsin.

next day he opens his eyes up from coma and his kidneys start working. In two weeks, he was out of the hospital and walking.

Some accident could happen anytime. Some bleeding could happen—this and that. But these are all repairable. The main problem: give normal liver to the patient. If you have end stage liver disease—cirrhosis—the easy operation and the best operation is liver transplant.

At that time, liver transplant was tough. The operation was so stressful. I don't think I slept in 60 hours. I slept in the intensive care unit. I slept with the patient. You cannot say tired in this business. There is no way you can get tired. You don't have right to complain because you start with the patient. Patient need you. If you do mistake, patient will die. They trust they life to you. You don't have a team. I was the team. I took the risk, yes. Only God can help me. I put my hands up and pray to God. Maybe I was lucky. Maybe God loves me. Sometime you need help from above. Maybe I train well. No one see liver transplant. Then, they hired me to do liver transplant. I thought, if something happens to the patients, they can send me back to Turkey.

Tell me about growing up in Turkey.

I was born in 1940. I have a sister four years older than me. My father was judge. My mother was teacher. I grew up in small town in Turkey and I reached the 11th grade at about 14 to go to high school. I come to Ankara, the Capital. After I finish high school, I go directly to medical school. My father wanted me to be a doctor all the time. My mother, she wanted me to stay in the academic community.

Oh, actually, all my life, I tried to be an engineer, an architect. I went to engineer school exam and I couldn't pass. I never thought I would be a doctor. I took the medical school exam and get the results. I pass the exam and I accepted to med school.

When I start anatomic class, I saw the human body. I saw how good mechanically it is, how smart is the creator, you know? The bones, the muscles, the nervous system, then, I amazed. And especially after I start at the clinic and seeing the patients, and then when I start seeing surgery. The first day when I operate it would hit me. It's like heroin. I never have any heroin. But the surgery, that's it. I'm going to be a surgeon and nothing else. That clear. First day I scrub and go to the operating room, that hit me.

In 1963, I graduated one of the top ranking students in my class. Then, I got my MD diploma from the president in his hand.

The president of the University?

President of Turkey! Yeah, yeah—the Founder of the Republic. Anyway, after I graduate, I start surgical education. This was 1963. I finished my surgical education in '67. I became a general surgeon.

I was interested with babies and my university—they called Hacettepe

University —like a semi-American university, although the staff of that University trained in the United States, and then come back to Turkey. It was a very big children's hospital—very busy. That university send me to United States for education in pediatric surgery.

I was at New York City at Mount Sinai for one year, and then moved to Pittsburgh Children's Hospital—'67-'71. Four years, I was in the United States. Three years at the Children's Hospital. I finished my formal training in pediatric surgery, and '71 I go back to Turkey. At that time, I'm married. I had two boys.

I learned Dr. {Thomas E.} Starzl moved from Colorado to Pittsburgh. He is the first one who did liver transplantation in the world. And, at that time, he was the only man can do liver transplantation. When I heard he's in Pittsburgh, next day I took the plane and I come and talk to him. I told him I am very interested in learning liver transplant and he accept me as a visiting professor. Then, I got my sabbatical from my university and couple months later, July first, 1981, and I start working with him.

When I was working in Turkey, I was interested in liver disease, especially in children. My hospital, one of the largest in Turkey or in Middle East, we have a lot of referral—a lot of liver disease. It was more challenging, more difficult. I was doing a lot of research. I did a lot of liver transplantation in dog.

But to do liver transplant, you have to have good training. You cannot do yourself. At that time, 1980s, the only way you can learn, go be near to Dr. Starzl. I decided to get my sabbatical and learn more, because when I was practicing in Turkey I lost a lot of kids with liver disease.

At that time, 1981-'83, I work with him. That was the time liver transplant flourished. My father died in 1984. He saw me after school. I think he was very happy.

Life Magazine published in 1982, and we reached the success {of} 80%. Before that time, 1981, the success rate of the liver transplant was about 18-20%. They find some medication in Switzerland—immunosuppressant medication they call cyclosporine. That changed, and we can treat the patients without their getting rejection.

Was rejection the number one problem?

Yes. And the second was the technical problem. Doctor Starzl did a lot of operation before cyclosporine. He did about 170 operations and there were a lot of technical problems, a lot of rejection problems. But he did first liver transplant in '63. I was lucky to work with him. He is one of the geniuses in the field of surgery. Anyway, that his picture {Points to wall}. I have a great admiration to him.

In 1983, I finished work with him. I learn. And I was going back, by chance, I guess, to Dr. {Folkert} Belzer,† who was chief of surgery here in

---

† Pioneering kidney transplant surgeon who died in 1995.

Madison. He was looking for someone who can do liver transplantation. He called Dr. Starzl. He says, "Do you know someone who can do liver transplant?" And Dr. Starzl gave my name and he wrote an excellent recommendation. Dr. Belzer called me. He says, "Why don't you come here? Let's talk."

I say, "Okay." And I come to talk.

I was still member of the med school faculty in Turkey. He says, "Let's talk business. Can you do this operation? I need someone can do liver transplants successfully."

I say, "Look, I never lie in my life. If I close my eyes, I can do it because I was professor of surgery before I come and start working for Dr. Starzl."

I don't know how many thousand operations I did. I was young. I did two or three hundred operations a month for ten years. A lot of surgery. Plus, I worked with Starzl. I was confident.

"I can do it."

He says, "You're hired."

I came back with my wife to Madison and we looked around. It's a beautiful town and we decided we have to continue our life in different country, in different city, and different university. It was a good decision. I find my second home here—beautiful university, beautiful hospital, wonderful people to work with. I got full support from Dr. Belzer.

I did ten operations, and then I give my results to State Medical Society. They looked at my results and they accepted them. My results at University of Wisconsin were good to support the state medical system. Medicare patients, they were paying, and we start program here.

The first year I did five. The second year, I did 11. Third year, I did 20. So far, we did almost 1,400 liver transplants. We are five liver surgeon now. I celebrate my 1000th liver transplant about four years ago.

The first time when I see this transplant in Pittsburgh when Dr. Starzl perform, the patient was a 14-years old boy in liver coma. He was dying. We were in the corridor and Dr. Starzl says, "I have a liver in Atlanta. You want to come with me?"

I say, "Sure."

We go to Lear Jet and then, we go and take out liver and come back and deliver liver to that guy—that kid. I never seen anything in my life. Patient was bleeding all over. Patient was not breathing and was intubated. Patient's kidneys was not working and patient doesn't have any muscle tone or anything. I thought this kid going to die, definitely.

He had Wilson's disease, and in my experience, at that time, I was professor of pediatric surgery, I never see any patient recover. I thought, *Why we doing this?*

And next day, the patient was awake. I saw in two weeks, he went home.

Then, I come home and I told my wife, "Look, I saw a miracle. It's impossible. I'm praying to God. I wish I can do this operation myself." After I saw that it's possible with a few more operations with Dr. Starzl, then I say, "Why not? Maybe I can do it." I want to do it once. If I can do one, then I can die in peace. And then, I remembered those words when I did my thousandth operation. In every patient, I talk about this one. It is possible now. Now, we do the transplant like an appendix operation or hernia operation. It's a simple operation.

When we started doing that, TV was coming, and newspaper—another liver transplant in Madison, Wisconsin. Hundreds of new medications, you change your technique. Thanks to Dr. Starzl and Dr. Belzer, many things have changed. And then, we start doing more and more.

Doctor Belzer come to Wisconsin in 1974 from California. Before he come here, he did a lot of research on organ preservation. In 1987, he invented some preservation solution, which we call Belzer Solution or University of Wisconsin Solution, that increase the time preserving liver outside of the body up to 24 hours.

So that increased the number of donors?

Yes. We don't have to do this operation very fast. In the beginning, you have to do fast operation. You don't have time to wait too long, otherwise it would never work and patient may die. Everybody is working hard. We have to go fly to California, get delivery, come back and have to go to work very fast. I cannot teach my fellow residents.

But with the University of Wisconsin Solution, we can keep liver alive outside of the body up to 20, 24 hours. But we have to prove that works. That's the reason we did a lot of research. And finally in 1987, I try extended preservation. I went to Beaumont, Texas, take some liver from young guy in the car accident, diffuse with Wisconsin Solution, bring it back.

Instead of doing surgery in middle of the night, I go home and get some sleep and next morning at 7:30, I start surgery, like we were doing liver transplant as elective surgery. That operation did work.

We did 18 more operations like that and we have a 100 percent success, and then we published in *Lancet*, important medical journal, and some company start making this solution, and almost all liver centers still using this solution. That was one of the advances, having good liver transplant program; not only clinical, but as far as research-wise, also.

What is the main reason people need liver transplants?

Some babies born with no bile duct in the liver, and this patients may need liver transplantation in the future. About 60% of my pediatric liver transplants are due to biliary atresia.[‡]

In adult, the biggest indication are hepatitis C in our state, and alcohol-

‡ Biliary atresia is the congenital absence or closure of the ducts that drain bile from the liver.

related liver disease. And there are some with some other metabolic liver disease, some cancer, but mostly hepatitis C.

In some disease, you may treat some liver disease. But if there is cirrhosis or end stage liver disease and there are complications, such as severe jaundice, bleeding, and fluid accumulation in abdomen or hepatatic coma, the liver doesn't work. Ammonia will accumulate in the blood and that may poison the brain. The only way to save patient's life is liver transplant.

Just couple of things you can do. But this a very radical treatment. Like a heart transplant. The heart is not pumping. But liver, there is no machine for this and if you give them a good liver, patient flourish. Usually if you don't do anything, in about 12 to 18 hours, patient die. If you do something, change the plasma or do a shunt operation, you can extend it a couple days.

We don't want to just go treat the patients here. We want to be the best university, as far as the teaching. The biggest center is UCLA. The problem is donor. Whoever has more donor, they do more transplants

We have one of the best results, as far as the patient success comes in pediatric and adult patient, and I'm proud of that. But I'm more proud that I trained a lot of people and this is one of the best liver transplant training centers in the world.

Your legacy?

No. No. This does not belong to me. It belongs to the team. If anyone wants to learn liver transplant and all transplants—not only the liver, kidney, pancreas, intestines, all other transplant related surgery—our 2008 program is full now. Too many people wants to come here. We have a hard time to select our fellows. You see that big group picture there. There are almost 40 people I trained and they are working all around the United States. Now, everyone is a liver surgeon.

It must be very rewarding.

Oh, it is, yeah. Take someone never seen liver transplant and in two years make them liver surgeon. It's a lot of fun, also. Some are very excited they cannot sleep. Now, I saw some of my students, now they are professor of surgery, director of transplant program in some centers. I remember the day when they start doing surgery. That's good satisfaction.

My first patient I described to you died about six, seven years after that surgery of non-transplant related problems. But my second patient, she is doing wonderfully. She grew up, finished her school and married, and has two kids and is still working. We talk from time to time.

You keep in touch?

Oh, yeah. Sometimes I forget what I did last night, but I do not forget my patients. Sometimes, I saw the patient's face—I never forget. But name, I usually forget. Not only that, I remember their liver. How they liver looked like. Yeah, everyone's liver is different. The liver disease are different.

Transplant is different. When you accept someone as a patient, you make him some contract. It's more close than marriage. If you have a wife, you can divorce. But you cannot divorce your patient. If I do operation, they will see me till I die or until they die. Transplant needs lifelong commitment, and lifelong follow. There is no other way. Surgery is only one part. Following is important because this patients will get anti rejection treatment till end of their life.

Yesterday, I saw a patient, a young woman. She nine years old when we first met. She had severe problems and she was in intensive care unit almost two weeks. I start remembering how sick she was. Now, a young woman and she come to be checked and everything was okay. I really feel good.

Hernia operation—there's some complication. Gallbladder operation, a lot of complications. But liver transplant, you doing something positive. You're taking sick organ and replacing it with new one. That is right now the easiest operation. Now, we can do this operation within three to four hours. Patient usually staying 7-10 days in the hospital.

One team go and take out liver. Bring it. Another team opening up the patient. Then, they call me and I go another couple hours, to the important part of the transplanting liver, and other surgeons come and check everything and close.

With this way, we can do three, four liver transplants in one day. If there's enough donor in our community, we can do at least two, three hundred liver transplant with this manpower. At least 20 people are working there.

Unfortunately, availability of the organs are biggest problem now. About 20,000 people in United States still waiting for liver transplant and only 6,000 patients may get liver transplant every year—about 30%.

When you take out liver, you have to replace with another human liver right away. That comes from someone who dies. Brain death, but heart is working and family donate organ to us. Someone may donate half of the liver to loved one, such as to children, to father, mother, sister, brother or your friend. We can do this operation also in this institution. We did 20, 25 of them.

In the beginning, I was doing a lot of research with preservation. I was transplanting fox liver to the puppy for different species. I brought liver one day from California, and somehow we did not transplant that patient. Patient die. That liver I transplant to baboon—human liver to baboon. That worked, initially. But when I get too busy with the transplant training, patients, we are doing some clinical research—graph studies, etc.

Is there a potential for using animals, pigs?

In the future, yes. We did use three, four patients with it. Take out liver from pig. We hook up the machine and we got the patient's blood through the machine, pass through pig liver and filtrate it, and then give back. In the meanwhile, that pig liver clean up patient blood. We did four of them and three of them we find transplant to liver and then, we transplant the patient. Then, these patients did survive.

Any ill effects from the pig?
So far, no.

What is your main concern about using animals?
Infection and rejection. But mainly it's infection. You have to go get a new liver every eight hours. We're not doing anymore. The one we did about 8-10 years ago, there was some transgenetic pig, but then there were a lot of concern about infection. The best is still human liver. But in the future, we don't know.

Are there other operations you've done, other than liver transplants, that stand out in your mind?
I don't like easy stuff. I want to attack always the hard things. In 1984, I did the first Siamese Twins separation, conjoined twins. It still the first and only one in the state of Wisconsin, successful one. In 1984, July, I got a call Saturday night from Meriter Hospital. They say our patient just arrived—joined abdomen each other. I go to hospital right away. And about two months before this happened, they sent the patient to Children's Hospital, Philadelphia, and the family told me, "Can you do it?"

And I said, "Sure, I can do it. No big deal." We did a couple of tests and next Sunday morning at 7:30 at Meriter Hospital, I did surgery. But somehow the press knows and there was a TV station, CBS, ABC, NBC, whatever, was there and they were live coverage of this Siamese twins separation. I divided in three and a half hours and the twins did go home in nine days. Now, they are 20, 21 years old and they are both healthy, two girls. And time to time, they come and see me. They look normal.

Most of the operations, you have to do in your head before you go in. If you know where you gonna cut, how you gonna suture before you finish. If you plan everything, you have a confidence, nothing can go wrong.

I know that I cut this one under the skin, there is a tissue here and here. I have to be careful here. I have to talk to anesthesia and that has to be ready. If you plan everything, like you're playing chess, second step, later, fifth step, 20 step later. If you can see that—that is the game of mine. Good surgeon finished operation before start surgery, and then no big deal.

I did the first baby liver transplant. I did the smallest baby. I try to challenge. I try to push. I'm so happy I did it. I have a lot of international patients also. I did the first liver transplant in Japanese citizen—small kid. They come here. I took one liver from Madison to Brazil—Sao Paulo. We transplanted the first international, oversea liver.

How did you develop the confidence to do these things?

Confidence or stupid courage? First, you have to have good training. I trained one of the best hospitals in Turkey. Then, I come to Pittsburgh. My chief was one of the best pediatric surgeons. These are the giants of surgery.

Then, second time when I come to Pittsburgh, I work with Doctor Starzl. Any place he goes, two years, I go with him day and night. I follow him like a shadow. I was like his slave. He says sit here. Then, I sit. He was my maestro. Watching Dr. Starzl was like that. It was not surgery, but art.

Then, I come back to Madison and I work with Dr. Belzer. Dr. Belzer, one of the biggest teacher and biggest researcher, and one of the biggest first generation transplant surgeon. I'm the second generation. I trained well. That give me some confidence.

Now, if you go to the operation room with the confidence, I can do this. If something happens, I can do that. Walk in with confidence, and your success will be higher, definitely. But if you're scared—if I cut this, what's going to happen?

But I did over 40,000 operations. OK? I did almost 1,400 here. Two hundred in Pittsburgh.

In this business, you have to believe something. There are too many examples. Scientifically, you say coincidence. Some people may say luck. Some people may say God. I don't know.

Let me tell you. Some woman had liver problem. Liver ruptured, somehow. They call 911. The ambulance come. They resuscitate the patient. Come to emergency room from someplace in rural area. And then they send the patient by helicopter here right away. During the helicopter trip, that woman heart stop five times. They were pumping.

They come here and I have no idea what is going on. But some of my surgeon friends call me in operating room and say come and look at that. I found a dead liver and we have to change right away. And we go talk with the family. They say, "You're kidding. She was okay. No big deal. Why did this happen?"

We told them, "Whatever happened, this patient has dead liver. They have to change." They discuss. Finally, they accept it. But at that time, the patient heart stop, again. Two hours later, they call us. There's a liver available, same blood type. If it not God, what it is? I call one of the surgeons.

"We don't have time. You have to take out the liver and send it to us."

He send it to us in two hours. In the meanwhile, we took the patient to the operating room. On the way from intensive care unit to operating room, the patient's heart stop again. And then, we were pumping and anesthesia say, "You crazy. You cannot do this operation. Patient is already dead." No. We did it. I start surgery before the liver arrived to hospital. I take it out and replace with new one and patient then home in 11 days. You call coincidence or miracle or God. I say it's God.

Have people back home ever tried to convince you to come back to Turkey?

Yes, but I decided to finish my career here. I go and help every medical school. When I go back, I give a talk in each faculty. I kept my relation with Turkey, all the time. You can see these are all the presidents of all the Turkey. This is the founder of the Turkish republic and that is the current president. All of these, they invite me to the Presidential Palace.

You've actually met all of these presidents?

Oh, yeah. {Points}He gave me 2000 Doctor of the Century Award. I took my mother to that ceremony. It was a presidential ceremony at the Presidential Palace. My mom was so happy. This is the picture taking in that ceremony. My older son. He is MD-PhD. He's in Boston. He did ophthalmology training at the Harvard. And he's {points to the other son} second year law school student here in Madison. I became United States citizen in 1992 and all my family still here and living happily.

Last year, Prime Minister come to Chicago. I go met with him. I am trying to share all the information. All my life I stay at the university. I enjoy teaching. Every surgeon can do surgery, but not everyone can teach. You have to be patient. You don't have to get nervous. You don't have to be rough. I consider all of my fellows, my residents, my friends or my sons or daughter.

It was very tough to teach my sons when they were 16, to teach driving. But I was telling them to go slowly. Look at right side. Look at left side. Then, stop and then go. I was excited. But you know, teaching surgery is like that. I enjoy to working with young people.

I decided because I'm 65, I have to stop. I do more and more {transplants}, but the thing is my administrative position. Yes, I give it {up}. But I left that job to a younger generation. This is the program. I build it. My kids, my children, will take from here and then go out there.

For how much longer will you do the operations?

Honestly, if somebody tell me, "Stop, you cannot do it." But I know when the time comes. If you learn from every operation and if you try not to do mistakes for other operation, you can improve. In this age, with this white hair, I have enough experience now and always thinking not to do same mistake. Practice does not make perfect. Perfect practice makes perfect. I can be helpful to my patient. It's pity if I stop right now because too many sick people waiting. Too many young people I can work with.

I have a wonderful life. But it's pity to just go to Florida, get some retirement home or some place with golf. I'm not going to be a good golf player, but I'm a professional liver transplant surgeon. It doesn't come easily and it doesn't grow in the Christmas tree. It takes years and hours, and bloody days and night.

The last three weeks, I did three liver transplants myself. I was busy. The new patients I saw, maybe 30-40 patients. The follow up patients. I talk with my residents. I make rounds or go to meeting, this and that. I'm working full-time and I enjoy.

How do you handle the stress?

Stress? We don't use that term. We use fun. If it's not stressful, it's so easy. Sometimes, you lose a patient. It's sad. Sometimes, we do mistakes. We try to learn from that mistake and we openly accept it—that's the key. When you do mistake, do not blame someone else. Just stand up as a man. Say, "It was my fault." But next time, try not to do it. Some people says, "Oh, I never do this. I don't have any complication." No! I did that—no one else. Someone say, "No, my assistant cut this…" No. If they're not good, don't let them cut. If they cut, you walk in and you say, "This is my responsibility."

We did almost 1,400 liver transplants. Me or none of my surgical colleagues ever sued for liver transplant, since I start doing liver transplant here in this institution. We go explain everything. As long as family are happy, you have a very good connection. If they think you're trying to help, and actually, so far, we didn't do any stupid mistake.

Losing a patient is always bad. You feel very sorry. Some days you cannot sleep. But you accept that. That is your job. You're trying your best. Sometimes best is not enough. Sometimes we need luck. Sometimes, whatever you do, the patient may die. We are dealing with sick people. My patients, if I don't do liver transplant, usually they are going to die. We always sit down and explain to our family, to patients' family and patients, also.

Sometimes, you're invited to the funeral. You go to the funeral. Any of my patients are like part of my family. But what can we do? But the next day, we have to be strong again for some other sick people waiting for us.

All patients are my friend. And good friend means, I do not go out. I don't play ball, which I never play ball in my life, anyway. But if I have to play, then I play with nice people. But their life is different. My life is different. I'm a surgeon.

What do you do in your spare time?

I spend it with the family. I cannot do all of this without my wife. She is a very understanding woman. One of the way to handle the problem, go home and talk with my wife. We walk, and bike together. Now, after I play tennis, I have pain all over my body. Walking is a better sport for me, instead of playing soccer or tennis.

I wish I can spend more time with my wife, but she does understand that. Surgery is part of my life and I have to live it. But I don't have too much hobby. Surgery is my hobby and my family.

Now, when I look back, I wish I could have more time with my kids. How lucky I am. They're going to school and they are successful students. My son is an ophthalmologist and he's doing an MBA.

I say, "I don't know anything else, except medicine. If you ask, am

I happy to be a doctor? I say, yes. If you go and be MD, you can do too many things. You can do research. You can work 10 hours per week. You can work 100 hours per week. You will have a good social life. You decide it." My oldest son accept that idea and went into medical school. And my youngest one, he told me that he even doesn't want to come near to hospitals.

Any of your kids actually watch you perform surgery?

Yes. Both of them. Yeah, actually one of the highlights in my career when my oldest son go to medical school here. And in surgery, when he was doing rotation, they gave him to transplant and one night I was doing a transplant, then he come and assist me and I was so happy. You saw your son who you took fishing or hunting or take to soccer game or football game. What you do with your son, too many things. It was a highlight of my career as a father. I show my sons what I am doing. You want to show your kid what you know best.

My youngest, when he was in college, he come one night and then watch me do the surgery. I try to show him what is the best, and he didn't say anything. He did not come anymore. That surgery affect him very badly.

Too much blood?

Maybe, maybe. I don't know. No reaction and he still doesn't say anything. He says, "Oh, that's good." Maybe some day he will write his memories. As long as he's happy, I don't care what he does.

I will continue doing what I am doing and in the future, we don't know what life is going to show. I still can do many things—still very tough operations. Again, I feel privileged human being. How lucky I am that I can treat sick people. I think God loves me. It's an unbelievable satisfaction and feeling.

I remember when I start. We come from long, long way. It was beautiful journey that I really enjoy each minute of that. But what I do best, surgery. I'm still too good and my last operation is my best operation. I will do surgery till I die, if I can.

Postscript: Doctor Kalayoglu retired from the University of Wisconsin in March, 2007 and is now Chairman of the Department of Surgery at Memorial Hospital, Istanbul, Turkey.

Chapter Thirty-One

The Vision Thing

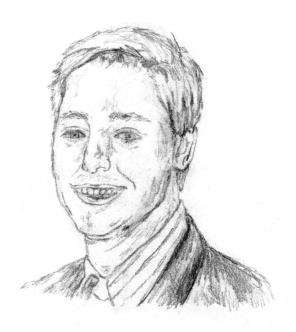

"You don't do things that are sudden—a lot of it is just figuring out how to move under high magnification."

Kevin Flaherty, MD
Ophthalmologist, Wausau

Doctor Kevin Flaherty grew up in the shadow of his physician father, who rose to the top of the medical hierarchy at the American Medical Association. But the younger Dr. Flaherty, in his early 50s, has developed his own passion for medicine. Restoring eyesight for patients in central Wisconsin isn't enough to satisfy his need to contribute. That's a lesson he surely learned from his dad, which drives him to participate in medical politics.

In his spare time, he enjoys collecting antique toys, cast iron mechanical banks and art. He also loves to travel. And that's a good thing, because he's frequently going out of town to attend various medical meetings.

On this day, Dr. Flaherty, Speaker of the Wisconsin Medical Society's House of Delegates, just gaveled the body to recess. During the lunch break, he sat down with me before giant windows at the Monona Terrace Convention Center in Madison, which offer a panoramic view of Lake Monona.

Doctor Flaherty loves his job, but he says an eye doctor's view isn't always pretty.

~~~~~~

There are things physicians see that are not very appealing or attractive. For me, those have been the severe traumas, like where someone comes in with a ruptured eyeball. I've seen a lot of injuries from paintball guns. They're very nasty. That's completely avoidable visual loss, and it's just such a tragedy. It's usually people 12 through 16, and they have irreversible visual loss. Eye protection is critical.

All you can do is take care of that patient to the best of your ability. The most common cause of visual loss is trauma—the young adults and children. Someone's using a weed whacker and the string breaks off and slices through the eye; the cornea, or a dog bite in a child where you've got huge portions of the upper and lower lids completely gone because the dog has chewed it off.

Dog bites are usually during the summer, on hot days. If you look at the incidence of dog bites, they're much more common on the hot, sultry days of summer. Just like people get a little short and irritated when they're hot, dogs are the same on those summer days. I've seen a number of dog bites over the years and usually the dog is sort of sleeping, or gets teased, or they take something from a dog.

I remember one girl very clearly. She was fooling around and teasing the dog, offering him popcorn and taking it back. And the dog just had enough and took a big chunk out of her eyelids. That case was particularly challenging because it involved the tear drainage system, where the tears, as they flow across the eye, drain through these openings in your upper and lower lid. We had to reconstruct the tear drain system so the tears could drain away from the eyes, so she wouldn't have a problem with constant tearing.

Sometimes these procedures require second stages or other procedures, like skin grafts. You need tissue, because you need to have upper and lower eyelids to protect the eye. Without an eyelid, the eye will ultimately fail. You need that protection. The lids are more than just cosmetic. They protect the integrity of the eyeball, and that's so important. They lubricate the eye by blinking.

Wear safety glasses. Even lawnmowers—it's really important. If you're pounding a nail, you should know that the number one occupation for losing vision is carpenters. There are a lot of one-eyed carpenters walking around because they're pounding nails or using table saws, and they don't put safety glasses on. It comes back and hits them in the eye. It's a common injury—and completely preventable.

What about congenital blindness. Will doctors be able to cure blindness, some day?

The problem with doing a whole eye transplant is there's no good technology to allow central nervous system nerves to regenerate. That's the same reason that people who have spinal cord injuries can't have that cured because their central nervous system won't go together again like peripheral nerves will.

There's lot of research being done to get central nervous system nerves to regenerate. I think that'll happen. When that happens, theoretically, you'll be able to do an eye transplant—sewing the muscles together, sewing the optic nerve together. The time may well come when you can have the eye completely replaced or maybe an artificial eye can be devised and connected to the neural network in the brain; the visual cortex part of the brain to see. That's not on the too far distant horizon.

The future of ophthalmology is very exciting. We have technology now that we're starting to treat diseases that we used to not treat before—age-related macular degeneration, which is the leading cause of blindness of people over age 65 in America. We're on the threshold of really dramatic changes in that field.

We now have medicines that we can inject into people's eyes to stop new blood vessels from growing. There are new diagnostic tools. There are people implanting chips into the retina to try to allow people to see when they have visual loss from macular degeneration. I also believe they'll be artificial corneas. We won't have to rely on donor corneas.

Lasik,* which is very popular right now, is very safe and effective when it's done on the right patients. My bigger concern, long term, is whether these eyes are going to be the eyes we're going to use for corneal transplants. Our exclusionary criteria has traditionally been that if anybody has had previous eye surgery, we exclude them as a potential donor. With the increase of refractive surgery, we're limiting our potential donor pool in the future, and this may be an issue in the years to come.

Right now, the problem is that artificial corneas tend to get spit out and rejected by the body as not being part of the self. Theoretically, they'll be able to take a cell from your cornea and, perhaps, grow a new cornea, so they'll be no risk of rejection. Give that cornea to someone who's blind from corneal disease.

With lens implants, the technology's changing. We've got lens implants now that we're just starting to implant where they can see close and near at the same time. Some of these new lens implants, you'll be able to correct

---

* Lasik is laser eye surgery that changes the shape of cornea.

distance and close vision simultaneously, so I think the future is very bright for ophthalmology, no pun intended.

Tell me about the early stages of your training. There can't be much margin for error when working on the eye.

It's a step-wise procedure. When you do your first cataract operation, you don't do the whole operation. The operation would be broken down into parts. At the beginning you might just be allowed to do the prepping of the eye or maybe anesthetizing the eye—giving a shot around the eye or making the initial incision in the lining in front of the eye, or making the groove or incision or removing part of the front of the lens.

Your senior resident, looking over your shoulder, would say, "Okay, now you're going to do this." You do a little bit at a time and so each time you do a bit more of the operation, until eventually you're doing the entire cataract operation.

There are a variety of things you can do to facilitate your ability to operate under a microscope. There's some lab course where you go in, under a microscope, practice tying sutures and trying to figure out where you are in space, so you know how to move slowly. You don't do things that are sudden. A lot of it is just figuring out how to move under high magnification, and how to make small movements. You go a bit at a time. That's the case with all the other operations, too.

After I took my ophthalmology residency, I did a fellowship in corneal transplant surgery. It's a process to start doing more and more corneal transplants, until you're very comfortable doing different transplants for different disease processes.

The most common procedure I do is cataract surgery. I still love doing cataract surgery. The operation I do now is completely different than the one I learned during my residency, where we learned to make large incisions. You removed the entire lens of the eye.

Nowadays, we're making really tiny incisions, three millimeters in length. We use ultrasound energy to break up the cataract lens. And the lens, after it's broken up, it's aspirated out of that tiny incision. The lens implant is folded and inserted through that tiny incision and the patients see almost immediately.

You get so excited when you talk about this.

It's very gratifying. There are few things as personally satisfying as caring for patients. More specifically, in my case, operating on someone and restoring their vision is a wonderful ability to have. There are no shots, no stitches, and people's visual recovery is very rapid. It's not at all uncommon for people to see 20/20 the day after the surgery.

The anesthesia we use is just ointment or drops, so the whole surgery is done with drops or ointments in the eye, but no shots whatsoever. No needles; no injections. That keeps them very comfortable and we can do that surgery.

It's continually evolving. What's neat about medicine is the way the technology changes, to allow us to better care for our patients. You take someone who can't see, do a thirty minute operation, and restore their vision. The joy that brings to their lives and the improvement is just astounding, especially when you take someone who's got dense cataracts in both eyes. As soon as you do one eye and they see, their world is open to them again.

Are you seeing an increase in cataracts?

Yeah, there's no question about it. The older people get, the more likely they are to develop cataracts. The other risk factors for cataracts include ultraviolet exposure and, possibly, diet. But if you look at the world distribution of cataracts, the closer you get to the equator, the higher the incidence.

We, as a society, are living much longer, so there's a much older group of people having cataracts. The oldest person I ever operated on was 102. I really didn't want to operate on her. I'd seen her about a year before when she was 101 and she said, "I really can't read and do things." I sort of tried to talk her out of it. I was thinking, *Do I want to do cataract surgery on someone who's 101 years old?*

So I said, "Why don't you come back in six months and we'll talk about it again." And sure enough, {laughs}, she came back in six months and she again said, "I just can't read. Can't you help me?" Eventually, I relented and I took off one cataract, and she came back and absolutely was seeing better and pleased.

We see a lot of the elderly population. Another patient was about 96 years old. This woman lived in a small town. She was quite an independent woman, very bright, living alone, and still driving her car. She had difficulty with night driving. I did cataract surgery on her.

Two years later, when she was 98, she went to the Division of Motor Vehicles to get her driver's license renewed and was given an unrestricted license—an eight year license. Her license wouldn't expire until she was 106. She even thought that was too long.

What was your main concern about operating on a patient that old?

The biggest challenge is when people have other problems, like severe arthritis or positioning problems, or back or neck problems. The way we do modern eye surgery is that the patient is monitored and there's very little stress involved. They lie still for a half hour or less in a comfortable position. Sometimes the most challenging part is getting them positioned comfortably, so the surgery can be done. The eye surgery is generally very well tolerated for the patients. I've never had a patient die on the table.

The ages are so variable. Some people—their chronologic age might be quite elderly, but it seems like their biologic age, or their tissue, is still not representative of their chronologic age, so there's a lot of individual variation in patients. Some patients, at 60, are in much worse shape that other patients in their 80s. People are very different in how well they've aged.

When did you decide you were going to become an eye doctor?

I really had the idea that I was going to be an ophthalmologist before I started medical school. I was influenced here in Madison, when I was an undergraduate. I majored in molecular biology.

There was a professor in the Department of Botany, Dr. Becker, who was very involved with some of the religious stuff around school. He had a bible study and Christian fellowship session at lunch time, and I would go to that frequently. He had a speaker come in one day who was an ophthalmologist, who talked about all the things that he had done in the rest of the world, traveling around to Africa and India, doing eye surgery on people who were blind from cataracts. He emphasized that this was something you could do to impact people's lives without depending on a lot of ancillary support staff. You were quite independent doing it. I was just fascinated by that. I thought that it would be great to be an ophthalmologist and be able to do eye surgery on people and restore their vision.

Following my graduation from Madison, I was encouraged to go to a big city for medical school, so I went to Loyola University in Chicago. At Loyola, I became good friends with the Chairman of the ophthalmology department, Dr. James McDonald. He had started a group with an acronym of FOCUS, which stood for Foreign Ophthalmogic Care for the United States. They started going to Africa and started a clinic over there. As a medical student, I told Dr. McDonald that I'd like to go to Africa some day, and do that.

After my medical school, Dr. McDonald was eager to have me be an ophthalmology resident at Loyala. I was honored that he wanted me to stay there. I was familiar with the program and knew the people, so I chose to stay at Loyola for my residency, but I wanted to do a rotating internship some place. I ultimately went to Spokane, Washington for an internship in a program that had family practice residents, internal medicine residents, and OB residents. I did a lot of OB. I did a month of plastics, and a couple months of general surgery. Then I went back to Loyola for my ophthalmology residency.

As it turned out, I did have the opportunity to go to Africa during my residency. I went to Nigeria twice with Dr. McDonald and some ophthalmologists from the Chicago area. This was a wonderful time to go for a couple of weeks and do volunteer eye surgery, where you could operate on so many people with so much need.

Since then, I've had the opportunity to do volunteer ophthalmology in other places as well. Several times, I've been down to St. Lucia. When I was in medical school, a physician, who was also a priest, was running the hospital down there. His name is Doctor Jack McCarthy. He's from the Green Bay area. I spent six weeks as a medical student doing a tropical medicine rotation in St. Lucia and got to know Dr. McCarthy.

I ended up practicing with his brother Chuck, in Wausau, for many years. He started a group that does missionary work in the Caribbean, and I've gone with that group several times to do volunteer eye surgery in St. Lucia. When I went to the Caribbean, I took six corneas with me and did some of the first corneal transplants on these Caribbean islands.

Fortunately, in Wisconsin, we have the highest number of organ donors per capita in the country. In Wisconsin, people are very generous, so my patients all eventually, got corneal transplants. The average wait is about two months for corneal transplants in Wisconsin, which is a lot shorter than in some places. In some parts of the world, for cultural or other reasons, they just don't donate tissue, and that's a real problem.

How much of a difference in vision can a transplant make?

Vision can be very poor before the transplant. It depends why the cornea needs to be transplanted. Typical reasons for transplantation are any of the inherited corneal diseases that are found in the elderly population.

The young patients can get a very unusual condition where the cornea gets very steep and bends light poorly. They get tremendous glare, and the cornea doesn't work very effectively. There's scarring from it. It gets thin. The apex of the cornea gets very high, so they can't wear a contact lens and glasses don't work at all.

After corneal transplant, it's not all that unusual for patients to get to 20/20 or 20/25, with some correction. Astigmatism, the amount of irregular curvature of the cornea, we always battle by suture removal and proper suture placement, and adjusting the shape of the eye as the sutures are removed. But it's a long procedure before they see well. Typically, they take six months to a year to get the best vision possible after corneal transplant. It's not like Hollywood, where they take the bandage off and they can see perfectly the next day. Now cataract surgery can be very much like that. People see dramatically well the next day.

Aside from your practice, you've become a medical leader at the Wisconsin Medical Society and in your specialty society. Your dad has been extremely active in the AMA. Did he encourage you to get involved in medical leadership?

I went to my first AMA meeting with my father. When I was a resident, I saw how the AMA worked. It just seemed natural to get involved, and so I did. I'm very proud of my father and his accomplishments. He's done probably more than I'll ever do. Being chairman of the Board of AMA—you don't get much beyond that. Growing up, I guess I just felt it was part of the responsibility.

Tell me about your upbringing.

I was born in Milwaukee, when my dad was a medical student. My sisters were both born there. We moved to Texas when I was about two years old. My father was in the Air Force, and we lived in Amarillo. One of my earliest memories of living in Texas was on the air base. The jet fighters would always come by and there'd be sonic booms every day. It would shake the house and shake the dishes. It was very commonplace. I went to Kindergarten in Amarillo, rode a blue, Air Force school bus.

When I was going into first grade, we moved to Madison. We four children were all born in five and a half years, so we're very close siblings. We moved to Madison so my dad could finish his residency. He had been a general medical officer in the Air Force, after his graduation from medical school. I know the sacrifices it takes. My dad was away at meetings sometimes when I was growing up. My mom was affectionately known as St. Joan, and there's some truth to that.

I've had an excellent role model of a physician leader in my father. I strive to give back to the profession and to always do what's right by my patients, keeping them foremost. I've been involved in the Wisconsin Medical Society for 18 plus years now, and intend to stay involved for a number of more years, the good Lord permitting. I don't think it's genetic, but seeing my father's involvement, it seemed like the right thing to do to me.

Is it hard to balance your professional and personal life? You have a big family.

I have a wife who's quite understanding, but yes, there are tensions. She says, "Why can't others do this?" She sees partners of mine who are not taking time from their practices to go to meetings that I think are important. I try to commit myself to doing things the right way. When I'm home, I try to be completely focused with my family.

When I'm here {Madison}, I try to work hard for the benefit of the physicians and the Society. I tend now to ask permission before I enter in new ventures and I try to be very inquisitive about how much time they'll take. When I get involved with one thing, I see if I can pull back a little bit from another thing, too, to try to keep the number of days and the amount of time gone from my family to a minimum. I'm fortunate that I'm in a very supportive group that's willing to cover for me when I'm not there.

What kind of time demands does your job require?

We start early, and go until six or 7 o'clock. It depends on the day. Then, the call situation can be tough because of the size we are. We take it a week at a time and it can be miserable. Fortunately, it only comes every ninth week. I'm certainly not complaining about my lifestyle. We'd all like to have more of our own lives and more time for things we truly appreciate, but there's a lot to be said for that physician/patient relationship. Patients want their own doctors, and they want their doctors to take care of them.

In ophthalmology, I see patients for years, and I see all ages of patients. We'll see families that are all nearsighted or farsighted, or all have high astigmatism. Now that I'm almost 50, I'm having some trouble with close vision, so I wear reading glasses. I wear contact lenses, and glasses, sometimes. So much of our vision is inherited.

I'll see whole families—kids, the moms, the dads, the grandparents. They all have different eye needs, but I'll see the entire spectrum of ages. That's what I love about ophthalmology. I'll take care of everyone from babies with blocked tear ducts to the 100-year olds and everything in between.

Some of my colleagues in surgery, such as in OB, they have it much worse, in terms of sacrifice with personal lifestyle. My general surgical colleagues, my heart goes out to them with how busy they are. I can see why they want to reclaim more of their lives.

But ophthalmology is a great specialty. I love what I do. The eye is amazing. That's why so much of the brain is devoted to it. There are 12 cranial nerves. All these nerves are related to the eye. It's such an important sense. We get so much visual information.

When you think that waves of light strike an object outside of your body, you see the reflection at that wave length and you perceive it as color, as shape, as motion. You can recognize the face of your wife, your child, and it all comes from your visual system.

CHAPTER THIRTY-TWO

MIRACULOUS MINDS

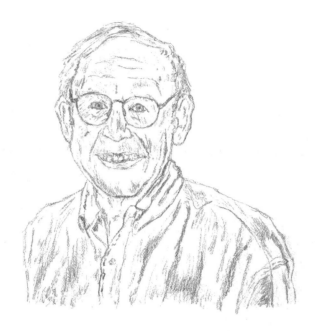

"He's memorized 9,000 books and can pull those back, page by page. He says that he reads one page with one eye and one page with the other."

Darold Treffert, MD
Psychiatry, Fond du Lac, WI

One evening in the late 1980s, a blind and severely impaired man sent shivers through my body when I witnessed his musical ability. Had he levitated, I would have been no less astonished.

I had arrived after sunset and had difficulty finding his farmhouse in the pitch black. I was on assignment for Wisconsin Public Radio for a story I was doing on Leslie Lemke, a musical marvel. He lives in rural, central Wisconsin, with his caretaker sister. When I introduced myself to Leslie, then in his mid 30s, he could only mimic what I said. In fact, he sounded like one of those computer generated voices.

"Hello, Leslie," I said.

"Hello, Leslie," he responded. This echoed response went on, no matter what I said. It was kind of spooky. That inability to hold even a simple conversation made what he did next all the more remarkable. He began playing the piano, and singing, too. How can this guy who can't even converse, sing?

Then, he went a step further. When Leslie played commercial jingles, he would mimic the announcer. In this mode, he could speak complete sentences, based on what he had heard on television. It was eerie to me, but this is what Dr. Darold Treffert calls it: "Savant syndrome is left hemisphere damage with right brain hemisphere compensation, coupled with higher circuitry."

Okay.

I still couldn't help wondering whether he was faking his disability. Apparently, it's not an uncommon reaction. But the guy is for real. In fact, Leslie's one of a few dozen people in the world known as prodigious savants, some of whose skills were later portrayed in the movie "Rainman." The medical consultant for that movie was Dr. Treffert, who remains active on various mental health issues.

"Any friend of Dr. Treffert is a friend of mine," said Leslie's sister, when I called to request an "interview" with Leslie.

Many years later, Dr. Treffert, now in his mid-70s, and I, are once again discussing Leslie, and where savant research has gone, though we've talked many times over the years.

Why did you become a psychiatrist?

After medical school, Dorothy and I picked up everything we owned and we put it in the back and on top of a '47 Studebaker. I wanted to go somewhere else to do my internship, and went to an Oregon hospital. I was on duty in the emergency room and a patient came in. She had repeated stab wounds all over her body and she was flagrantly psychotic. And it just occurred to me, that of all the other things that came into the emergency room, the splinter in the knee, hives, and bee stings, we pretty much knew what to do.

But this was such a mysterious situation. She had harmed several of her children and stabbed herself. Here's somebody who was as flagrantly ill as somebody in the intensive care unit, and it just piqued my interest. That's what I wanted to do, because we knew so little about that illness. I had always been intrigued by those things that we don't know a lot about.

Even when you were a kid?

In third grade, I wanted to be a doctor. I don't know why. My parents always supported the idea, but they also realized that that was a long road. I was born and raised in Fond du Lac. I never intended to practice medicine in my hometown. I was born at the hospital where I practiced, which is a little unusual.

My dad and mom lived in Fond du Lac. He worked for Giddings & Lewis Machine Tool Company. He was a foreman there. He had an eighth grade education, as did my mom. But he was really good at what he did, in terms of the machine shop. He would have gone further in the company, but they told him that, "We really need to have people with more credentials."

He accepted that, but he always told me, "Darold, now you get that diploma. Whatever you do, you've got to get that piece of paper, because that'll open doors that otherwise won't." And so I did. My dad was very supportive and encouraging about getting an education, but if I didn't, that was fine, too. He wasn't pushing the issue.

I was a good student. I had a good time, too. I enjoyed my years, and I got a $500 scholarship to Bethany Lutheran College in Mankato, Minnesota. To our family, $500 was a big deal. I was intrigued with psychiatry. In fact, my buddies called me Sigmund there. I went to Iowa City for premed and UW Madison for medical school. For residency training the University of Wisconsin had something called the career plan, where if you agreed to work with the State of Wisconsin for two years, at the end of your training, they would pay you a living wage. That was an attractive incentive, so I went through the psychiatry program there. At the end of that time, it came time to be assigned for those two years of indentured service, and I got assigned to Winnebago Mental Health Institute in Oshkosh, and specifically to start a children's unit there. I didn't know how to run a children's unit. But there weren't any children's units around the country, which was a good thing, because then we could set it up the way we wanted. It turned out to be a really good program.

The superintendent of Winnebago had come up to Wisconsin from Louisiana, and decided that the climate here was a little too harsh, so they asked me if I wanted to be acting superintendent. I was 29 at the time. I said, "Well, sure. I'll try it." I was on staff for 17 years, but I was superintendent for 15 years.

Of course, running a mental hospital is a very interesting occupation. I got this emergency situation at the hospital that I had to go back for one evening. I just had on my street clothes. I didn't look a heck of a whole lot like a mental hospital superintendent, I guess.

I was walking from one building to another, and one of the patients came up to me and says, "Hey, I haven't seen you here before. Who are you?"

I said, "I'm Dr. Treffert. I run the hospital."

He gave me a very knowing and a very reassuring look and said, "Well, you'll get over that. I thought I was the governor when I came in here."

That sort of helped keep things in perspective through that whole tour of duty. Anyway, the children's unit, my first day on the job, I met my first savant. We had gotten these youngsters together—about 30 of them who were under 18—at the hospital on this unit. Most of them were autistic, though not all of them were. But there were three little fellas who were of special interest to me because one had memorized the bus system of the City of Milwaukee. If you gave him the time of day and the bus number, he would tell you what corner that bus is going by. We had another little guy who could put jigsaw puzzles together with a sewing machine rhythm and accuracy, without looking at the picture, just from the shapes. And, we had a third little guy who was sort of a history almanac. Every morning when I came in, he'd say, "Dr. Treffert, did you know what happened on this day in history?" And of course after a while, the night before, I would look things up. I could never stump him.

I became interested in this phenomenon of people who had severe mental impairments, but had some island of genius or ability that was so striking because of the disparity between ability and disability. In those days, they were called idiot savants. I developed an interest in that, and began to do some research in that area.

Autism had just begun to appear on the map. As it turned out, Dr. Leo Kanner, who was the first doctor to describe early infantile autism in 1943, was a visiting professor for a time while I was in medical school. I was very impressed and influenced by him, and his interest in this. He was a very kindly gentleman and a very wise man, and so I followed that interest.

How much did you know about savants when you first met those three kids?

I knew zero about it. That sent me to the library to start finding out what we knew about this condition. There was very little written about it at that time. There were some things in the literature, but probably, 25 or 30 articles total. Savant Syndrome had first been described in 1887 by J. Langdon Down, who was better known for describing Down's syndrome. But, for the next century, there would be sort of anecdotal reports in the literature. He described ten cases in his 30 years of experience.

And, to some extent, I identify myself with Dr. Down because he gave this lecture at the end of his 30 years, and described Down syndrome and a bunch of other things. He said, "There's this one little group that I want to talk about." And he described these ten patients, all of whom had the same characteristics known as savant syndrome now: music, art, calendar calculating and mechanical skills.

Well, after I became superintendent of the hospital, I had other things to do. I developed an interest in major mental illness in general; not just in children, especially the legal rights of the mentally ill, and began to write fairly extensively in that area.

I also was in a small private practice, in what I would call the general practice of psychiatry, everything from children to people in their 80s or 90s, in the general hospital setting.

I've had private practice and public practice, and liked both. I got into the rights of the mentally ill, along with alcohol and drug abuse. I maintained my interest in autism and savant syndrome, but was not really actively involved in that until June of 1980 when Leslie Lemke came to Fond du Lac to give a concert. My daughter, Joni, was at the concert. She came home, bounded through the door and said, "Dad, dad, I saw a small miracle."

I said, "What did you see?"

"I saw this guy. He's blind—very mentally handicapped, with cerebral palsy. Never had a music lesson in his life, but he's playing this music, beautifully. He can listen to a song and play it back just on a single hearing."

I said, "Well, that is a miracle, but it's also something we call savant syndrome."

The next day at the mental health center, one of the television stations had been at the concert, made some tapes. They didn't believe what they saw, so they brought them to me, as the local mental health expert. "Is this a fake? Or is this real? If it's real, how in the world can that happen?"

I said, "Well, it is real and it's something called the savant syndrome."

It turned out that some AP writers were in the room at the time and they picked up the story. They carried the story on the wire about Leslie Lemke and May's miracle, his mother, May. Walter Cronkite used that as his Christmas story that year.

That's Incredible must watch Walter Cronkite, because they did a program. And Donahue must watch That's Incredible, because he did a program and had Leslie and myself on that program. It's the only time I've seen Phil Donahue at a loss for words, because May took over the program.

Then, "60 Minutes" did a program in October of 1983, which a lot of people still remember, because as I go around the country talking about savant syndrome, they remember Leslie, George, and Alonzo, and especially, Leslie. That program really was the country's introduction to savant syndrome, because I had a chance to talk about what savant syndrome is. Somehow, they took miles and miles of footage and condensed it to 18 minutes.

Well, it turns out Dustin Hoffman was watching that program. When he saw Leslie, he said he was moved to tears by this blind boy with this handicap, playing this beautiful music.

I had been sent the script for the movie "Rainman" because they wanted me to be a technical consultant to make sure the program was accurate, which I found hard to believe. Hollywood wanted to be accurate? But they really did, mainly because they didn't want to offend the parents and families of mentally disabled people. They wanted to come across well and not look like they were making fun of them.

Dustin Hoffman was scheduled to play the brother and not the savant. But after he saw the *"60 Minutes"* report, he wanted to play the savant. He did, of course. *"Rainman"* made autistic savant household terms, and did more for public education about savant syndrome and autism than all the other things that had ever been done.

There were some major changes for the script, but I must say the story was inspired by {savant} Kim Peek. Barry Morrow had met Peek just by chance at a convention, and he was so startled by Kim's memory of zip codes and phone books and that he wrote this script for *"Rainman."*

In the original script, there were some scenes that were sort of embellished. Those kinds of things got changed. The other major thing is that Kim Peek is not an autistic savant. He has some autistic features. There was a conscious decision made to portray an autistic person because there had never been portrayal of autism on the screen, and so that was a major change in the script.

"Rainman" is not the story of Kim Peek. He inspired the movie, but it's not his story. It is a composite of a number of savant skills in the character of Raymond Babbitt. But all the skills that you see are based on real people. The toothpick scene is real. There have been cases of that instantaneous, eidetic imagery, and the ability to immediately count how many items are on the floor, almost before they get there. Computing square roots, but not being able to tell the difference between the cost of a candy bar and a sports car, is a very real phenomenon.

The movie is really about two conditions. One is autism, and the other is savant syndrome, which is grafted on to the autism. The spectacular abilities—memorizing the phone book, the toothpick scene and others—those are part of savant syndrome. But, "Judge Wapner— I got to see Judge Wapner" at an exact time—those are parts of autism. The point is that not all autistic people are savants and not all savants are autistic.

Dustin Hoffman did a marvelous job of portraying autism and savant syndrome. He spent some time with autistic people. Savant syndrome is a condition in which people with autism, or some other developmental disability or central nervous system disorder, have some island of genius that stands in contrast to their overall handicap. But it can be autism. It also can be just more generalized brain damage, or it can be, we're learning, Alzheimer's or certain other forms of dementia. For example, people can develop skills, unearth skills that were not evident before, which is the so-called acquired savant, which itself is a fascinating area because it talks about what I call the little "Rainman" within us all. And the trick is how to tap that without having a stroke or some other kind of catastrophe.

But {musical savant} Leslie Lemke is not autistic. He has some autistic mannerisms, but his basic difficulty is some central nervous system defect that he was born with, closer to mental retardation than autism.

Kim Peek has some unique brain architecture. For example, he has no corpus callosum, which is the huge structure that connects the two hemispheres. That may account for some of his abilities. He has some autistic mannerisms too, but he is not autistic. Now, he has a lot of motor impairments. For example, he can't button his shirt or tie his shoes or brush his teeth, and he thinks very concretely, although that's changing.

If you ask him anything you want to know about the history of Beethoven, Mozart and Rachmaninoff, he will tell you when they were born, when they died, pieces they composed, when they composed them, when the piece was first performed, when it was last performed and what present TV commercials draw from those particular pieces of music.

On the other hand, if you ask him, "What is happiness?" or, "What is love?"—the abstract kind of things, he'll say, "I don't get into that." He will do some math, but he's not a lightening calculator. His memory is the most massive memory I've encountered or have even seen described in the literature. There are a couple of cases in the past, but Kim is really unique, and we're spending a lot of time now trying to do some specialized imaging on him. Not so much architecture, but functional imaging to see what might be happening there to explain those incredible gifts he has.

As it turns out, Alonzo Clemens was also one of the savants on the "60 Minutes" program; he is a marvelous sculptor. He was having his premier showing of his work in Denver, Colorado in 1986. One of the galleries wrote to me and asked me if I would come out for that because they wanted to give the proceeds to some charity. They wondered if I knew of any such savant charity. I didn't, so we created the Savant Syndrome Fund, which started modestly with that contribution. We set up a clearinghouse for information about savant syndrome, so that teachers, students, parents, families and therapists could request information. I wrote some things that could be sent out.

Well, that was going along fine, and then came along the Internet. We started the website.* And of course that is just a natural place to disseminate information. That website was getting about a thousand hits a day. Then it was announced that Kim Peek and NASA were going to work together, and I think we had 17,000 hits that day because people are just intrigued by that story.

The website is where I spend a lot of time now. We're in the process of enhancing it with some streaming video, because I can describe Leslie, but there's nothing like seeing a minute or two of him working. Video is just a natural for savants.

We're doing that, and we also want to really make the clearinghouse more visible and more available, because I get requests every day from families, teachers, and others. Teachers, in particular, ask, "Do you have clips or anything that we can look at that I can use to demonstrate to my class

* See the links section of www.whitecoatwisdom.com for Dr. Treffert's savant syndrome site.

what savant syndrome is?" I have a little editing suite downstairs, and I crank those things out.

Did you feel comfortable with the national attention after 60 Minutes?

I was, but only because there wasn't anybody else who knew more about it than I did. That's not a boastful statement. It wasn't anything that anybody really paid much attention to, so I knew as much about it as anyone only because I paid some attention to it and culled the literature. I was simply sharing my own observations and conclusions about it.

By that time, I had spent my year and a half writing the book {*"Extraordinary People"*} and reviewing everything that had been written about savant syndrome. I could do that because there wasn't that much. I've got a couple file drawers full of papers, and some books. But I think at that time there were no books on savant syndrome.

It always had the "Gee whiz, look at that," kind of quality—and then we'd go back to our more mundane things. You can't stop at gee whiz. Then, we go on to the rest of our studies of the central nervous system. Until we can explain savant syndrome, we can't explain the central nervous system. We can't just leave it as an outlier out there. There has to be an explanation. It can't just mysteriously happen.

It provides a unique window into the brain. The fact is that everything we know about health, we've learned from the study of disease. Everything we know about how to stay healthy, we learned from studying people who are sick. So, I think we can probably learn a great deal about normal central nervous system function from these situations that are sort of anomalous. Savant syndrome is one, but there are others, as well.

It sort of escaped our attention, because people went back to their microscopes and CAT scans and sort of left it out there, like a UFO floating around, except it's real. It's something that you can't say, well, maybe this happens. That's where I've been sort of tenacious. I can't explain it, but other people will, with the technology that we're developing now. We're coming closer to being able to explain it. The CAT scan and MRI do remarkable jobs. You can see the amygdala[†] and hippocampus[‡] and pick them out. That's remarkable. But it's architecture. The resolution is sharp compared to when I started in psychiatry. We had skull films and that was it. They didn't tell you much, unless it was a fracture of the skull.

The illnesses I deal with, which are major mental illnesses—schizophrenia, depression, and savant syndrome—are not disorders of architecture. They're disorders of function. The parts are all there, but the parts are not all functioning. If your car won't start and you look under the hood, all the parts are there—the battery, the carburetor and everything. But if the carburetor's not mixing fuel and air right, or the timing is off, the car isn't

† The amygdala is the center of emotional or affective behaviors and feelings in the brain.

‡ The hippocampus is the part of brain that plays a role in memory and navigation.

going to start. We keep looking for architecture, but I don't think that's going to provide the answer.

With the PET scan, you can look at the brain at work and see music, for example. Savants all can have right brain skills instead of left brain skills. Art, music, calendar calculating, mental skills, and they all play by ear and have perfect pitch. But if you do a PET scan on a musician who plays by ear, you'll find activity on the right hemisphere. If you do a PET scan on a musician who reads music, you'll find activity on the left hemisphere, so it's not a music center of the brain. It depends on which strategy is being used.

With the savant, we're able to now look at those areas of activity and see how they're functioning. I think we're going to find out, and not just about savant syndrome, but about major mental illness and some of the other conditions that we see, probably even Alzheimer's itself. There are architectural changes in Alzheimer's, but those are changes that are results of Alzheimer's, probably not the cause of it.

We now have a technology called fiber tracking, which is the capacity to actually look at the fibers of the brain as they are connected. It's sort of like taking the top off of your computer and looking at the circuit board. We're going to find out much more from those techniques than anything that we've had so far. And there are people who are now interested in that—neurologists, and neuroradiologists, and ophthalmologists, because of this peculiar association of blindness, musical genius, and mental handicap.

A lot of the savants that I've had a chance to study, at least with CAT scans, and with MRIs and neuropsychological testing, have left hemisphere dysfunction. What appears to happen is that in the savant there is a left hemisphere dysfunction from autism or other brain disorder. There's a lot of good evidence of left hemisphere dysfunction in autism itself, which is part of why there are five males for every female in savant syndrome. But there's a fair amount of evidence of left hemisphere dysfunction in autism and about one out of 10 autistic persons has some savant abilities.

But what happens is that there's left hemisphere dysfunction from disease or developmental disability, whichever it is, depending on the savant, with right hemisphere compensation, because the skills in the savant are right hemisphere—art, music, unconscious calculating, mechanical skills and calendar calculating. These are done in an unconscious, sort of preconscious level, which, by the way, is the same circuitry that geniuses use. We're now beginning to study what is the link between prodigy genius and savant syndrome, other than the handicap.

There's left hemisphere dysfunction, and right hemisphere compensation coupled with damage to the cognitive higher-level memory circuits with compensatory habit memory, which is sort of unconscious memory—memory that is very deep and very narrow. That's what savants have;

this so-called habit or procedural memory. They may not even comprehend what's going in there, but they're able to retrieve it.

Now, I'd always thought that this compensatory process was one which developed because of brain damage, and the right brain compensated for the damage, much as somebody who's blind might become much better at hearing because they're concentrating on a different sense. But it may not be so much compensating as it is that the right hemisphere has been released from the tyranny of the left hemisphere. The left hemisphere is described as the dominant hemisphere. Is that true with each of us?

It's simplistic to talk about the right brain and left brain as if they are two entirely separate systems. There's a ton of cross representation in the central nervous system, but the fact is that the hemispheres do specialize in certain functions.

I had followed this savant thing for so long, and had been finding these left hemisphere defects in some of the savants I was working with, and then I came across neurologist Bruce Miller's work in San Francisco. He had 12 patients with a form of frontal-temporal dementia, which is sometimes confused with Alzheimer's. The end result looks much the same, but it's different. But he came across a series of patients who did not have any prior artistic or musical skills, yet some of these developed at a prodigious level, as dementia proceeded—the so-called acquired savant.

There's a lad out East who got hit in the head with a baseball at 10, and suddenly began to be able to calendar calculate and now remembers the weather every day of his adult life.

There's a woman on the West Coast, who was a fairly well known artist with her right hand. She had a stroke, which paralyzed her on the right side. She had to use her left side, and it changed her style completely. But she's much more skilled and gifted with this left hemisphere. She doesn't recognize the painting that she had done earlier on.

There's a fella in England who had a stroke. He survived the stroke, and had a subarachnoid§ bleed, actually. But after that, he became a poet and a sculptor, though he was somebody who, in his prior lifestyle, before the stroke, had no interest in either of those.

I started thinking more about the reservoir within all of us, because these are people who didn't learn that. It was tapped, either because of the interference with the left hemisphere, or else the release of some of the dominance of the left hemisphere.

There's no single theory that can explain all savants—no over-arching one. Savant syndrome is sort of a spectrum. There's something called splinter skills. These are youngsters who may be autistic. They memorize license plates or vacuum cleaner motor sounds, or whatever. There's a little lad here, who if you take him into a vacuum cleaner store and plug in any vacuum cleaner, he can tell you what year it is and whether the vacuum

§ Subarachnoid refers to bleeding between the membrane and the brain itself.

cleaner is about to go to pieces. That, among autistic youngsters, is probably about one in ten. I've seen a fair number of autistic kids who have these so-called splinter skills.

Then, there's something called the talented savant. These are people who are beyond the splinter skill to honing some particular activity—music or art, particularly, and sometimes math.

And then, there's a group called the prodigious savants. Now, these are people whose skills would be spectacular, even if they're to be seen in a normal person. They're very rare. I used to say there are fewer than 30 living, but now I'm up to 50. There's closer to a hundred, because with the Internet, I'm learning about more cases. I just learned about several in Taiwan that I didn't know about before. And of the prodigious savants, I've probably met 15 of them.

Having known these savants and studied the syndrome for so long, have you become sort of accustomed to learning about things most of us laypeople find inexplicable?

I continue to be astounded by it. I thought I would sort of get used to it, but it continues to boggle my mind as much as it did that first day that I walked on the unit. It's that striking. It is that discordance with what we know, or think we know, about the central nervous system. It doesn't make sense that somebody who has that much disability can still have that much ability. And Leslie—! I still stand in awe of his ability when I hear him play. I am still amazed by that, and by the artwork that Alonzo does.

Part of it is because they are progressing. That's some more good news about savant syndrome. It's more than a frivolous skill for them, because it's their language. It is their way of relating to the world. I have a number of savants who are very skilled artists or musicians, who don't speak a word.

There was a program on Dateline the other night that I was on with a young female pianist. She's blind, and has very little language. But with her music she's communicating. She's talking.

When Alonzo Clemens was in a residential setting for a while, as a teenager, and he was making all these little animals out of clay, they said, "Now Alonzo, we're going to take your clay away because you have to learn how to comb your hair, brush your teeth and tie your shoes. And if you can do that, you can have your clay back. You're not going to make a living making those silly little animals out of clay."

Two weeks later, they came into his room and looked under his bed and there were a whole menagerie of little animals he had sculpted from the tar that he had scraped off the roof—because he had to sculpt.

It's a conduit toward normalization for these people. If we use that, they develop more social skills. They develop more language. They develop more daily living skills. What I continue to be amazed by is the progression.

Like with Leslie, it's astounding that he can listen to a piece of any length and play it back after a single hearing. That literal memory itself, is remarkable. He will do that now in the challenge part of the concert.

So if you say, "Leslie, I want you to listen to this and I want you to play it back," he will dutifully sit there, and will dutifully listen, and then he'll dutifully play it back. But when he gets to the end of it, he gets restless, and then he improvises and does his thing. He improvises because he wants to move beyond mere memorization to improvisation. Then, he moved from improvisation into actually creating.

Leslie has a song called *"Down on the Farm in Arpin."* He loves nature and he did this piece about what it's like for him. And he has another song called the *"Bird Song."* It's the birds that he hears as he whistles and plays and mimics the birds. He moved from repetition to improvisation to creating something.

What, for us, is something which we marvel at, for the savant, is an actual tool. Part of what we're trying to do with savants is take whatever their particular skill is and channel it, and use it. It turns out that some of the math geniuses are terrific computer programmers. Their coding just flies, as they say. They just do it in a way that other people would have to spend a lot of time learning how to do it.

Are these talents therapeutic for them?

Music is important to them—not just for the sake of the music—but to increase their language. With Leslie, for example, he'll now repeat things, but sometimes spontaneously start a conversation.

It's true though, that as some of this improvisation and creativity came on to the scene, some of the literal memory seems to be lost, either because it's not of interest or because there is this more substituting kind of behavior. But that's not a huge trade-off. It's worth it. Instead of just saying, "Hi, I'm Dr. Treffert." He's likely to say something or ask me what I've been doing, or ask me about the weather.

But Mary also has something called, "Can you stump Leslie?" to demonstrate how wide his repertoire is. Some songs are obscure, and Leslie has to dig a little deeper. Some of them he has simply never heard of, nor have I. He'll start playing a beautiful piece of music. Mary doesn't know if that's what it is. The person in the audience is the only one who knows.

She'll say, "Leslie, are you sure?"

"Yeah, that's what it is."

She'll say, "Leslie, are you making it up?"

"Yeah, I'm making it up."

We had Leslie give a concert in the fall of 2003, during Abilities Week, which focuses on abilities, rather than disabilities. He gave a concert. We all like feedback. We all like applause and we all like appreciation. Leslie loves applause. He likes appreciation. That's fine. But there's more to it than that.

We come with certain templates in the brain—there's a music template, a math template, a language template, and there are other templates.

With music and teaching, even in grade school, language really excels at a much higher acquisition than for kids who aren't exposed to music, so there's some real crossover between music and language and math. Some people say music is just unconscious counting anyway, especially piano.

You can use music therapy with people, post-stroke, which is more than just interacting with them and soothing. There is some evidence that it is, in fact, a neural kind of networking that develops from this crossover.

From what I've seen in the musical savants—I get e-mails every day from somebody who tells them about their son or daughter, asking, "Do I have any suggestions?" Whether they have any musical inclination or not, get them a keyboard and let them start. It's amazing how they progress.

I've gone from understanding the savant to the so called acquired savant, to now looking for the little "Rainman" within each of us, which is something we need to pay attention to, and it gets me into an area that's very foreign to me. It's what I call ancestral or genetic memory. It sounds a little UFOish or Eastern, but in trying to explain the savant, we have to explain how people can know things they never learned. The prodigious savant starts with a body of knowledge and information and ability that he never learned—genetic memory, the genetic transmission of knowledge.

In the animal kingdom, we've sort of become used to the fact that the swallows of Capistrano somehow know how to come back on that particular day, and that instinct of how the pigeon can find his way home. In the animal kingdom, it's sometimes some really complicated instincts. Bird sounds, for example. Some bird sounds are extremely complex, and yet as a tiny bird, they haven't learned that from mother. It's there.

This whole idea that we come with these templates, which I call software attached, when we're born, is something I am spending a lot of time thinking about now, because you can't explain the prodigious savant unless you can explain how somebody knows something they never learned, especially the very severely impaired, because they haven't learned music. They haven't learned math—but they know it.

This gets into this whole area of all of us having a lot of software, but we don't have access to it. Well, the question is, if it's all there, how come we don't use it? Well, I've got a computer downstairs that's got all kinds of software on it. But I don't know how to get at it. I don't know how to use it. And if I tried to access it all at once, it would crash, so I just leave it alone and just use those I'm familiar with. But in terms of these more obscure chips I know are there, I don't know how to get at them. I don't know what to do with them after I have access to them.

We have some of that in reserve as a kind of survival back-up. The acquired savant sort of reinforces that idea. That whole area of ancestral memory has put me in touch and corresponding with people who I never thought I'd be corresponding with. We even get out into extra sensory perception, because some of the parents report cases of instances of what is called ESP, in some of these savants. And these are credible parents.

For all these things there could be reasons, there could be explanations, like all ESP kinds of things. The only criticism I've ever gotten about my savant syndrome work has been when I wrote an article in which I reported what parents reported, and I said that some parents report these ESP experiences.

I got a rather scathing letter to the *American Journal of Psychiatry* about my sort of supporting ESP, which has no scientific basis whatsoever. I tried to say, "Look, I'm simply reporting what people say, that's all. I'm not saying it does or doesn't occur."

But this people remembering things they never learned—there are people out there who believe that ESP is an explanation of autism or of the savant. I talk about genetic memory, which is very scientific. It's all embedded on the chip. There's nothing mystical about that.

There are people who believe the air is full of all sorts of information, from centuries ago, on art, music, and all kinds of things, that just as we sit here, this air is full of signals from I don't know what, a thousand FM station and 2000 AM stations and how many television stations? I don't know that unless I have a tuner and I tune into that.

And they're saying, "No doc, it's ancestral memory. It's this huge accumulation of information and these people have the capacity to tune into it. That's what savant syndrome is about. To me, that's a little hard to accept. So that's where the ESP and all the other things come in. These are people who are really interested in it, and are convinced. I don't know. But I'm not into that and I'm not going to get into that, in terms of my inquiry. I'm not saying we're all little Mozarts or Picassos, but the acquired savant sort of convinces me of that.

When I was in practice, I would occasionally use sodium amytal with patients. These people would say I know there is something on the tip of my tongue. I know something happened to me and I know I just can't get at it, but I know it's there. It's making me tense.

Okay, well let's see. We'll do this sodium amytal, and I did a fair number of them. These people would have incredible memory of events that they had no access to when they were awake. Some people say that everything experienced is being recorded. It's just that we only have access to a small amount of it.

Warner Penfield, with his work with brain probes, was looking for the site of epilepsy. The patient is conscious, the dura is laid back, and the brain has no pain neurons itself. But the dura does, so you anesthetize the dura with a local anesthetic and you put the probe down to find out the exact spot that triggers the seizure. Then, that can be excised.

In looking for the spot, he would put the probe down and the patient would, say "Oh my gosh, that's my fifth birthday and there's Aunt Mildred and Uncle Harry," and wherever the probe went would come this remarkable memory. All that tells me is that there's a great deal more storage in each of us than we have access to, and the place that that is probably most easily found is in our dreams because one may have a dream, and you wonder, "Where in the world did that come from?"

I'm not talking about a nightmare or something, really some kind of psychoanalytic insight. I'm just talking about waking up and saying, "My God, I haven't thought about that in years!" I simply extrapolate from that to say there's much more capacity there than we have, and maybe it's a survival mechanism.

What are the practical implications of this? There's a book called "*A New Drawing on the Right Side of the Brain*," by Betty Edwards. What she does is take people like me, who can't draw anything—can't even draw a straight line—and spends a week or so with them teaching them how to draw. She says learning how to draw is no different than learning a foreign language or learning music. There is a way to go about it. You're accessing a different part of your brain than you typically use. With drawing, it happens to be the right side of the brain, and so she has these seminars where she will take people and teach them how to draw.

Okay, so you learn how to draw. But what she does is she takes executives, for example, from companies and will work with them for a week, teaching them how to draw. The thing is there are certain skills and some articles on where the ah-ha! experience is a right brain experience and that's been demonstrated in other kinds of things, including vision, in the sense of seeing the big picture.

Up until the last few decades, we looked for executives who manage, management by objective sort of thing, bean counters, and being able to see the bottom line. We're looking for a different thing now. We're looking for people with vision; the kind of guys who can see the bigger picture. That's a right brain skill.

We're a left-brain society, and it's served us well. I'm not knocking the left-brain. It's a great hemisphere, and it served me well. It got me through "*Grey's Anatomy*" and through medical school and my boards—God bless the left hemisphere. But I think that it's spent to some extent at the expense of right hemisphere stuff, so we tend to say, yeah, we need music and art. Those are for the gifted and talented kids, but we've minimized creativity. We've minimized the vision thing, particularly in seeing the bigger picture, being able to be a problem solver. There are people who can walk into an organization and problem-solve. We've tended to see that as soft and fuzzy thing. You can't make any money doing that.

We've changed our thinking and there is some migratingness, what I call rummaging around the right hemisphere a little bit more. There's some work being done at the University of Wisconsin, working on the monks and their meditation, trying to see how their brain waves differ from the brain waves of those of us who don't spend much time meditating. There is a difference, and there is something to be said. I'm not selling meditation here, but I think the idea of changing the focus and getting out of our standard routine kind of thinking is good, and sometimes one is kind of startled at what you find.

A lot of people, after they retire, are kind of amazed at some interest that has developed or some capacity. It's more than they just have time on their hands. It allows them to shift out of the left hemisphere into this more curious kind of thing and they're startled to find a whole new area of interest or capability.

Part of understanding Savant Syndrome better is getting us to understand these various compartments that we have and getting them to integrate better. It will provide some better insights into memory, as well, and into connectivity between hemispheres.

Kim Peek can read a page in eight seconds and then have it on his hard disc. He's memorized 9,000 books and can pull those back, page by page. He says that he reads one page with one eye and one page with the other. I'm not sure. We're going to test that to see, but that may, in fact, be the case because he has this incredible ability to read at incredible speed.

If we can learn something about that memory circuitry, and what that means about the connectivity between the hemispheres, that might give us some insight into normal memory. It provides kind of a unique window to the brain, and there are people who have much more technology available, or many more resources than I have, who are picking up on this now.

When I did the *"60 Minutes"* program, I was asked, "Will we ever understand this?"

I said something that is still true. "I think we'll better understand, but there may be an inherent inability of the brain to understand itself. The brain can understand the kidney and the liver and the hand, but I'm not so sure it can transcend itself to explain itself."

There's going to be a lot of mystery still because I'm not sure the brain can figure itself out. Maybe it can. But I think we'll need to learn a lot more about it. It's such a marvelous instrument.

We tend to think of ourselves, when we're born, as having this beautiful piece of equipment, with a blank disc, and what we become is on the disc. But I've come to believe that we start with a lot more on that disc than we ever imagined. And that speaks to potential. That speaks to possibilities and tapping into that, and there we can make some real strides.

Have any of these revelations regarding brain development affected your personal interests?

I've come to respect a little bit more my ability to see the bigger picture in a lot of things. I've always thought of myself as sort of a troubleshooter, in terms of walking into situations that needed to be solved, and being challenged by that and being pretty good at that.

I've probably worked more not at painting, not at art, but in expanding my own boundaries of inquiry, even within this area. For me to dabble around with ESP in any sense, before, would have been out of the question. Or, for me to think about, is the mind bigger than the brain? I would have said, well, it's an interesting question, but I've got work to do. Now, I find myself treading into some of these areas.

If I have any of the savant skills—not in art, music or math... Thank goodness, one of my professors gave me a D instead of an F in algebra. Algebra class—everybody else always got it. I never got it. I always ran up, guessing answers, so that disqualifies me in three savant areas. So what's left? Well, mechanical skills. I do think I have some ability there. Actually, that comes from my dad. He was a great problem solver, mechanically. People where he worked said, "Something about Wally. He ran the tool shop. He's the only guy in that whole organization that if you wanted a tool, he didn't have to go look up the number." He had these numbers, thousands of tools, in his head. He had this huge inventory.

I prided myself, if something wasn't working, in being able to get it working, or find even sort of a wired together solution from parts down in the basement. In that mechanical area, I have some abilities.

The other, I guess, way that it's affected me personally, is that there's more to savant syndrome than neurons and synapses. There are these families; the fathers and mothers and siblings who are so proud of their kid. "Yeah, he's got disabilities, but have you seen this or that or whatever?" The power of that kind of belief and determination, and prayer, is to bring about these changes. I've learned as much about the human spirit as I have about the brain in this whole odyssey, because I've run into these fantastic people who are dealing with these youngsters all the time. I try to balance that and not just get hung up on the synapses and neurons. May Lemke and Mary Parker take care of Leslie, and they had a huge part in that equation.

But I'm still involved and still do some forensic psychiatry. I spend a lot of time now on the savant syndrome, but I have another life, which is another whole area, which is called mellowing. I still do a lot of writing and public speaking in that area, which has nothing to do with savant syndrome. Mellowing is an outgrowth of my work at Winnebago, and in prevention in the mental health area, which is something I call lessons from listening—40 years of listening. From that, I was starting something called "A Sane Asylum." That's where the "worried well" would go before they got worried sick.

Listening to people and their predicaments, aside from the savants, there are some real lessons to be learned. Psychiatry is a very interesting occupation. It's just rich with experiences, and causes you to look at your own priorities and getting people to sort out what I call the urgent things from the important things. It may seem like an obvious message, but it isn't.

Give me an example.

Two lessons stand out. One was a suicide note—not a patient of mine, but it was from a little girl. She was a straight A student in school and she got a B on her report card for the very first time on the last day of her 14th year of life. On her 15th year of life or birthday, she hung herself because she got a B on her report card. She left a little note that said, "Mom or dad, I never said anything to you about having to get good grades, in fact, we rarely talk about it. But I know that you do not want or could not tolerate a failure. And if I fail at what I do, I fail at what I am. Goodbye."

She had no sense of anything between what one is and what one does. So the first lesson in mellowing is that there is more to me than what I do, or what my kids do. I see that in grown ups. I see that in doctors—who are impaired physicians who are so busy doing and have their whole being tied up in what they do. When things don't go so well, there's nothing in the bank to draw on.

I learned three things that sort of stick with me from medical school. One is that the first step in treatment is to make a diagnosis. And that's true. So often we jump in before we make a diagnosis. The second is, listen to the patient, because he's giving you the diagnosis. Before you run to the lab with PET scans and all this MRI stuff, listen to the patient, if you haven't listened the first time.

I had a patient in my training who still leaves an impact on me because he was hard of hearing. He couldn't hear, and nobody could understand why he couldn't. He went through a $10,000 work–up, and since they couldn't find anything, they put him in psychiatry. It must be in his head that he can't hear, because all the parts are there and everything is working. And so I sat down with him and obviously, he couldn't hear me, so I had to write.

I wrote, "How come you can't hear?"

He said, "Because I don't have any ears."

He had selectively hallucinated away his ears. But nobody asked him why he couldn't hear. That changed the course of what was wrong with him.

I remember another patient who came in who was on psychiatry, who had come in because she was quite depressed. And in those days I did a very careful neurologic examination—and we probably don't do those much anymore. But I systematically went through each of the cranial nerves, asking questions and so forth. And I asked her, "Have you noticed any difference in smell?"

And she said, "Yeah. Funny thing you should ask."

I said, "What?"

"Well, this weekend we were going up North and we put the motor in the trunk. The gasoline fell out and it was in the trunk, and I could see it there, but I couldn't smell it. It occurred to me so strange that I couldn't smell that gasoline."

She had a midline meningioma. It was a midline brain tumor, which selectively affected the olfactory nerves, and so she couldn't smell. We removed it and her depression cleared up. One thing that we really need to resurrect in the profession is listening to the patient. We don't have time. We have all sorts of gadgets that distract us. They're remarkable and I'm not knocking them. But that's what I hear. The doctor doesn't take the time to listen.

Sometimes people will say, "Don't you miss your patients?" Yeah, I do miss my patients, and I think some of them miss me. But it's time to make that transition because of the sort of on-call responsibility. After 37 or 40 years, it's nice not to… If you went on vacation, you had to spend a lot of time getting ready to go and a lot of time catching up when you got back. I don't miss having to do either of those right now. So to me, that on-call thing has been a little bit of a parole.

There were three of us—three psychiatrists for probably 20 years. The hospital bought our practice, about three or four years ago. And that was a good time for me to step back from day-to-day practice.

We made rounds on our own patients. We didn't turn somebody over on the weekend. So if you're in town seven days a week, you go to the hospital seven days a week. I'm not complaining. That was a choice. I liked it. And I continued to do it. But that's the way we practiced. That also means that if you go out of town, you're sort of leaving your patients with people who don't know anything about them. In psychiatry, that's hard. It's hard in all specialties, but in psychiatry, that might be a little more difficult than others.

The thing is, now I have more time than I did before, which is nice because I don't have the day-to-day patient responsibility. I want to get the fresh new explorers going, and I hope that, at some point, there will be some sort of a Savant Institute. I'm working on that too, because I get a lot of inquiries from people who would like to have somebody seen or evaluated. There's plenty of that still to do, so I'm still going to keep doing what I'm doing. It's the old story. I'm as busy now as I ever was. They are things that I like to do and don't have to do, so I consider myself fortunate.

I don't look upon it as work. It's challenging and invigorating. It's good for the central nervous system anyway, keeping those synapses firing. Some people do it with a lot of reading and crosswords or whatever. I'm much more involved in doing it this way, in terms of the interaction with people who are interested in the things that we're doing.

Warner Penfield[¶]—he struggled with the question his whole career as

¶ Canadian neurologist

to whether the mind was bigger than the brain. He spent his whole life looking at the brain, and he wondered, is there more to us? Is there more to the mind than the brain? And we're talking about spirits and about all kinds of things that are not under the microscope. And interestingly, at the end of his career, he decided there was more to the mind than the brain. But at the end of his career, he said that he had gone as far as he could with his limitations, mind and age. What he was looking for were some fresh new explorers. And that's where I am.

I give lectures to high school students and college kids, and at the end of those, I'll get some remarks. They're always well received. It's a fascinating topic, and the video clips are riveting. I got a very nice write-up, here in Fond du Lac, of some kids who said that maybe that's an area they might want to go into—and so the fresh, new explorers. That's really the objective of the website and the objective of this whole savant thing, is to get other people interested to carry that on. That's happening.

CHAPTER THIRTY-THREE

PRACTICING MEDICINE… AND A FOREIGN LANGUAGE

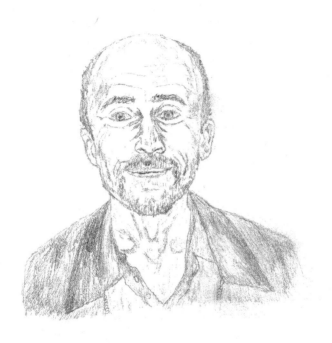

"Petra, we have to do something about Misha's English."

Miroslav "Misha" Backonja, MD
Neurology, Madison

I landed the biggest story of my journalism career, thanks to a Madison neurologist. But he was neither the source for the story, nor the remarkable patient's doctor. Nevertheless, without Dr. Miroslav Backonja {BAHTCH-cawn-yah}, I never would have gotten to tell the world about a man who, on several occasions, temporarily awoke from a vegetative-like state after nine years.

We hadn't talked since that story went national and international in 1990, but Backonja, now in his early 50s, remembered me. And like in the old days when he readily helped me with a variety of news stories, he quickly agreed to contribute to this book, as he has quite a story of his own to tell.

Foreign-trained physicians like him pursue one of the most challenging

*and demanding professions one could imagine, and then begin practicing it
in a language they don't speak fluently!*

*In his free time, Dr. Backonja enjoys biking and running, despite the
pinched nerves in his foot. But pain is something this guy knows well, and
communicating that knowledge to others is a big part of what he does.*

*On his cluttered bulletin board is an Albert Einstein quote: "Everything
should be as simple as possible, but not one bit simpler."*

*"Being an educator, one of the tasks I have to do is to make things simple
for people to understand," explains Backonja. "But then on the other hand,
you can't make it so simple that it loses the meaning. A lot of times it's very
difficult because the nervous system and neurological disorders are very complex, and they're dynamic."*

*He walks that line every day, which is further complicated by the fact he
is not a native English speaker.*

I was born in Banja Luka, which is now Bosnia. I did not know English.
When I came here, I totally got immersed in English because I had to
take the ECFMG* exam. I had to study in parallel, English as well as medicine. The test was 90% medicine and we had only one hour for English. I
passed the medicine part, no problem, but I flunked the English part.

I had to study an additional six months for English as a second language course. It's just one of those things. If you want to swim, you get
in the water. You swallow a lot of water. When I started to speak English,
I spoke with a strong South-Slavic accent. My chairman at that time, Dr.
Henry Schutta, native of Poland, himself had to learn English. He was a
great scholar. He and his wife became good friends of my wife. He would
host the departmental Christmas parties at his house and he would always
take my wife on the side and talk to my wife in confidence.

"Petra, we have to do something about Misha's English."

I ended up taking a course. It was in reality speech therapy. I took four
months of training to pronounce sounds that I did not grow up with—all
the "ahs," "oos" and "thes."

For a couple of more Christmases, he said, "Misha still needs to learn
English." And then my last year, he didn't bring her to the side. And I
asked her, "What did Dr. Schutta say?"

"He didn't say anything."

"Phew. I must have passed." {laughs}

Coming to the University of Wisconsin, it was much less of a surprise
to hear a person with an accent. I didn't think it was ever a problem. Even
if I do not speak well, at least I listen well. I always was certain that with

* Educational Commission for Foreign Medical Graduates.

patients it wasn't a problem, and if so, I repeated myself, or rephrased whatever I needed to say. I find that talking to patients is 90% of my job. It's patients' education, especially when it comes to pain management, having patients understand the problem.

Sometimes, it's like talking to a kid. Unfortunately, even a lot of children have pain problems, from people who have very little education, all the way to talking to the professors and colleagues. Being able to communicate with all of them is the essence.

A lot of my colleagues say your patients have to convince you that they have pain with a lot of pain behavior. But what I learned quickly in pain management is most patients do not accept the fact that they are having problems. They just ignore it. It's denial.

A young man in his 30s was referred by another pain doctor. I opened the door to the exam room and you could just feel his anger. I looked at his records and talked to him and everything was clear. He had an injury, after that, a surgery, and it got worse. He overused his other arm and gets problems with the other arm. He gets surgery on the other arm—it gets worse. He gets all the appropriate treatments and so he was trying to go back to work, light duty and couldn't do it. The next exam with the other doctor said that his condition was nerve pain related to injury; terrible pain.

I sit down, and after I was done, I had to tell him what I think it is and what needs to be done. He was pacing and he allowed me to examine him. He sat down, stood up, sat down. I was thinking, I am going to tell him what I need to tell him. I mean, he is disabled. He is somebody who, like had an amputation at the elbows, and then I thought this guy is just going to blow up.

I said, "Well, you have injury to your arms and you have this pain, pretty much like someone who has amputation. You have hands, but you can't use them."

He stood up, cussed, and then, phew. Big sigh of relief.

He says, "Well, thank you. You're the first person who told me what's going on." The problem was his doctors wanted a cure. They wanted to help him. But nobody realized that after a certain point, you have to call a spade a spade and pronounce what it is. You can't let him say, "Well, you don't have it."

You have to tell him, "No, you do have it. But there are things you have to do to make it better, to keep a quality of life and function."

I told him he could make some use of his arms, and here's what he needed to do. But he never realized what the problem is and he was not working in a productive way. He was fighting it.

It turns out that most of the time I have to convince the patient that there's a problem. Only when they accept that they have a problem are they able to engage and do what they need to do to treat it and manage it—the same thing for many other neurological problems. So, in a way, I find that being able to talk to patients in a way that they are able to understand it, is very important.

How difficult was that, considering you aren't a native English speaker?

I took a couple of night courses of English during medical school. I took a course in French and Arabic, too. Medical school has a lot of kind of dragons to slay. You start taking exams, and throughout your career you keep taking exams because it's a powerful field that is evolving so fast. There's so much to learn.

What did your parents think of your interest in medicine?

My mother was proud I was able to enter medical school. And my father, my impression was that he probably was expecting me to go into the profession. My parents went through World War II because of one of the battlegrounds in Europe was former Yugoslavia. And my father was in the military, but then after the war was in commerce. My mother was a grade school teacher. They came from villages in the mountains of Bosnia.

The University of Zagreb is a very old university, going back probably 400 years. But one difference as compared to here, at least when I was going to medical school 25 years ago, was that our exams did not only include written, but also included oral exams. That was nerve-wracking because it was a lot of times being examined by professors of the old school. We're talking about being trained in Austria-Hungaria, people at the turn of the century, who had very interesting ideas of authority. They were the ultimate arbiters of knowledge.

It was well known that one of the professors would say, "God knows how to get a grade 5. I know everything that could be rated as 4, and you cannot get more than 3 on a zero to five grading scale." Even if you cram fast and know everything, the best you can do is C {laughs}, so you can imagine what that does to any enthusiasm.

I have an uncle and an aunt. Both of them are physicians. If anybody had any influence on my decision to pursue a medical career, it was my aunt. She was a very imaginative person, very inquisitive. Some of the first ways of thinking, as I was growing up, were actually, under her influence. She liked to spend time with us children, so she would read us books and tell us stories when we were younger. And then, as I grew up, we kept a real good relationship. As I was learning things in high school, I was talking to her about scientific issues, and she was always fostering my inquisitiveness. I guess that was clearly a positive feedback that led me to be interested in science, medical science, in particular.

Another person who was a great influence was my art history teacher in high school. She really instilled a lot of curiosity about the humanities. She trained me to put things in perspective, like nothing happens in isolation. Art only happens in the context of history. There are things that happen before and things that will follow. It's like biology in many regards, but just a different dimension.

I was interested in science during grade school, so my high school actually was already science-oriented. {Former} Yugoslavia had a school system that's very influenced by the German system of so-called Gymnasium, which was the general high school education, preparing the person for college, while other high schools were bent more to the trades.

Medical school starts right after high school, but lasts six years, so it's different from the American system. You're still green under your ears coming out of high school, so it was a big immersion into the pre-clinical sciences.

Banja Luka, where I went to high school, was probably three quarters the size of Madison, which for the Balkans is relatively big. But then I went to the big city of Zagreb to medical school, which had a million people. It was a way to grow socially and personally.

I have uncles who live in Milwaukee, and I visited them during my medical school, so I had the opportunity to kind of get exposure to people who were educated here. The educational opportunities here really had a lot of appeal to me, so I was contemplating to come and do specialty training here. I had a couple of colleagues who went out of the country to specialize, so I was already thinking in those terms.

But then, when I was visiting my uncles, I met this young woman from Milwaukee, and we corresponded. Then, the question of coming to here became much more certain, because we got married. It turned out that her parents were also friends of my uncles. I finished medical school in Zagreb and then, as soon as I was done, I came here to the United States.

As a foreign graduate, I had to slay another dragon before I could do my residency. At that time, it was not only that you had to take your equivalency exam, there was a list of 70 countries at medical schools that would not be recognized, unless you go through "like a fifth year." So it was like an externship, as opposed to an internship. I had to find a place to do that because not every American medical school or residency programs or hospital was offering that. It was a bit of homework to find a place that would do that program. It took me two years after I came here to do all those exams.

I did my externship and internship in Omaha, where there was much less exposure to people from foreign countries. I did that year in family practice and it didn't really have a lot of appeal for me. During my first year of internship in family practice, I realized that neurology, as a specialty, had more appeal to me, and so I decided, halfway through, to change from family practice into neurology.

There was a bit of fascination about the complexity of the nervous system on one hand. On the other hand, I had another person that was very inspiring—a physiology professor from Zagreb. He was very flamboyant, but a very good scientist and a good teacher.

He said, "Everything you guys need for the exam is in the book, but I'm not going to talk to you about that. I'm going to tell you what really matters about neuroscience." It was a tour de force. He used a lot of analogies to explain some of the complexities to us. He was using an innovative mathematical model to explain how a nervous system works, and it was so enthralling, so that was sort of cooking in me.

But the unfortunate part that happened over there was the war in the early 1990s. I couldn't believe it, because I was there a year before war broke out, and I really didn't see any hint that it was going to happen. Looking in retrospect, it was incredible how little it took for people who lived together to become {pauses}—I'm still struggling for the past 10, 15 years when this war started, how to describe it. But I think one word comes back—being so stupid. After seeing other parts of the world, such as Rwanda, and other places where people live together and just turn on each other, it's clear that no one holds the license on being stupid. It can happen at any time and any place.

The problem turned out to be first political, and then ethnic, then religious. Things just blew up. My brother's married to a Croatian. My first cousin's married to a Muslim. My best friends were—I didn't care—they were Croats and Slovenians. For people to turn around and start shooting each other . . . I stayed in contact with some of my friends throughout the war. Some of them had no option, and were dragged into the war. It was hard for me from a distance. It's ironic that the country fell apart because people couldn't live together.

My medical school had a number of people from Arab countries, so I had a number of friends who were Arabs. The best man at my wedding was Lebanese. Unfortunately, I lost contact with him after the war in Lebanon broke out. A couple of my colleagues and a couple of my relatives died in the conflict, so that definitely sealed any idea of going back.

So you established your practice here. Tell me about the early years of your neurology practice.

When I started my internship, we had a couple patients who were very complex and had difficult neurological problems. One was a young woman who had a disorder called Guillain-Barre Syndrome.[†] Her presentation was almost like a textbook. Usually patients have a viral illness, and then develop symptoms which were neurological. She had numbness and tingling in her hands and came to the emergency room. The emergency room doctors told her she was hyperventilating.

---

† Guillain-Barré {ghee-yan bah-ray} syndrome is a disorder in which the body's immune system attacks part of the peripheral nervous system.

"Breathe in a bag and go home." So she was back a day later, saying my hands and feet are tingling even more.

And they say, "You're still having anxiety attacks. Here's a bag."

The third time, before she went to the emergency room, she called her primary care doctor. Then, they called us. My senior resident was smart enough to realize there was more to it, so we did the appropriate test, which was a spinal tap. That showed she indeed had a positive test.

Fortunately, for her to come in so early—ultimately, to come into a hospital—so she ended up on a respirator that night because she progressed so fast. After six weeks, she recovered almost completely. It's one of the neurological emergencies, because if you miss something like this and send a patient home, it can literally, in a matter of hours, progress to the point where you're losing the ability to breathe, and die. That was pretty dramatic, and a lesson to be learned.

Now, with modern treatments, you can prevent people from going on a respirator, saving them the trouble and extreme illness. Then, the patients can recover much faster, just seeing how colleagues in neurology just sailed through to making a diagnosis and a treatment plan.

I learned quickly that the University of Wisconsin Medical School offered a lot. But the first year with all the call on neurosurgery was pretty intense. As part of neurology training, we do a rotation on neurosurgery and I did my first rotation in the middle of summer, where you have a lot of accidents and neurosurgical consultations.

I had another person who was really an important influence. He was a neurosurgery chief resident. It was really fun working with him. He was very calm for a neurosurgeon. There's always action, yet he was always composed. One thing that amazed me was that he had stamina. We would be on call all night long and he would come in the morning, do rounds and operate. I would just crash.

My primary area is neurology, which is non-surgical. But during the neurosurgery rotation, you can see the brain in front of you. You forget that. Blood is just a substance you have to wipe off, and the brain is a thing you have to understand and fix the things you need to fix.

All the emotional stuff that comes with blood and guts just falls to the side. You know that blood is there. You have to figure out where it's coming from and how to stop it—the same thing with a patient who's having a seizure. It's very dramatic, having a stroke or things like that—the other neurological problems. What goes through your mind is, What do I need to do to help this person here and now? At the end of the day, you definitely do feel what you go through. We're still people, after all. When you get home, a lot of times, you just crash.

One thing that's interesting about neurology, it follows a set of rules. Neurological emergences, one example being stroke, if one follows and recognizes a certain set of principles, all of those neurological emergencies can be identified quite quickly by primary care. And it is incredible, looking back over the past 20 years since I've been doing neurology, how much the science has advanced. When I was studying in neurological sciences, we had only a limited number of treatment options.

For example, you would treat Parkinson's disease with a medication called L-dopa. Most other neurological conditions were not treatable. There was an old saying, which has plagued neurology for some time. It was, "Diagnose and adios." We didn't have many things to offer to our patients, and it's really incredible to witness the revolution in medicine. The biggest revolution, probably next to oncology, is neurology—neurosciences.

Now stroke has become a neurological emergency. It's a brain attack. There are probably multiple testimonies in the lay press, as well as medical press, that patients who have a catastrophic stroke can literally walk away with very little neurological problem at all, if any. In most of the cases, there are new medications that can treat many of the conditions better. For example, with epilepsy, you have a much wider choice of medications—safer, better tolerated.

I ended up sub-specializing in the field of pain management. That probably didn't exist until 10 years ago. It's obvious that chronic pain, in particular, is a neurological problem, and so a lot of treatments we use in treatment of chronic pain are neurology-based. So it's a privilege to be a witness, and, in some ways, a participant in developments in the field.

My initial experience in family practice, of treating the patient as a whole, has really turned around and come back to help me. I loved the family medicine experience of being able to treat people from delivering babies, which I was doing left and right, all the way to taking care of people at the end of their life-cycle in old age. The basic skill of treating a patient as a whole person, which is the premise of family practice; has really made me a better physician.

My primary area of specialty is what's called neuropathic pain, which is pain which comes from nerve damage. So probably a better example of that is pain after shingles. I treat patients with pain problems, from low back pain to belly-aches to headaches, including migraines, including some of the very unusual pain disorders.

I am taking care of a woman who has congenital insensitivity to pain. She was born with a condition without small nerve fibers. In addition to not being able to perceive pain, she also does not have other small nerve fibers that control function of many organs—including the gut, sweat, and things like that. She could not perceive pain and she would injure herself constantly. But what she has is some very annoying tingling sensations that is call paresthesia—don't feel pain on any part of the body, no sensation at all. She would actually scratch herself, and because she didn't feel any pain, she would scratch herself raw. She cuts herself many times and burns herself, and she didn't feel pain.

Pain has very important biological function. Example, for this woman or people who have leprosy—there's actually infection that infects the nerves and kills the nerves that give pain. You've probably seen pictures of lepers, because they're all mutilated. It's actually self-mutilation. They burn themselves. They cut themselves. They break their bones. They walk on their broken bones because they don't feel pain, so pain protects the body.

In an acute setting, pain has a protective function. But what's interesting is that's not what we have a problem with in the clinical setting. What we have a problem with is the chronic pain, where pain is not serving its primary, biological function. What we end up with is a disordered system, where a system that is supposed to protect us now becomes a source of a problem. It failed to reset itself to go back to its normal function, and be activated only when there's an injury signal.

We're now learning that, in this case, nerves that are activated continue behaving as they are being activated. In most circumstances, if you're not touching your peripheral nerve endings, they're totally quiet. Unless you touch it, all the nerves, let's say in my hand, this is all quiet. As soon as I stop, it goes to sleep.

What happens in patients with nerve injury pain is one of the most dramatic examples. Those nerves keep firing because they're being activated continuously. So we can now understand—what was a puzzle for a long time—why would you hurt when the wound is healed? What's the problem? We're learning now that these nerves, and not only the peripheral nerves, but also parts of the central nervous system—the spinal cord pathways and areas of brain that are supposed to turn off after injury signals from periphery—haven't stopped. But they continue to go on.

One area I started recently to do is looking at the interaction between the immune system and the nervous system. It turns out that probably part of the answer is in the interaction between the two because, ultimately, what guides the repair is the immune system.

We find evidence now that not only the peripheral, but also in the spinal fluid, that so called pro-inflammatory cytokines, are turned on. They keep propagating inflammation while anti-inflammatory cytokines, which are supposed to turn off inflammation, are decreased. There's this imbalance which keeps pushing the inflammation. That's probably one of the explanations. We have to figure out what it means and how it works.

In the case of migraine, there's no injury to the nerves. But we're learning that some of the similarities of the nervous system being turned on without turning off when it's supposed to turn off. In migraines, it shouldn't be turning on at all.

Is it hard to assess what level of pain patients are suffering?

We are using, as a hard scientific fact, just what patients feel. A lot of times it goes against the grain that a subjective thing being considered objective. But it's the only thing we can go on. It turns out it is objective. It's as objective as a blood test or chest x-ray. If you ask very specific questions, you get answers that are as good as a blood test or an x-ray. And it's a pattern we rely on. If you look at the x-ray—if you're a physician, everything's a pattern. Usually, there's not a single piece of information—it's a pattern of information that you get. It's actually one big story of neurology—everything in neurology is a pattern, so I guess one of my talents is pattern recognition. {laughs}

In addition to things as simple as talking to patients and getting their reports of sensations, their ability to describe and rate their sensations, we also use other tools such as MRI, where you can look at the brain activity. Actually, doing MRI alone doesn't tell you anything, unless you match it with what the patient is telling you. It gives credence and credibility to both.

Ultimately, everything is in the brain. Patients say, "You think it's in my head." It's not that I think—I know it's in your head. If it's not in your head, you don't have a pain. Like every other experience, for you to know that you're talking to me has to be in your head. But it's different the way I think about it being in a patient's head, as opposed to what they're thinking. They're afraid I'm thinking they're imagining. In addition, empathy, in some regards, makes the pain doctor.

Another young woman had very severe pain. She taught me what patients who have severe pain have to go through. She was playing soccer and got a sprained ankle. For most people, you put ice on and stay off it for a few days, and go your merry way.

But she ended up developing a condition called RSD {what was called reflex sympathetic dystrophy}, and it became so severe to the point that she ended up being hospitalized. Then, she began having severe reactions to medications. So instead of getting benefits, she started getting complications from her medications and treatments.

She was an A student and starred in soccer. She had a lot of friends. Teenager. I mean, the world was just opening to her. Now, she ended up spending a lot of time in the hospital and being bed-bound. She responded dramatically and she was someone who had pain 24 hours a day. I saw her like a couple of weeks later in follow up after a successful pain treatment and I thought she'll just be thrilled and run out and do whatever she did before. She was totally frightened.

I ask her, "What's wrong with you?"

She said, "I'm scared."

I said, "What are you scared about? I thought you were scared when you had pain. Your pain is down. When you have so little pain you can step on your foot. You've gone through rehabilitation."

"Well, I'm scared of the world. What do I do now?"

Then, I realized that she built a wall around herself to just go through the day with such severe pain. She had to walk in such a way that she wouldn't step on her foot. Even if she would get excited, that could make her pain worse. For something like a year and a half, she was living in a shell, and pretty much the rest of the world just became non-existent.

She forgot what being a young person means—kicking a ball, running around, having parties. None of that existed for her. Now, after the pain subsided, it's becoming an opportunity for her to do again and she doesn't know what to do. It demonstrates to me what kind of scar severe pain can leave on a person. They're already scarred, and to stick the knife in even deeper, it's just not fair, point blank.

I told her, "Why don't you write your experiences down?"

It would probably be therapeutic. Psychologists know that keeping a journal is very helpful. I kept following her for a number of years and she did very well. As part of that condition, she still had some residual problems, but she was able to resume a normal life. But it took quite an effort. She had supportive friends and family. It was her leg that was injured, but those misfiring nerves, and probably her immune system, weren't working right. But it's the person that was hurt.

Again, most of the time, real pain, as opposed to imagined pain, has a very different pattern. And that leads to another category of pain. How do you know who really has pain, and someone who is out to do you for drugs? Drug addiction is a big issue—social, medical, otherwise. One of the biggest tip-offs is—"guess what?"—patients who have pain talk about pain; patients who have a drug problem, what do they talk about?—they talk about drugs. {laughs} A lot of times it's a tip-off to me. If we find we spend more time talking about drugs—wait a minute—the patient does not have a pain problem. They have a drug problem. A patient who is bothered and tormented by pain, there's a whole baggage that goes along with it. The whole person is affected.

There's the hum of the air conditioning, but you just ignore it. If you have pain, you do not ignore that. After surgery, especially the first couple days, you wouldn't take a breath because it hurt. Even though a person has a foot pain, if it's chronic pain, it doesn't mean you only have to work on the foot and the rest of the leg. We also have to work on the brain.

It's incredible to recognize research that was actually done with rats. You can make the morphine, as an analgesic {pain killer}, work 100%, or make it zero percent, just depending how you affect, mentally, a subject, a rat, just by changing their environment. There were different cages where morphine worked 100% and there was another cage where it worked zero percent. We see that a lot of times in our patients.

Medicine won't work, and if you turn things around, everything works. It's an important part of multi-modality approach to pain management. It's not an either this or that. It's not a pill or an injection. It's medication a lot of times. Sometimes, it's injections. Most of the time, it's physical therapy and all. It's also always having a person be part of it.

What's your day-to-day practice like?

I see patients and do patient care every day. Most of my appointments are clinical. I also see research subjects. I collaborate with colleagues in psychology doing research on functional MRI—brain scans. The high point would be putting it all together, learning from patients, learning from these other aspects, and then from research solving problems, and then seeing the results.

A lot of times, the line between what's meaningful—and especially when a person goes from losing simple functions, like an injury to a single area, where you might feel numb here and there—as opposed to somebody who has a spinal cord injury, where you get paralyzed from the waist down and lose the function of the legs, but also control of your bowel and bladder. Those are the things we take for granted. Going to a bathroom for those patients is not an option, all the way to the patient who suffers severe strokes and debilitation, and, in the case of paraplegia, needing care 24 hours.

In a way, it's a product of an advancement of medical science in general, and neurology as well. It raises a lot of ethical questions. We can now keep the body alive when we know the person is gone. When does life stop? Or, when does meaningful life stop? It really kind of puts neuroscience in the limelight of helping patients to face the fact. Ultimately, like when somebody has a catastrophic illness in a hospital, usually a neurologist is called in to pronounce the state of what's going on with the person back in his head, when the brain is damaged to the degree that it's just a piece of tissue. You can take a picture maybe. There's tissue there, but there's nobody there.

What can happen is that an injury is such that the part of the brain that makes a person a person—the frontal lobes, temporal lobes, are the lobes that say, I know it's me. You remember who you are. You can lose part of the brain where you can go blind, but you still know who you are. You can still recognize things, enjoy things.

But there are certain areas called thalamus, when you have a biological, chronic pain problem. We have an increasing number of circumstances where we face these consequences of people surviving what, ultimately, ten years ago was considered not a possibility for survival.

There are a lot of patients who suffer grave bodily injuries, not only neurological, but in other aspects—people living without guts, or half a lung. I imagine that things will get much more complicated when we get therapies that can maybe change many other things—how long we live and what kind of disabilities can we continue living and working in. It goes back to putting us as a species, in a very interesting position. You can see how doing this can take over your life. It turns out our job never stops.

How did I go through all this? I just do it. I didn't know I was doing it. I don't think I would be able to do this job if I didn't understand what patients are telling me. I might not understand it completely, but one of the first axioms in this area, is to take it as a patient is telling you it is.

CHAPTER THIRTY-FOUR

LIFE LONG RESCUE MISSION

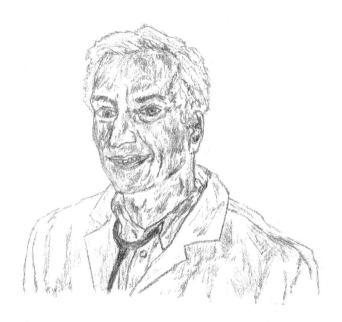

"In the medical field, there are no geographic borders."

Ayaz Samadani, MD
Internal Medicine, Family Medicine and Pediatrics,
Beaver Dam

The son of wealthy land owners, Ayaz {eye-AZ} Samadani, MD, grew up in a region of India that is now Pakistan. His station in life was such that he would never have had to work, though he chose one of the most demanding professions, nonetheless. Doctor Samadani attended medical school in his home country, followed by further training in England and Africa. A "rescue mission" to the United States was next on his itinerary–but it's lasted for more than three decades!

Somehow, he ended up in Beaver Dam, a south central Wisconsin community of 15,000 people, where he has practiced family medicine. Beaver Dam, home to 21 Protestant churches and three Catholic ones, is an odd destination for a Muslim physician. But for Dr. Samadani, religion, language, nation of origin or wealth, are simply circumstances of one's life that make patients more interesting; not any more difficult to treat.

Samadani not only became a community leader, but a leader in the Wisconsin medical community, as well, rising to the top of the profession as the first Pakistani American to become president of the Wisconsin Medical Society. He is in his mid 60s.

Samadani explains to me how he initially became interested enough in medicine to become the first doctor in a large family.

I used to volunteer as a Boy Scout in eye camps, run by British surgeons. They visit India, and need schoolchildren to volunteer to take patients from one tent to the other. By holding their hands, I took them to the surgical suite. This simple procedure {cataract surgery} that they had in that tent intrigued me. They were wearing a green, little sticker on their eye.* And when they came back, they were able to see.

When I was in college, I was sick with a simple sore throat and an earache, so I went to a doctor.

He said, "What do you want to be?" I wanted to be a physician.

After he examined me, I said, "Here's your fee."

He says, "Well, you're a future doctor, so I'm not going to charge you."

That made me think that it's such a noble profession that the greed isn't there, so this would be the best way to get educated.

I grew up in pre-partition Pakistan, which was part of India at that time, but we had land on both sides. My grandfather was chief engineer for a Muslim state in India. He was instrumental in development of several towns. I grew up mainly on those farms. Initial childhood was mainly in the small town, which the cornerstone was put by my grandfather.

We were eight—four brothers and four sisters. My father and grandfather always believed in education. They said if you have to travel or go abroad, it was open to us. My grandfather and his children, they all went to a university in India, which is still very famous and one of the top universities, so standards were set up very high.

What did your father do for a living?

My father managed the farms. We had people who lived on the farm and they worked. He spent his time engineering the whole outfit, how to grow the properties, how to manage them and make them profitable.

In spare time, we did a lot of hunting. In those days, we had friends with the railway who will put us in a caboose and we will travel about six miles out of town and they'll drop us there out of nowhere, and we'll hunt

---

* Indicated which eye to operate on to remove cataracts.

all day. On the way back, they'll stop the train in the same location and pick us up. There was not too much refrigeration, and most of the animals like deer, we'll keep alive till we have a feast or something. But the birds we will distribute. I remember sending five to ten birds to each government official—our friends. {Smiles}

My father was very fond of music and we had one of the best spiritual, musical artists. It was very common for them to come year after year to the functions where they would have five days of musical festival. That was all sponsored by our family. There will be one day of Farsi-Persian language, two days will be Punjabi, so it's a mix.

When I was like 12 years old, I left that city. He {his father} did not want me to be there. He sent me and my older brother out of that area to a different school. That was keeping up with the family tradition, too, to go away for education. He had a suspicion that we may not do that well in {local} schools. These teachers, they didn't make that good a living. I moved to a bigger city where there was a family school, much better high school and a college. I went 12 years at that schooling.

At the airport—when I was going to England for my higher education——that was the last time that I saw him. He died from a heart attack. He said, "When you grow up and your children leave the house, you'll remember me saying to you, whatever you do, do the best."

After graduation from college, I went back to the area nearby where our house was. By that time, there was a medical college there and I got admission to the medical school and spent another five years boarding in the dorms. I got all the education and college activities right there.

In my immediate family, there are five kids—one son and four daughters. My older daughter had three times admission to Northwestern medical program, and all three times, she decided not to go. She ended up as a PhD in biomedical engineering. Other daughter is a mathematician. Another is in sports diplomacy—works in the United Nations, in New York. The children's inclination was toward education and our daughter who became a physician, she had a special interest and stamina to keep awake all night and not have weekends off. If there are 25 hours in the day, she'll find another hour. She chose a profession which was extremely challenging to the human race, as well as to females. She became a neurosurgeon.

A daughter who's a brain surgeon?

Yes, she doubled me. She did a PhD and an MD, so she's twice the doctor I am.

Your kids live all over the country. Did you encourage them to travel?

When the children were in college or schools or were away from home, I had an 800 number, so they could call at any time. They had joint credit cards. But the values were explained to them from day one—no drinking, no alcohol, no drugs and no girlfriend, no boyfriend. That held till the end.

It was not that we had to tell them day after day. It was built into their character.

We came to England in 1964. After I graduated, I had visited several countries. The countries were not the barrier. I love farms. I love solitude. I love big cities. I can be adjustable, so our family is very fortunate that we have a very close relationship and understanding. We communicate.

I was the first doctor in the family. It was a big step to think about a profession and a job because after my grandfather worked for the state, he didn't let his children work for any corporation or state or government. He believed that independence is the best, so all my uncles and father managed the lands.

We grew up in those environments, so getting a job was not important. Later on in life, when I became a physician, I got my diploma and I remember receiving a letter from my cousin's sister. "You are the first physician in our family. The art is given to you by knowledge, but the healing power still comes from God. Always keep in mind that you get to heal people. Don't ask for money."

You said a job wasn't important and you didn't have to work. So why did you?

When I got my first job, which was more for recreation and traveling, my brother was working as a captain in the merchant Navy. I had special interest in traveling and seeing different countries, so asked him if I could go on his ship after I graduated from medical school.

He said, "Why don't you join as a doctor?"

So I joined the ship and traveled to Africa and Madagascar, India, and the Far East and Middle East. I enjoyed that and even at that time, it never occurred to me that I have to work for a living because most of the time, all my salary was spent in buying gifts. I didn't save anything.

After that, I went to England for further education and spent five years there and did my post graduation in pediatrics and infectious diseases. And I got married. When you get married and have a family, things became different. Then, I have to work for myself and support the family and buy a car—the usual things in life.

It was a very rainy day in Blackpool, England, where I spent two and a half years doing pediatrics and neonatology. It rained for seven days, continuously, and it was dark all the time. There was a British Medical Journal sitting on my desktop and in the back, it said, "Sunny Arizona. Pediatrician required."

Without telling my family, I caught a flight to two or three places. I sent an application to Arizona, Miami and Washington, DC, not knowing much of the States. I elected to apply for these jobs overseas. But I did not end up in Arizona, or sunny states, because a friend who was in Blackpool had moved to Chicago. He asked, "Why don't you move there?"

When I went to Chicago, I was right away recruited to be an intern at one of the small, private hospitals. They even sent you the ticket to travel and received you at the airport and chaperone you and put you up in a hotel.

It was 1970. I came by myself and had an exchange visitor visa because I had no intention of staying in the United States. I wanted to go back. Soon after I arrived, there was a war between India and Pakistan and my father had just expired, so there was a certain change and shift in life in Pakistan, and my mother told me it would be better if I stayed outside the country.

I thought it would be good if I applied for a change in my visa status and that was granted. I became a resident. My consultant, a very renowned surgeon at that hospital, became a fatherly figure. He said, "I'll give you a job in the V-A, in Hines, Illinois." But my interest was people and talking to them, and be one-to-one, rather than do surgery. I wanted to make them better in a different manner.

Wisconsin was suggested to me as a very good state for bringing up the children. California, at that time, it was attractive to a lot of physicians, but the culture of drugs and hippyism and different color hair, did not appeal to me. We had three children at that time, very young—all under three—and we decided to come to Wisconsin. When I came to Wisconsin, I was a resident in that hospital. There was a friend from the Philippines, much older than I am. He said, "Let's go to take the Wisconsin medical examination."

I said, "That's fine." I appeared for the exam and passed.

Then, we were looking for a job. It happened that I came about five times to this Beaver Dam area. Every time I came, I loved the location, the lake, the fall colors were just beautiful. The moment I went back to Chicago, I said, "No, I'm not going anywhere in a small town. I'm going to stick in the big city."

I suggest to my friend, "Why don't you take that place? There is an opening, so you just start your practice and your family is going to come from Philippines. You'll be much happier. Just go there."

He came to Wisconsin, and I introduced him to the people. When he started his practice, he didn't last but two months. He didn't like it. These people came back to me and said, "Now, we want you because you referred that person to me and now you have to come." I came as a rescue operation, and here I am, 35 years later, the same place.

We did not have very much in common with the people we were settling with, coming from a different culture and big cities and different religion. But my wife believes that happiness is within you, so create your own atmosphere. We've been very fortunate to have very good friends. My first acquaintance and a friend I met at a wine and cheese party. His folks are from England. That was the beginning of our social life.

How was it interacting with patients in Beaver Dam?

Getting used to the patients is very easy, actually, if you have these skills and knowledge and wisdom. Wisdom is actually to use the knowledge. You can study and become a scholar, but if you don't know how to use it, then it becomes a burden.

Was there any pressure for you to come back to Pakistan?

There's a saying in Pakistan, that if you're out of place and you did a beautiful dance, nobody will notice you. So if you want to do a beautiful dance, you should come back home and do it here. You were educated here, so why don't you come back? I felt, at times, this is a very poor nation, not financially, but in the sense of the medical field. They do not have access or means to get to the doctor and the doctors also have limited means for serving because they don't have access to the diagnostic material we have in this country.

After training in England, and the United States, it was difficult for me to practice medicine in Pakistan because I'm used to this diagnostic aid. I was examining a patient and wasn't ordering routine lab work at that time because we always depended on the clinical judgment rather than lab support.

But here, because the atmosphere was such that demanded laboratory work, to substantiate your diagnosis, I also learned "defensive medicine." The culture was if something goes wrong with the patient, it's not the course of illness; it may be the fault of the doctor. It became clear to me that you have to do a practice of medicine that is more attuned to Western culture and will not be practical in Pakistan.

But I've been very actively involved in Pakistan health care. I was on the advisory board to the president for health care improvement in Pakistan. And with the natural disasters in the past—flooding, or even in good times, visiting hospitals.

With the recent earthquake, all the physicians of Pakistani descent and to a larger extent, the Muslims, have participated in getting their resources together. You can help in many other ways, just not being there. The other avenue of help is medical education. At the University of Wisconsin, I participated in global health initiative programs and chalked out a program for the faculty and students to travel abroad, and similarly, for faculty overseas, to come to the United States and spend some time learning programs, such as "teach the teacher." Those are the programs which are helpful in promoting and improving the health care system in Pakistan, or any other country, for that matter.

Tell me about your practice here. What is it like?

Family practice. I enjoy that because every patient brings a different story to me. It's not their ailments—those are simple to treat. Sometime, I get to talk to them about what they have done in their life.

I have delivered babies. I have delivered mothers and daughters and one time they were delivered within an hour of each other. It was in the paper that Dr. Samadani delivered mom and daughter.

Another time, I was at the ice cream shop and I bought ice cream for my kids and there happens to come children whom I delivered. They have a large family, so soon I found out there were six or seven of them, so I had to buy extra ice creams for them. Those are pleasures.

My patients are very simple or complicated in a disease way, but in talking to them as human beings, they're amazingly, simple and straight forward. We were dining one evening and this lady comes out of the door of the restaurant and says, "Hi, Dr. Samadani."

I looked at her and said, "Hi, how are you? Are you doing fine?"

She said, "Yeah, but you don't recognize me, unless I have my clothes off."

My wife didn't appreciate that joke.

That's a real thing that happens in my life, so I enjoy practice. We had a very good relationship with the patients and my motto is if they have come to see me, they should not be waiting in the waiting room. They have to be in the exam room right away. That's where we do not waste any time. If I see 20 patients or 40 patients a day, there's no limit. Depending on their illnesses, if they're severe and need attention, I'll see them. It doesn't matter how long I have to stay.

If there is no patient, I'll take time off. It's not fixed. If they need secondary or tertiary care, I have never hesitated to call upon a colleague or a specialist and send them to a place where they'll get the best treatment. Sometimes, they will go there and be hurried into an operation, and I hesitate with such referrals. I want them to understand. I want them to think beyond the operation. What is afterwards?

I work five days a week—Saturdays and Sundays off. My half-day is when my appointments are low. I mean you take time off for the family. If they have a commitment and you have to be together, you make time for that.

The burden is most on the wife. She has to understand what the medical profession is. Sometime there will be a party at home and the doctor is called. I've been called so many times and by the time I have returned home, the dishes were in the dishwasher and everybody's gone and the food's been eaten.

So many times at night you're in bed asleep and all of a sudden you get a phone call and you disturb your wife. Then, you get out and spend two hours outside and come back and crawl back into the bed. Those are the situations they have to get used to. I can get up many times during the night and go back to sleep without any problem. Usually, I keep my phone on a very low volume and my beeper; I prefer a beeper call because I'm a very light sleeper. I'll get up and get dressed and go, and sometimes I'll come back and my wife won't even notice that I ever left, except a couple of times.

I went to the emergency room to see a patient and somehow the patient got delayed and called back. My wife picked up the phone. "I want to kill myself right now." It was 2 o'clock in the morning, in a dead sleep and {my wife} said, "Wait a minute. Let me say something to you."

She remembered that she had to keep him engaged, so she kept talking to him. She picked up the other phone. She paged me that "this patient wants to kill himself and he's on the phone and I don't know what to do."

So I told her, "Give him hope. Give him something to look forward to," and that's what she did. He did not commit suicide. We've had moments of concerns, right on the edge and moments of pleasure. That's what makes the doctor's life so intriguing. I just love every day of it. Every time I come to the office to see my patient, I want to learn more about my patients.

I enjoy working. I graduated in 1964, so it's been many years and people ask if I am approaching retirement. I'm 63 years old. I'm in good thinking, clear mind and body and exercise. I am very active, so as long as my brain, body and functions are in harmony, I don't think there is any restriction or any rules for retirement.

I eat very little. I always believed in a small meal. I cannot tolerate seeing too much food on my plate. I will take maybe twice, but very small portions. Number one, I don't want to waste the food. Second, I want to really enjoy it and maybe taste it a little bit.

But three meals are necessary to me because of the metabolism. Breakfast is essential. Overnight, starving six to eight hours creates certain hormone changes in your body and if you don't eat after that interval, and you miss still the next meal, all the food taken will be thoroughly absorbed, rather than bypassed. I stay about the same weight and it does not matter what I eat, but it matters how much I eat. I eat three times regularly, exercise and I stay the same. Get out and walk. You have to work throughout the year to be in shape. You have to have endurance and stamina built up.

I swim at least twice a week. If I can't swim, I walk. I walk 30 minutes if it's indoors and 30 minutes I devote to the weight exercise, upper and lower body. If I'm not doing the weights, I'll be outside walking 55 minutes to 60 minutes—I'll do three miles. That's a good pace walking. You will not sweat too much, but your heart rate will go up. If you do that regularly, you will have no problem digesting those three meals.

America eats too much. You see obesity has increased so much in the developed world because people have an abundance of food and second, we're served too much food. It is expected that if you go to eat out that you're served large portions. Compared to England, France and Italy, you will see that the food servings are much smaller portions.

Then, also the contents, what are served are different. If you eat green vegetables, tomatoes, cucumbers and cheese, verses potatoes, meat and bread, along with alcohol, the mechanism is different. You don't want to conserve all the calories consumed and convert it into fat and store into the body, especially if you don't exercise and watch TV.

In your free time, you do more than exercise. You were the first Pakistani American to become president of the Wisconsin Medical Society. How important was that achievement?

The Achievement was important, but to me glory is not. When I moved to Wisconsin in 1970, I participated in strategic planning. I was always interested in policy development. What is the shape of the future? I participated and it took me almost 30 years to climb up to that level.

You can keep integrity within yourself and you be portrayed as a professional. Recently, I was really surprised at the younger physicians. I'm not blaming them as a whole—but at the hospital, we had a note from the chief of staff that nurses have complained that some doctors are showing up in dirty clothes, odor in their clothes and dirty hands. Perhaps they have come from field work or whatever they were doing and were called in during an emergency. That's a different story. But to come for the rounds in that kind of apparel is not a dignified manner of a doctor showing up for seeing a patient. Certain requirements go with the profession.

How I got {to be president} was maybe an accident. It was not that I was longing for it, that I wanted to be a president. It was suggested to me at certain level. This was by your colleagues who have spent some time with you and knew the nature of your personality. There is a path and if you take that path you can achieve any goal.

Your presidential theme was organ donation. Why?

Organ and tissue donation was important to me because we had a liking for the spiritual. This guy who was our favorite musician was very young and had diabetes mellitus. I was arranging for him to have a kidney transplant, as he was on dialysis. During this process, the gentleman passes away en route to in the United States. To me, it was one little shocking thing that stimulated me. I could see 83,000 people on the waiting list {for an organ} or every day the list was increasing. People were dying with the need and people were dying without giving their organs for donation, being buried in a non-productive way.

The medical society backed me and gave me the material, as well as the personnel. We increased the awareness and we also increased the donors. That cause is very dear to me and I'm still working on that.

My sister's husband had a kidney transplant as a complication of diabetes. Kidney transplants are done in Pakistan, too, but the problem there is quality control. Dialysis machines are all infected with hepatitis C virus and it is very hard to scrutinize or see which system is perfect.

The donors are not selected. It's a different atmosphere there at the hospitals because they tend to get the donors who are not the family members or friends, and their background is not thoroughly checked. That's why he came here. He's two weeks here, post op, and doing very well.

Why don't people donate?

The information is still not available to them. We still haven't done the job properly of asking people. Once it's explained to them, we make a request, then the job becomes easy. We can increase the numbers of donors. We should continue to go through the media.

But you cannot stop death. The time is fixed at the time you were born, so you cannot die early or any later. I live from moment to moment and I believe that death is imminent.

It's not good to predict anybody's life. I've seen people with cancer and they come back to the office, and say, "Doc, I went to see so and so and he told me I've got three months to live. Here I am, four months later, still alive. What do you think?" On the other hand, sometimes it's true, too. Patients come in and say, "My dad was told he had two months to live and he's gone in a month."

The best thing is to give them odds, but every individual is different. They react differently to treatment. They react differently to the chemotherapy, to radiation, to surgeries. We cannot generalize.

But you ask for God's blessings. You ask for His prayers that you spent the time productively. I strongly believe that spirituality has all the parts in healing. I have the knowledge. I was trained and I have the experience. But the healing part, which is to make people better, comes from God. It is the prayers.

I have seen patients who have listened to the prayers and responded in a much better way. It works. It's your own faith, as well. The diagnosis comes to your mind by God.

You've lived all over the world. Is it more challenging to treat patients who don't share your faith or speak your language?

Our education was in English and it was a choice in the high school, whether you take English or Hindi. But in medical school, everything was English.

During my travels, after I became a doctor, I was exposed to different countries and different languages and patients. I never felt that the language or the country was a barrier. When I started, I used to see a lot of migrant health workers who spoke Spanish and I took a few lessons in Spanish, but mainly I learned some words from my patients. For example, in East Africa, where they speak Swahili, people have the same illnesses. If they got their finger chopped, we put it back.

In Saudi Arabia—prior to all the oil—there were pretty poor conditions there. There were no lights, no education, no medical facilities. I was called upon to visit a home. I walked through several corridors and there was no sunshine in the house. When I went to the back room, there was a lady with a young child, walking age, but with bowed legs. Both legs were completely bent. Immediately to me it came that this child has rickets—no sunshine, poor diet, resulted in calcium and vitamin D deficiency. There was no language needed that time either.

In the medical field, there are no geographic borders and there are no limitations. Language, religion, your race or color, does not matter because it's a very noble profession. It's beyond any other profession and beyond any other restrictive covenants of the world.

X

Grave Matters

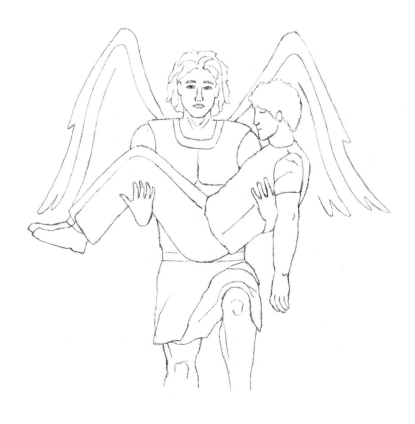

"Too often we underestimate the power of a touch, a smile, a kind word, a listening ear, an honest compliment, or the smallest act of caring, all of which have the potential to turn a life around."

—Leo Buscaglia

CHAPTER THIRTY-FIVE

DYING RIGHT

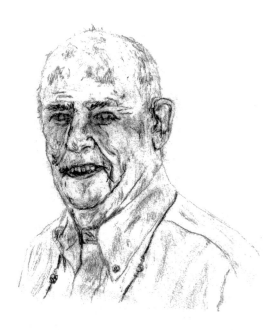

"People who are being kept alive unaware of who they are, where they are, lying in their own stool and urine—it's not the way people are meant or want to be."

Philip Dougherty, MD
Internist, Menomonee Falls

Philip Dougherty is a soft spoken doctor who's as comfortable talking about death as he is talking about wine making, his long time hobby. In fact, he wants you to become comfortable discussing death, too.

He worries because people who refuse to consider their end-of-life options when they're well, may leave their families in an impossible situation, should they become unable to make their own health care decisions. Who can possibly know what life and death health care decisions to make for their loved one if the subject is never discussed? And that, Dougherty knows, is a recipe for what could be a long, expensive and torturous conclusion to one's life.

But more importantly, it makes an already difficult time for loved ones that much more stressful because they're the ones left to sort it all out.

Dougherty's wife and eight children know all too well his thoughts on the subject.

Dougherty explains how death issues became so important to him. Maybe it had something to do with that sick cat he had as a kid.

~~~~~~~~~~~~~~

My earliest experience with anything medical was with a white cat in the family. The poor cat had the mange, and looked to be so uncomfortable and in such bad shape. I told my dad we really should put the cat to sleep. And my dad said, "Okay, go ahead and do that."

So I put the poor, damn cat down the basement and put him under a box with a hole in it and slowly dropped chloroform through. And the cat just went absolutely wild. I can't imagine how we could ever do that. But the cat was obviously being tortured and wasn't going down, so we finally gave up and let the cat out of the box, and the cat ran off and was never seen again. I don't know where the hell the cat went, but that was my first medical experience—a sad one.

Where did you grow up?

In a small town in central Illinois called Oglesby, named after a Civil War general. It's a town of about 3,800 people and the countryside is corn, as far as the eye can see. It's peculiar, in as much as there were three other lads in the community, all of whom went into medicine, which is a lot for a small, rural community. My father was a pharmacist in this community and perhaps I got some interest in medicine from him. I was very strongly directed. When I went into high school, I enrolled in a classical pre-college curriculum and went right on into college and then, into medical school.

I went to the University of Illinois in Chicago and that was a rather sad experience, as the whole class was canned from the school because they thought we were all cheating on an exam. That was the farthest from the truth. They reinstated us and I was able to graduate along with 180 others.

Peculiarly, of 180 people in that class, there were 13 women. I participate in the ethics programs at the Medical College of Wisconsin, and I am amazed to sit in the classroom and see all of the young women.

My father, being a pharmacist, was very proud of my desires to be a physician. My father had actually passed away when I was finishing my second year in medical school, so he never had the pleasure of seeing his son graduate or be called "doctor." But I know he is around and knows it now, anyway. The strongest feelings about going to medical school came from my mother and father.

My mother was always very proud of my scholastic abilities, so I had a lot of support, emotionally, in that way. Speaking of support, you might be interested to know that in 1952-56, I was at the University of Illinois. It cost $200 a quarter.

The single person who most influenced me about going into medical school was a Benedictine monk in high school, Father Damien. He taught biology and embryology and subjects of that sort, and he encouraged me and fostered my own interest. I was fortunate to go to a Benedictine high school, which was an all-boys school at the time...the priests there, the monks there, certainly were superb, very motivating. As it turns out, I was the only one of my class of 86 who went into medicine.

The {monks} thought I was bright. They thought I could make it into medical school, that I had features of humaneness and kindness that would allow me to be a good physician. And they encouraged me all along the way. The sciences seem to come my way very easily—not without study. I did have good grades and was accepted into medical school with ease.

There were books that rather strongly influenced me. One was the *"Life of Louis Pasteur,"* and it was a popular book at the time. We're now talking about 1939, 1940, I was a young lad finishing grade school, and the life of Louis Pasteur seemed so exciting and so wonderful.

The other was the life of Father Damien, the priest of the Hawaiian Islands—Molokai. I've been to Hawaii once in my life to visit Father Damien's grave, his church and clinic, where he took care of the people with leprosy.

What was medicine like after you graduated from med school?

There were no plastic syringes. All the syringes were glass. All of the needles were reused needles and sharpened to get rid of any burrs that may be on them. There were no such things as plastic bags of intravenous fluids or blood. It was all glass. They, of course, had to be sterilized and so forth.

We were amazed at the boldness of the young nurses who started appearing in the hospital wearing slacks. Never would it have ever happened in the early days that they would be allowed to appear in slacks. And, not only in slacks, but without their caps—a reflection of their dignity. The people who showed up for work in slacks were almost seen to be hussies of a sort, but we soon got over that.

When we graduated from medical school, there were three antibiotics available: penicillin, sulfa drugs and streptomycin. And we used them to treat everything because we didn't really know what the capabilities or the proper use of those medications was.

I recall so well the plight of the poor people who came down with polio. And the place I interned, St. Francis hospital in Illinois, was a referral site for people with polio. And to see the poor people in those huge iron lungs—they were so loud. The noise was just unbearable. It's amazing that anybody got any sleep when they were in them, and terrible consequences of people being put in them. You could get maybe three iron lungs in a room of this size. It was a pneumatic pressure—it would build up and let go, build up and let go, so it was compressing, physically, the chest, of these poor people whose muscles would no longer allow them to breathe on their own, sometimes permanently.

A big deal was made of a fellow named Fred Snipe. Snipe was a celebrity of his own sort at the time because he got married while in an iron lung. Now, whatever he did with his wife outside of the iron lung, I have no idea. But certainly, it made all the papers and all the news reels at the time. And then now, to see the wonderful development of the ventilators, that are so neat and clean and small, portable and quiet.

When I went into medical school, I recall at the interview before I was accepted, telling the interviewer that I wanted, likely to be a general practitioner. And it was only after I was in medical school for a while that I began to recognize what the subspecialty of internal medicine was like. From there on during my internship, I was motivated by several men in that community who were internists and I felt like I wanted to do what they wanted to do.

That was the time of the Second World War and we were still dealing with the doctor draft, so we knew we had to serve two years in some branch of the service. It was either volunteer or run the risk of being pulled out of whatever you were doing, either residency or practice, at some other time. I finished my internship and volunteered to be in the Navy because they're so clean.

I went to Great Lakes,* where they assigned me. I was told we were here for six weeks and we will teach you to be gentlemen, which infuriated me. Nonetheless, I spent the six weeks there and then I got my orders; my orders were not to go to a ship or a Navy hospital. I was assigned to the Marine Corps, so I spent two years in the Mojave Desert crawling around in sand and dirt. And temperatures during the summer months of 120, 130 weren't at all unusual.

Yes, we had what was actually a little outpatient clinic. The hospital itself was small. It had 13 beds. And we as physicians were told if any patient was going to be here more than three days, you transport them out of here to Camp Pendleton, which was about 150 miles away. In true Marine Corps tradition, we had two ambulances and we would put a patient in the ambulance and send it out to Pendleton and then a half hour later we would send out the second ambulance because we were never sure the first ambulance would get there.

The Marines, of course, have great esprit, and whenever a major conflict would erupt anywhere in the world where Marines might be sent, there was a constant stream of commanding officers going up to the division headquarters and saying, "Our division is ready and we're anxious to go and we want to be the first ones to go." And it used to drive the medical

* Chicago-based Naval Academy.

officers crazy because if any unit comes out of the base to be sent to a conflict, they take a medical officer with them. We could never understand why these Marine officers were running up wanting to be the first ones to go, and we wanted to trip them on their way, so we wouldn't be sent off to some battle. As it turns out, I never saw any conflict.

While I was there, a young fella joined us who had just come from Milwaukee. And another fellow and I had expressed interest in internal medicine and he said, "If you guys are interested in internal medicine, you ought to go to Milwaukee and check out Milwaukee County Hospital because they're developing a new internal medicine department and they've got some cracker jack young physicians there." So we did.

My background was Chicago with Cook County Hospital, which is in a terrible environment and was an awful looking place. I can still smell Cook County Hospital. But nonetheless, to walk into Milwaukee County Hospital grounds on a beautiful day in October, with the leaves all turning colors, I thought, *This can't be a county hospital*. But it was, and we met these young people who were developing new fields, nephrology and gastroenterology and all of the ologies you could imagine. We were so impressed and they were so gracious, that this other fellow and I decided we were going to take our residencies at county hospital in Milwaukee. I never regretted it.

We had to talk about the patients who died and why they had died and be critiqued by the other residents who were sitting there. We brought that same discipline to the hospital here in town, much to the dismay of some of the physicians who felt they were being picked on. It was a matter of being used to be criticized, and being used to standing up and admitting mistakes. It's a very healthy thing that I think continues to this day over there.

Do you remember when you lost your first patient?

I was an intern. People dying, on the one hand, it is always a disappointment and you're sad. It makes you feel as though, what else could I have done? Should I have gotten somebody else to do something? When you lose a patient, especially one you feel was a friend and has been with you for a long while, that's like losing a member of your family. It's very hard to stand at the foot of the bed and not have tears in your eyes. You embrace the family and the relatives.

How did you develop the rapport to deliver that very sad news?

It doesn't come easily. The classical circumstance where you're confronted with that is when it's an unforeseen death. People being brought to the emergency room and the family arrives and to have to tell them that their loved one has passed away. There's no easy way to do that. I always did that with a nurse with me because somehow nurses seem to be able to assuage some of that fear and some of that sadness more than a male can by himself. I never felt that I had to learn how to be nice, how to be comforting and understanding. It just kind of came to me, naturally.

A program at the Medical College of Wisconsin, in which they teach the sophomore medical students palliative care, is a milestone in the development of teaching medical students the kind of concern, helping them understand and to be nice people. A lot of them wouldn't need that kind of training, but a lot of them do. Young physicians of today will be and are more understanding, more empathetic and more capable of identifying with the sorrows that come with the passing of a patient.

When I talk to patients and groups about end-of-life care, I tell them my own story about my grandparents, how both of them passed away at home, passed away after lingering illnesses. Both of them were cared for by their family. Both of them were in circumstances where we would come to visit, and whoever was with that individual at the time, would say, "Well, grandpa hasn't had anything to eat for three days. We tried to get him to drink water and he won't take sips of water."

There wasn't the compelling need to call an ambulance and run people to the hospital. There was more concern about comfort, and comfort for the rest of the family who were trying to understand and realize that grandma or grandpa is going to die.

That still takes place and people still grapple with the concept of how much care should we be giving patients. We can virtually keep people alive forever. But alive to what end and alive to what purpose, when being alive just means suffering and being unable to relate to the people around you or the circumstances you're in? It just doesn't make sense to me.

It's always a very difficult circumstance, meaning patients' families never want to be guilty of saying, "Don't do anything. Let's stop now." But if they have a caring physician and they have been made to think about it in advance, then they're better prepared when the time comes. They realize that futility does play a role and to do more, often would be futile, and it's time to let the patient rest and let nature take its course.

That's still a fight, and hopefully we're making some progress. Last year, for the first time, every medical college in the nation had a palliative care program taught to the young physicians, so we're going to have to get rid of some of the old docs who still want to be so authoritative and paternalistic. Once we have all these young physicians who've been better trained about kindness and humility, then we'll see much greater strides being made in handling death and long illnesses that accompany it.

Have you made any preparations with respect to your own death because of the experiences that you've had?

I have completed my power of attorney for health care. We have talked with all of our children about our deaths, so that they know what we want. They know that my wife and I don't want to have our lives prolonged needlessly, to the detriment of the family or finances of the family. So yes, we do talk about it and I wish everybody did, so there wouldn't be the terrible angst that develops when that happens suddenly and unexpectedly.

I have a son-in-law who is especially disdainful about talking about death. He sometimes will say when we bring something up relative to somebody dying, "Well, I've only been here ten minutes before you start talking about dying," because he thinks we talk about it too quickly and too much.

As important as the Power of Attorney for Healthcare is, it is more important that the conversation take place. It's fine for you to have a document that you've written out, but you can't cover all the circumstances that might pertain. The most important part about that whole process is that you have the conversation with your family. That way there are no surprises. That way, everybody knows what you want and knows how to handle it and it is just so much kinder, easier and simpler and you don't have to worry about necessarily, having a document in your hand.

How frequently is it a close call, where you're not really sure whether to go forward with more treatment or let nature take its course?

It's difficult, at times, to know when and where to put the brakes on. It's easier for some people to say enough than it is for others. Physicians are never trained to quit. They are trained to prolong life as much as possible. It's easier for me to do that than it is for some other physicians. It's an individual thing, and it starts with the physician's own family background and how his grandparents died and what the families' reactions were. Young people in medical school who may never have had a member of their family pass away are frequently incapable of understanding what that's all about.

It's not at all uncommon anymore for people to live well into their 90s, past the age of 100. So we're going to have to deal with some of those circumstances—the great number of people in nursing homes—is of concern to me. When I was actively in practice, I was medical director for three nursing homes. I made rounds one day at all three nursing homes, and back then I was seeing 89 people. Of the 89 people, 11 of them could hold a conversation with me. Now to me, that's a tragedy.

The institution, just by keeping the person there, is treating them. They are obliged to keep the patient warm, dry, clean. That is treatment. It is not necessary for an institution to give the patient injections of medications, not necessary to give the patient intravenous fluids, not necessary to put a tube down and artificially feed them. You can impose what could be called comfort measures. And if the patient is thought to have pain, you give them pain medication and if the patient is short of breath you give them oxygen. You do all the things that are necessary to keep the patient comfortable and you do nothing to interfere with the death process that may be coming.

Pneumonia used to be called the old man's friend, and how true it is. The old folks lying in bed, breathing poorly, and their secretions build up and the first thing you know, they've got pneumonia. Let 'em go.

I had a patient who was in a nursing home and who didn't know who he was, where he was or what was happening in his surroundings. And, he had a problem with recurring infections. I would treat it and he'd get better. A month or two would go by, and he would get another infection and I would treat it. Finally, I didn't feel that we could logically do any more for him. I told the son, "He has another infection and I don't think you should send him to the hospital. That's inappropriate, after all this time."

The son was incensed. He was irate. "What do you mean you're not going to send him to the hospital?" After a lot of discussion, I finally had to say, in good conscience, I cannot do this. I cannot send that patient to the hospital again. "If you wish, I will find another physician to assume his care," which I did.

I found a physician that would accept his care. He did hospitalize the patient and he died in the hospital under his care, nonetheless. I felt like I had fulfilled my ethical responsibility. I couldn't see clear to admitting him myself, but I found a responsible physician who did and the family was satisfied—still upset with me and upset about the circumstance. You can do a lot, but you can't do everything.

He had been in the hospital multiple times in the past 12 months. He was over 85 years of age. He was demented, didn't know where he was or who I was. I'm not sure he recognized his son at all, so I think ethically, physicians have a responsibility of being gatekeepers.

A lot of physicians don't want to accept that responsibility. They want just to do everything possible all the time. We have to be directive of our patients and their families sometimes. It's sometimes unpleasant for physicians to make those decisions, but it's part of our job.

Another one I had participated in was a woman who had a terrible stroke and was kept alive virtually, artificially on a respirator for approximately a week. Finally, it became apparent that she was not going to come around and she was going to die without the respirator. We had a family conference. They had brought along their pastor and a friend, and we all sat down. And they want to know what the situation is, what we thought the outcome would be. A neurosurgeon talked to them, saying that he could do nothing under the circumstances. And by the time—it took about an hour by the time we were finished—everybody was on the same page.

We all said she wouldn't want to be kept alive artificially this way; she's not getting any better. We've heard from physicians that it's a matter of futility, and so they all agreed we should turn off the respirator. Everybody went to her room and held her hand, touched her and the nurse turned off the respirator. You could see on the monitor, the heartbeat just gradually slowed down and finally, the patient passed away. It took about 20 minutes.

The family was all hugs. Everybody wanted to touch the patient. What a beautiful thing for it to happen that way and it happened because the family had been programmed by the physician that this is what we might be facing at the onset of the illness.

Hopefully, people are aware of the fact that they don't need to be aggressive in the treatment of these folks. Hopefully, the patient has had the opportunity to talk with their agent ahead of time and let it be known that in this situation, I don't want a lot of medical treatment. But that's what the advance directive, living will, power of attorney for health care is all about—empowering somebody else to make the decision for you. And obviously, that person has to be somebody you trust, somebody who will be there, somebody who knows you and that you know understands. If all those things are met, then it really isn't such a grand circumstance to have somebody in a nursing home or a hospital and seriously ill, where everybody knows what was wanted, and it's so easily done. The death then, becomes a beautiful thing, to see somebody just quietly pass away.

People who are being kept alive unaware of who they are, where they are, lying in their own stool and urine, it's not the way people are meant or want to be. And yet, when they get pneumonia, we run 'em to the hospital, give them intravenous antibiotics, give them all these treatments and bring them back, so he can once again lay in his own stool and urine. That doesn't make any sense to me at all.

As a father, I have let it be known, please, if I'm in that situation, just keep me warm and clean and dry, and let nature take its course. I think that's what most people, most older people, will say that they want. Young people may have difficulty saying that, but society is slowly coming around to believing that.

The trial lawyers have put the fear of God into physicians and we practice defensive medicine every day, every time we see a patient. We prescribe things because we're fearful that if we don't, we're going to have a problem and the first thing you know, we're going to be sued. I don't know data or statistics, but I just have a feeling that the public is becoming more aware that that's not proper to sue everybody all the time for what otherwise could be things that could be avoided.

I had a lawsuit leveled against me. I had seen a woman who had an aneurysm and she was beginning to have neurological symptoms. I said, "We've got to get you to see a neurosurgeon." She ended up having an appointment for the next day. It's the old sorry—too little, too late. That's what bothered me. On the way to the appointment, she stopped to get gas and the aneurysm blew. She did survive, but she's a vegetable.

In retrospect, if I had not let her get out of the office, if I had told her, "You're in immediate danger" and gotten her to see a neurosurgeon more quickly, maybe something could've been done. You can't have that happen and not be regretful. As it turns out, I was dropped from the suit.

Lawsuits weren't common during the early part of your career, right?

But the opportunity to make mistakes was greater back then because you were doing more. I probably put in the first cardiac pacemaker at the hospital. Jack Manley, the director of cardiology at St. Luke's, had been an intern of mine. Over the phone, he told me how to do this. We did an awful lot of things as general internists, in those days, that now has become the aegis of the sub-specialists. It preys on your mind. If it doesn't prey on your mind, you shouldn't be a doctor.

It makes you cautious, it makes you fearful. I wouldn't for a moment think twice about calling a patient. I still do. If I see a patient and I'm not sure what's happening, couple hours go by, my conscience just drives me crazy and I have to get on the phone and call them. "Tell me how you're doing and what's happening." You become very conscientious of things of that sort. It is not often today that we are doing things that could cause their death, but we used to.

What was a typical day in practice like?

I was averaging 80 hours a week. And that was for real. And the problem was when we started in practice, there was no hospital here, so we had to hospitalize people either at West Allis Hospital or in Waukesha hospital. Well, if you have an admission that you want to see in the morning and you have to go to West Allis, and West Allis to Waukesha, and then from Waukesha back here. Then, do the same thing at night after the office is closed.

Now, we were all in practice about 12 years before any of us thought of taking an afternoon off. Everybody was there all the time and there was never any concern because we were all doing it together. So that feeling, that esprit, that camaraderie, came out of what some people would call, drudgery.

What effect did that have on your family life?

I was viewed by the children as being the source of discipline. But I was soft and easy, and my children could not be the people they are if my wife and I had not had the life we've had. My wife is a marvelous soul and a nice person, and a good mother and a good wife. So the children never said, "Dad, you were away too long" or any of those things. They just have stories about how my poor wife tried to discipline them and no doubt said, "Your father's going to be home pretty soon."

Were you ever torn between your professional duty to your patients and your eight children, whom you wanted to see?

Yes, unfortunately that happened all too often. I regret, in retrospect, that I didn't spend more time with my children. As it turns out, it didn't matter, because my wife was so marvelous and able to keep them happy and controlled and teach them to be nice people.

Next month, we are celebrating our 50th wedding anniversary and we're both so happy and so grateful to the good Lord. And yes, I've done some good things for medicine locally, and have developed a reputation for being a kind and thoughtful, effective physician. But certainly the greatest accomplishment of my—our life together—has been our family. You would like them. And they have become our very best friends. And they come home and go to the basement—I'm an amateur wine maker—and they know the wine is down there, so they never leave empty handed.

We've had a marvelous sort of existence here in this community. Our children all went to school in this community. We all went to church in the community. When we would go to the bank, everybody in the bank, walking by, the tellers, would say, "Hi Doc." And to me, those are two of the most marvelous words ever. And it's always thrilled me and sometimes will bring tears to my eyes to hear people....

I saw a lady just recently, and we were at a grocery store standing in line and she said, "I always thought you were the Marcus Welby of Menomonee Falls," which was thrilling that people would think such nice things.

Even though at this point in my life, I'm leaning more and more toward retirement, I do work part-time and I continue to run into people who say, "I was just a little boy, but I remember you came to my house." I made an awful lot of house calls at the time. The first car I bought was a little Volkswagen Beetle. And people will say, "I recall seeing you in your little Beetle coming up the driveway to visit us and to see our grandfather."

How often did you make house calls?

It was a common thing and people would simply call in to our clinic in the morning and say, "Johnny's been sick with a fever and wondering if you could stop by." Well, stopping by got to be kind of a problem. First of all, just finding the home was tough, especially out in the country, where sometimes people would forget to put on the porch light. If you were on call on a weekend, it wouldn't be unusual to make 15, 16, 18 house calls in a weekend.

It's an honor to be invited into somebody's home to take care of a sick person, but fatigue takes over sometimes. And because not all those house calls were made at one o'clock in the afternoon. They were made frequently at two, three, four o'clock in the morning. And people would call you and you'd get out of your bed and get dressed, drive to wherever they were. I always had my phone number listed in the book. I could never understand not having your phone number in the book. The concept of driving in wintertime out in the country was hazardous, to say the least, because it wasn't well lighted then and cars would get stuck in the snow and we didn't have cell phones and all of that, so it was kind of chore.

Oh, it's very definitely a way of life. It's not a job in a demeaning sense. It's a profession—and there are other professions, but there are none so noble and none so gratifying to the person who is practicing it.

One morning in the emergency room, I was asked to sew up a little boy's head. And it turns out that his was the fifth generation of that family that I had had an opportunity to treat. Things of that sort just grab you and bring tears to your eyes because of the sentimentality and emotionality of the thing.

Physicians are especially graced to be given the opportunity to be put on a pedestal, and we are. I don't think there is any other profession in which generally, people hold you in such high regard and put such terrible faith in you, and to the point where they allow you to manipulate their lives and they follow your advice and they come to you for understanding and for hope. So it's just the most glorious profession in the world. I can't imagine anything else. The relationships with people—we do things to people {laughs} that are just incredible.

I can't imagine when I hear people talking about wanting earnestly to retire. I've got to quit going to this factory or quit doing this job. I tried to retire and I couldn't. I flunked retirement, so I can't imagine not practicing medicine, even a little bit that I do now. I lasted about six months in retirement and I had to begin looking for something else to draw me back in. And the people at the hospital were kind, and took me on as director of palliative care and I continued on in ethics. People at the clinic took me on doing what is called urgent care, people who call in and need to be seen. So I'm very content and doing a part-time sort of practice.

About two weeks ago, I said {to a colleague}, "John, I think I'm going to hang it up."

And he said, "You are not going to hang it up. Goddamn it, you're going to stay here with me." We were at a function with my wife and he said, "Don't let that guy quit."

We're 73 years old. It sounds old, and it is. I don't know how much longer, but the worst thing I can imagine is that somebody would have a problem develop and they'd say, "Well, I was treated by that older doctor, you know, and if I had a younger doctor, it wouldn't have happened." You'd live in constant fear of that sort of thing.

It still makes me ten feet tall when you come out of seeing a patient and doing the best you can to help them. To come upon a scene and quickly institute some sort of therapy, and have it all work out properly, is just an incredible thing.

When we were still working out of West Allis Hospital, I recall walking into the emergency room and seeing a patient who was in the midst of reaction. Treatment is so simple and so dramatic, and I was able to tell the physician who was on duty at the time, what that was and give him a hundred milligrams of Benedryl, intravenously. Within moments, the seizuring stopped. The patient woke up. Those battles don't happen every day, but those are glorious moments.

It's also a marvelous thrill for a physician to be present at the birth of a new child. But it's equally glorious for that physician to be there when a patient dies. That's a privilege... to be present at the death of a patient and to influence whatever you can, to keep that death a peaceful death, a comfortable death, and to help the family to understand, to feel comfortable with it, as well.

CHAPTER THIRTY-SIX

MEDICINE RUN AMOK

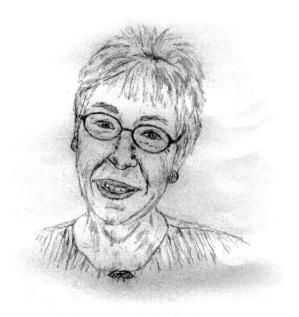

"Somebody could be 80 years old, and getting tens of thousands of dollars worth of equipment installed, while we have kids who don't get their immunizations."

Kay Heggestad, MD
Family Medicine, Madison

Anticipating one's demise may be one of the most difficult things in life. Perhaps, that explains why so many patients and doctors can't come to grips with it when death approaches, exhausting every futile treatment option, no matter the cost. Doctor Kay Heggestad has seen this time and again, and is sure there are better ways to die than being fed through a tube or accepting that last grueling round of chemotherapy, to forestall the inevitable for a couple more months. In many cases, Heggestad, in her early 60s, says doctors don't realize that they can be much more helpful to patients at the end of their life by providing comfort care.

For 30 years, Heggestad practiced family medicine before getting in-

volved with hospice and nursing home care. This later experience was a revelation, and she now regrets not having done more in her earlier years to relieve the suffering of dying patients.

Death also has played a significant role in Heggestad's personal life. She met her future husband, Paul Wertsch, in medical school during gross anatomy class. "Paul was at the next cadaver," she explains. "We ended up the last two people through this pathological exam. The doc who was running the show took pity on us and took us home for drinks after the exam. That was really our very first date. Had it not been for that exam, he would have been like any other guy in the class. We might never have connected."

As our conversation begins, Dr. Heggestad enthusiastically describes how rewarding it is to treat people who are on the brink of death.

One of the biggest successes I had was with a little lady who hadn't talked with one of her sisters just because they argued over something many years ago. They lived in {the same} town and hadn't spoken to each other. One of the big questions you ask in hospice or in long-term care is, "Is there anything that you need to get done?"

She said, "Yeah, I have some boxes at home that need to be cleaned out." Then, she started crying.

I said, "What else do you have to get done?"

She said, "I haven't talked to my sister in years."

I encouraged her to call her or write her.

The two gals got together.

It also turns out that her sister was actually one of my patients for 20 years, but they had different last names. Until the sister walked in, I didn't even realize there was a connection there. There was another sister who had also been out of the picture. The three of them got together regularly for lunch, talking and fun. She lived another couple months. One of the best things I've done in medicine was to get these people back together.

What exactly do you do when you're a hospice physician?

Hospice, by definition, for Medicare benefits, means a person has a life expectancy of less than six months. Everybody's different. A lot of people beat the odds and some people don't, so the emphasis becomes on comfort. You're not trying to cure anything anymore. If somebody has pneumonia, you treat it if the patient wants it treated, so there's a lot of talking involved in hospice. But if they don't want it treated, they've decided their illness is far enough advanced, they don't want to go on anymore, then you give them maximal comfort care. That's opioids, narcotics, if they need, because that helps with breathing discomfort, anti-nauseas. You don't quite worry so much about side effects. You treat them maximally. You get them off of drugs that make them sick, like potassium, and some of the hypertensive pills.

If the patient wants things to be treated more vigorously, we certainly do that. It lets the patients know that they're in charge. Often in the other world of medicine, the patients feel like they lose that autonomy. The doc says you come in the hospital and get IV antibiotics, and if you have gangrene in your toe, we're going to lump off your foot. In hospice, you can do all that stuff, but with end of life, in general, the emphasis is on comfort and treating what the patients want treated, and letting them know that they have a choice. They don't have to do all these things.

Let's talk about medical technology. Is it a double edged sword?

You don't know where to stop. For example, the coronary arteries can be stented with these little metal things that keep the arteries open, for fairly big bucks. But now they've come out with a new one that has a medicine in it that keeps the blood from clotting, at even more expense. I went to a lecture last week that said not only do they have the medicine in the stent now, but anybody who gets one of these really should get an internal defibrillator to boot. Somebody could be 80 years old, getting tens of thousands of dollars worth of equipment installed, while we have kids who don't get their immunizations.

You're trying to weigh all this. If she were my mom and she were 80, otherwise in good health, would I want her to get all this technology? It comes down to the autonomy of the person, again. If you want all this and you want to live forever or do you not? The people don't know what it's costing. It just keeps going on and on, and where does it stop?

How did you become interested in end of life issues?

I was in family practice for 30 some years. Hospice had already been out there for 20 some years, but a lot of us weren't really aware of hospice, unfortunately. My dad was sick in '84. We didn't think to call hospice and that's about the time it got started. Somebody came out and was drumming up money for the new facility, and I got interested that way. I started volunteering out there a couple times a month. I took some training from them just to see what it's all about. I went to do some home visits with them. At the same time, I was getting more and more fatigued with talking to people about smoking and diet because nobody was listening.

Also in family practice, it's very hard. You're covering the gamut of medicine and as a compulsive person, trying to keep up on everything from prenatal care and infertility workups, all the way through end of life stuff. It's very difficult, if you want to do a good job.

The other things that played in here was with the crunch of medicine, our visits were becoming shorter and shorter and I had less and less time to spend with patients. I was also getting very tired of taking call. I was having a lot of fatigue the next day, being up all night and then trying to do a good job the next day.

When hospice opened the inpatient unit out there, I already had been volunteering for them as a pain leader at times. It was a place where all the members get together and talk about their home patients. This would be interesting, so I studied up. I worked really hard. I got my boards in palliative hospital care. It was a new challenge. It was just exciting. So for a year, I did my family practice clinic, and hospice. I was at Wildwood Clinic a couple times per week and hospice a couple times per week, so I ended up working more than full-time.

Then, as the hospice unit got busier and busier, I jumped ship altogether. It was really a hard decision to make to stop practice and do just strictly hospice, but I loved it. I did it for four years, learned a heck of a lot. I could focus on the issues: symptomatic care, end of life care. I learned a lot of oncology through all of this.

But then I could forget all about obstetrics and how to do a fetal monitor and the doses to treat an ear infection in kids, so it was really neat for me, as being a little bit compulsive and being able to focus in.

You seem genuinely enthusiastic about it. But isn't it depressing treating patients who by definition have six months or less to live?

I never thought it was depressing. I certainly had times where someone I got attached to died and especially, if you really spent a lot of time with them, it was always hard. But on the other hand, I felt I was really doing good stuff because a lot of docs, don't know how to do this. They don't know how to talk to patients at this stage in their life. They don't know how to pull back. They don't have or want to spend the time sitting at bedside and just listening and holding a hand. That's one of the other things I really loved about hospice and what I'm doing now, is that my time is my own. If I want to spend 20 minutes just shooting the breeze, I can do that.

It's a team effort. It's not just the doc. It's also your social worker. The nurses take care of the patient and the nurses aids are probably the most important person in either hospice or long term care at nursing homes, because they spend the most time with the patient.

When I was in hospice, I told the patient we had two rules: Their eyes would get wide. "What rules?"

One, you're the boss. Not your daughter. Not your son-in-law. Not me. And secondly, pain and other symptoms are not allowed here. If you hurt, you have to tell us. If you're nauseated, you have to tell us. They want extra pudding? Well, the diabetes, we're not going to worry about that. If you want a glass of wine, you got it.

Then, being very up front with them about their illness and not giving them false hope. Not taking away hope, either, but saying if you want, we can do more x-ray therapy or we can give you more chemo. It's going to make you sick and the odds of this doing anything meaningful are minimal—being extremely honest, but only to the point that they want to hear. You give them the information by drips and drabs, and you get them on board.

How do patients react to the rules?

They're surprised because when they think of rules, they think of bedtime at this hour. I don't know that I saw any big response to it, but it had to be reiterated because people aren't used to it, especially older folks. And if you're a farmer, forget it. They aren't used to admitting pain. They've had their pain under treated for years. Docs are afraid to treat it, both for fear of the patient and because of worry that they're going to get in trouble with the feds or the narcotics agency. I'm not afraid because if you document what you do and have a good reason for doing it, you're safe.

Who's in hospice?

Hospice is 50% people with cancer and they do tend to be older. But the trend now is more and more people with other end of life diseases are actually in hospice too—heart failure, lung diseases. I had a five year old who had cancer. She died out there.

Is it harder, emotionally, for you, especially when you have to deal with five year olds?

{Pauses} Probably a little. I still have her stuffed toy here. {Laughs}

How do you deal with that? It's a little kid and there's nothing anybody can do.

But see, there's a lot we can do. We kept this kid pain free. We made it so her parents and sibs were able to stay in the room with her. She had lots of attention. The social workers talked to her at her level of understanding about what was going on. She understood. We gave lots and lots of comfort to her parents. People get the idea that end of life care is not doing anything, but it is!

We kept the kid symptom free and she was happy as she could be. When she died, I think she was pretty comfortable because the longer it got, the more short of breath she got, the more meds we gave her. She didn't die a terrible death.

When a child is that young, do you really try to explain that she's dying?

Even if you're only five or six years old, you know. They have a feeling that things are not good, that they're not going to be around. They start giving away their toys, sometimes. They have a sense. They're sitting in a place called hospice and there's nurses around. They don't have any false hopes that they're going to go back to school or be a football player.

What about your role with the parents. You have to somehow minister to their needs too, don't you?

We spend a lot of time with parents. We had parents of a newborn. The newborn was born with some sort of bleeding in the brain. I spend a lot of times with parents just sitting and encouraging them to hold the baby. The social workers often work with them on memory things, a special toy that they can keep, or locks of the hair.

They let them hold the baby after they've died. It's got to be the worst thing in the world to lose a kid. Some of the hardest ones we've had were dealing with parents, where the kid was 20, 30 years old. It's not supposed to be that way. They can be angry at the nurses, the doctors, the building, God, anybody. You just have to let them vent it out.

What is an appropriate way to tell somebody he's dying?

Generally, you're not telling them anything they don't know. You generally start out by asking them what they think is going on with their illness. How bad are you feeling? People pretty much have a good idea that things are not going well. They know they've lost weight. They don't have any appetite. They can see it themselves. They've been denying it, or for their spouse, they're holding it in. They don't want to tell them or something.

You tell them all the benefits that hospice has, all the people that will be working with them, and that all the medicines for the terminal illness are free. Then, you tell them there are lots and lots of things you can do for comfort. That's the aim.

Helping people die probably wasn't what attracted you to medicine. What did?

As I was growing up in Madison, Wisconsin, my dad always said if he was born in this county, he would have been a doctor, so I was indoctrinated from age five on up. He came to the United States when he was 19 from Norway; didn't know a word of English. Didn't know what a banana was. My dad was an excellent carpenter; he was still making stuff in his 80s and 90s. My bookcases downstairs were made when he was eighty-something. If he couldn't be a doctor, this was also fixing things and making things nice. He just held doctors in very high esteem. He thought it was the greatest profession there was.

Mom was an independent woman. She held jobs most of the time when we were growing up, secretary of the Eagles Club, had responsible positions all the while. She only got through tenth grade in high school. Dad got through eighth grade, but they were both pretty successful.

Was it unusual back then to encourage a girl to be a doctor?

I don't know if it was a purposely thought out thing or if that's just what he really felt. Dad was very proud of me. We'd go into pharmacies or grocery stores and he'd introduce me as "my daughter the doctor." It was so embarrassing, but so wonderful.

So at what point did you seriously consider medicine?

I started out in medical technology the first year of college. After a couple of classes, I decided that it sounded like more fun to be a doctor than a med tech. I switched to premed the second semester.

Were there many women in your class?

It was the University of Wisconsin, had the biggest class of women in some time. We had 14 women out of a hundred students. Back in '66, there weren't too many women in school. For me to get a seat in the school, I had to do not one, but two interviews and had to go in and talk with a couple of docs to get in. Found out only 15 or 20 years ago, that guys didn't have to have any interviews.

There was a certain pathologist who thought women shouldn't be in med school and he wasn't shy about telling us about it. I remember a dermatologist kicking us out of the room once because he was going to do a genital exam on a man and said, "Just get out. You can't be in here."

When they taught dermatomes—that's the section where various nerves, spinal cord nerves interface certain areas of the body—they had naked playboy bunnies with the drawings on her, to show where the various nerves go.

Honestly?

Really. It was a long time ago, so a lot of us women in the class, we hardly knew enough. We hadn't had our consciousness raised quite yet that we should be concerned about this.

I was pretty enmeshed in my studies. I almost missed the Vietnam War, I was so busy. I studied and kind of missed everything else. It was kind of tunnel vision on medicine.

As you're progressing through medical school, are you getting a sense for what type of medicine you wanted to practice?

Family practice was just getting going and was all the rage. It was really an up and coming thing and I really didn't consider much of anything else. I thought this is great. I can deliver babies and take care of little kids and old folks. There wasn't any question of what I wanted to do. I certainly didn't want to cut. This was perfect. That's indeed what I did and I would do it again as a choice of specialty.

How has your experience affected your own thoughts on end of life issues?

As I get closer to it, I'm not afraid of death anymore because I know there are good people who aren't afraid to take care of symptoms. That wasn't true 30 years ago. I don't get worried on the airplanes anymore. If it goes down, it goes down.

When you're dealing with death so frequently, how do you decompress?

I'm not really good at having fun. I've been taking tap dance class for the past 15 years and I'm still in the beginner's class, which is kind of embarrassing because the teacher just thinks that's where I belong. She's absolutely correct, but I love it.

I started taking Spanish last year. I'm in the third semester of Spanish and loving it. I'm having more fun with it than I've had with any other course before. I'm in class with a bunch of 20-year olds, so it's pretty interesting. The motivation for studying it was hospice, when I had that little five year old that we talked about. She was the only one in her family who could speak English. I also volunteer at a free clinic about once a month and 90% of the patients there are Spanish speakers, so the reason I started doing it is so I could be a better doctor.

In end of life care, not being able to speak their language is tough. But I would have done it anyway because I just love learning. Hospice experience has made me a better person. I have more sympathy with people who are in pain, certainly. I feel bad now—thoughts, feelings of the way I treated people back 20 years ago, not believing people when they said they had pain.

We now know that chronic pain doesn't look like acute pain. A person in chronic pain just looks depressed and apathetic and you have to believe a person when they say they're in pain, even if they don't look like they're in pain. I thought they were drug seekers or whatever. Of course, some of them are, but some were not.

I really feel more like making sure people have good control of their symptoms—that's the big one—more empathy with their emotional needs when you're trying to run people through an office.

Why are we so reluctant to talk about death and its consequences?

It's such a taboo subject. Years ago, people knew that if you got real sick you were going to die and people died at home. Now, with the technology, no one's supposed to die. I heard one of the doctors at University Hospital who said nobody ever dies there because you keep treating them no matter what. Keep them going. But death, people don't want to talk about it. They hate to go to funerals.

How do you go about initiating this discussion? There aren't that many Terri Schiavo *cases.*

Well, that's certainly a good jumping off point. You say, "Hey, if you got into a situation like that, how would you like me to deal with that with you?" You just bring up different scenarios. You talk about people who

---

* Schiavo was a 41-year old, severely brain-damaged woman who died in 2005. She spent almost a decade on life support while her husband and parents battled over whether to remove her feeding tube. Schiavo's husband eventually prevailed in court and removed the feeding tube. She died less than two weeks later.

have died before. You talk about Aunt Hilda who was demented for ten years, had bed sores and was miserable. If you were in that shape, what would you want us to do? You just try to bring it up. Or, you could start by telling them what you want. You could say, "Listen, if I get this sick, don't you dare do this or that to me, or I'll come back and haunt you."

Why should people draw up a power of attorney for health care?

The main reason is not so much the paperwork; though that's important, believe me, but to let your loved ones know what the heck you want done if you get into a situation where you're in a vegetative state. Do you want to live with a feeding tube for 14 years or longer, which you certainly could, or do you want the feeding tube removed?

This all implies that you can't speak for yourself. Many people, upwards of 50%, go through a time at end of life, it may be days or it may be years, where they can't make their own decisions, so the whole business of the power of attorney is to get people to talk with their family so they know what they would want.

When my husband's father had a stroke, he was in the hospital for six weeks on a respirator. Here's my husband the doctor, my sister-in-law the doctor, they didn't know what he wanted. They never talked about it, so it was very difficult. If their dad had said at some point, "If I'm in a state where I'm not going to come back to a reasonable state of health, pull the plug, stop the respirator, let me go," they would have done it at one week instead of at six weeks, and not go through all this pain and agony. The legality only comes in if there's someone who's going to contest what you want to say. The paperwork is just a safety device.

This implies talking about several different possibilities, anything from vegetative states to more importantly, dementia. People can go ten years with Alzheimer's and be non decisional. At what point do you want your relative to stop treating your pneumonia, stop treating your infections and let you go?

All those quality of life issues have to be discussed. It's hard for people to do this, so when there's a big television story, like Terri Schiavo, people start talking about it and it lasts about ten weeks and then they forget all about it again. There needs to be a constant push.

I begged and pleaded with my sister to do this for about five years and finally, we got her to do it. We took pictures of her signing her Power of Attorney because this was such a momentous event.

The biggest problem with the paperwork is if you don't have the power of attorney done, and you become unable to make decisions. Your family decides you need to go into a nursing home because they just can't take care of you anymore. Then, according to current law, the family can put you in a nursing home, temporarily. But to keep them there, you need to go for guardianship. Guardianship costs lots of money. It takes a while to get, and a guardian doesn't have all the rights and privileges of an agent, under a power of attorney. Not only is it costly, it's not as good.

Usually, the relative is named as the guardian, anyway, so you've gone through all this business just to get back to square one because you lost your rights and privileges and spent a lot of money in the process. Plus, it implies that the person never had the conversation to let you know what they wanted in the first place, so you lose all of that.

One story I have where this happened is my best friend's mom told him before she got sick that she did have a power of attorney. And of course, after she had her stroke and the Alzheimer's was diagnosed and she was no longer competent, they found out it was a power of attorney for financial affairs. She had never done one for health care. So my poor friend had to go back and forth from Milwaukee when she was hospitalized to meet with the lawyers, get all the paperwork signed. Now, he's her guardian and she's still in assisted living, still not decisional, but went through all this extra hassle for something she could have done for free, taking five minutes to do it.

People don't want to think about their own death. They also think that the paperwork's hard, and it's not. You can download the paper off the net. You can do it in five minutes.

The hard part is the talk. But if you get the legal thing done, you can talk your heart out after that. But there's a perception that if you sign it, you're giving away your autonomy and you're not. You're actually increasing it by telling people what to do. There's so much misperception.

Fear of dying—somehow that if you do this it's going to bring on your death. I don't know what the mentality is there. Hospitals are required to ask patients if they have an advance directive, either a living will or a power of attorney. They're required to ask the patient if they want to pursue doing it. But when the patient says no, they don't push it.

In your presentations, you make a big deal about the fact that people should write as many phone numbers on the forms as possible. Explain that.

The forms ask for your loved one's address. Well, if you need them, you're going to need them right now. You're not going to send them a letter. The doc needs to find them by phone or e-mail, at least. It is an emergency. If somebody needs your role as an agent to fall into place, you have to be able to reach them.

You need a power of attorney, they have the right thing, but you can't reach anybody?

Yes, most of the time. One of the problems is they have the power of attorney done, but you can't find it, or you have a partial copy because it's five pages long. I wish it was down to one page somehow. Once you have it done, you need to give it to the agent and an alternative. Tell them to keep it safe. Bring this up once a year at a holiday to keep it fresh in their mind.

Give one to your doctor and if you're at more than one clinic, give it to each clinic. Make sure that the hospital you're likely to use has a copy because that'll automatically pop up if you get there then.

Keep a copy for yourself, but by definition, if you need it, you're not going to know where it is, so you have to make sure agents know where it is. It's also a good idea to give one to people who aren't your agents, like other siblings, your best friend, somebody who is going to be around who will think of it when the time comes. Keep in mind that if your agents are your age or older, they may die or become demented before you, so you may have to pick another agent. You want to have at least two.

You have to keep a list of where you send all your copies because if you change your mind or your agent dies, you have to start all over and send your copies to the same places with a note saying this supersedes my last one.

Our society is aging, as is our uninsured population. Where is this going?

It's busting our system. I imagine when it gets pulled to the maximum, there's going to have to be some rationing. Somebody's going to have to make the hard decisions about anybody over this age with this condition does not get the lung transplant. Anybody who smoked more than 30 years can't have a lung transplant. Anybody who's been drinking this long can't have a liver transplant. There's got to be some personal responsibility in there. I don't think I'll be alive when that happens. It's gonna happen.

The technology just keeps going up, and people, especially those living in a place like Madison, they think they should never die. They also think that every baby should be a perfect baby. It's just not the way it is.

But isn't quality of life improving?

The older you get, the worse the quality of life is. I've certainly seen people on 12 different medicines and spending all their money on medicines. If they'd rather spend their money on medicines and eek out a few more months out of life rather than stopping some of this and enjoying life more, people have to decide that.

Most people at the end of life aren't hungry, anyway. To feed them, is actually a disservice because they don't want to eat. They also don't get especially thirsty. Their mouth gets dry, which can be taken care of by frequent swabbing of the mouth or rinsing the mouth if they can't swallow. After a week or seven, eight, nine days, these people drop into a coma and once they're in a coma, they don't feel anything. I don't think it's a real bad way to go.

I had one woman at hospice who voluntarily quit eating. She had a feeding tube put in because she had swallowing difficulty. She was perfectly rationale about it all, that she just wasn't going to take any more water or fluid because she didn't like the feeding tube. It hurt her. She was missing food. She had done everything she had wanted to do. It was hard because she was such a wonderful lady. I would have liked her to go on forever. She brought a novel with her. She read her book. It took her about two weeks and she was pretty much alert until the last four or five days.

Will hospice become more common?

It's all over the place now. Most people are at home and hospice comes to them. Ours here is at 200 some at home, and the maximum in-patient is 18. It's not just for the patient. It's for the entire family.

Is it the family doctor's responsibility to refer patients to hospice?

Doctors are part of the problem. They're very reluctant for a couple reasons. They don't want to tell the patient they have six months left to live or less, because that's the criteria for getting into hospice. They just don't want to tell them that.

One lady I was going to recommend hospice to, I thought, I've got to tell her today, so I had to come in on my lunch hour at the office. I had a 15 minute window to talk to her about this when I was very naïve and early in all this, and you can't tell somebody this in 15 minutes. We went an hour and a half {laughs} just to talk about the concept of it.

So docs don't want to get in the conversation because they don't have an hour and a half. They have seven minutes. Also, they don't want to admit that their usual treatments aren't working. Oncologists are probably the worst. Oncologists and neurosurgeons just don't want to say it doesn't make sense to give more chemo.

I've had people who were hanging on by a shoestring and the doc is still talking about chemotherapy. I don't know where this comes from because a layperson should be able to see this person's got a week to live and yet they're still pushing the meds. Part of it is the patient, too. If the oncologist says this treatment has a three percent chance of turning you around or giving you an extra two months of life, "Oh, 3%, great." They're grabbing at straws, not realizing how sick it's going to make them and maybe they should opt for quality, instead of another two months.

People with cancer tend to do pretty well and then suddenly, they get sick. It's kind of a flat curve, and then the bottom drops out. When they start going down that slide, you can predict pretty well, but until they get to that point, it's real iffy.

On the other hand, medical patients, especially chronic obstructive lung disease—emphysema—and congestive heart failure, their life expectancies are usually six months when they're in the final stages of that. But they can fool you. Their course is more of a roller coaster. They get really sick and then they bounce back a little bit. That can go on for a year and a half, two years.

But the good thing is that Medicare said you can be in hospice as long as it looks like it's going to be six months. You can keep re-upping them for as long as it takes. There's no limit, so as long as they still meet the criteria.

This lady I spent an hour and half telling her she needed to be in hospice, she got readmitted to hospice three times, kicked out of hospice twice. When I was talking to her about it, she was quite ill and she was at in-home hospice, rallied, they kicked her out. She got sick again, six months later. She was in. Finally, she didn't get out the third time.

It's got to be the greatest feeling in the world to get kicked out of hospice.

You're a hospice graduate. That's good. I've had a couple like that. You're not necessarily in for the duration.

Getting my boards in palliative hospice was exciting and I'm continuing to learn more and more about that. I'm amazed at how much I know now that I didn't know five years ago when I started. Although I'm not at hospice, being at a nursing home is very similar—a lot of palliative care needs and a lot of people are going to die there. I'm continually learning and I love my patients and I'm enjoying what I'm doing.

If I had to do it over, I would spend more time with the kids at home because we tried to do it all back then. We were both full time, up until last year, so the kids got gypped a little bit in getting our attention. We had live-in sitters from the time they were little until the time they didn't need sitters any more. At the time, we were both gung ho and we were both delivering babies, so if one of us was on call and the other had someone in labor, we both wanted to be away. That was always tough.

I'm pretty much semi retired now because my nursing home responsibilities are minimal, doing lots of other volunteer stuff, but my husband does not want to quit. He's active in the AMA and the Wisconsin Med Society, and quite rightly. He has to be in practice to be in these other endeavors, so he doesn't want to retire. I'll probably keep working until he decides to hang it up.

Why couldn't you just retire whenever you want to?

Nah, we're too competitive. We've been competing since day one and I have to keep going. We had the flu during internship and we lie in bed and see who had the highest temperature, passing the thermometer back and forth. Every exam we ever took, who had the better score, who did more of this, who could stay up the longest. We compete on everything. We've been together 37 years, so I guess that's not too unhealthy.

In your life in medicine, what have you learned from patients at the end of life?

A remarkable strength and bravery. People are just so wonderful the way they bring their family together and heal old wounds. A lot of people at the end are thinking about you, more than themselves.

One lady hung on for her sister's wedding. She pretty much raised her sister. She was only in her 40s. Transfusions, treated her infections with antibiotics, just went nuts treating her. A horrible disease. A lot of things you wouldn't do to a hospice patient. The wedding was going to be in Chicago. She made it all the way, actually stood up at the reception, pictures of her looking like a healthy person. Died that night in her hotel room, but she hung on for that wedding. It took a lot of work to get her there, but she made it! Amazing.

People, in the last few days, seem to have a little bit of control over when they're actually going to die. Other people waited for wedding anniversaries. I had several people who all of sudden said, "Call the family. I want all of them here tonight." The family would all come in and they would talk. The next day they would die.

They hang on for the turn of the New Year. One person kept saying, "Is it January first yet?" As soon as it turned January first, he went. He was waiting for that. I can't explain that.

XI

Tribute

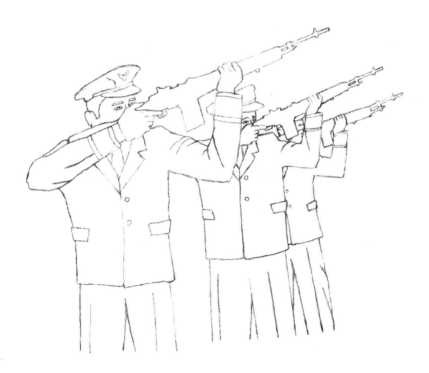

"The truest wisdom is a resolute determination."

—Napoleon Bonaparte

Chapter Thirty-Seven

Rolling Wonder

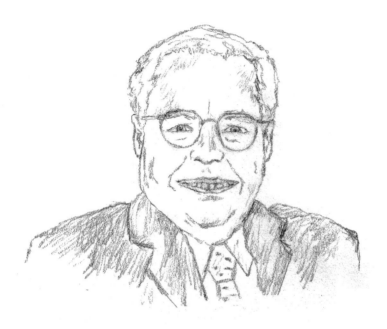

"When I tried to get out of bed, I fell flat on my face. Something terrible was happening to me, but I didn't know what."

Kenneth Viste, Jr., MD {1941-2005}
Neurologist, Oshkosh

Ken Viste was the first doctor I had in mind for this book. He was a natural–a great speaker, brilliant physician, fascinating man with a unique story. What's more, he had a long history of helping me, so I felt no real urgency to interview him. Intuitively, I considered that conversation practically in the bag, so I first tackled the other interviews of doctors I knew less well. Wow, what a mistake. Doctor Viste died on August 21, 2005, before I could record his story.

By the age of 14, when he contracted polio, a wheelchair became his constant companion. The only time I recall not seeing him in that chair during the 20 years that I knew him, was when we attended an AMA meeting together in 2000. We were outside at the pool at an incredible resort in Tucson, Arizona, complete with surreal mountains as a backdrop for the turquoise sky.

"You get some nice perks when you attend these meetings," Dr. Viste said to me, smiling broadly. We exchanged pleasantries, and then I turned away momentarily to gaze upon the magnificent scenery. Suddenly, I heard a big splash. He somehow had catapulted himself out of the wheelchair and into the water. By the time I turned, he was doing the backstroke. I didn't even know Dr. Viste could swim.

Viste was legend for the way he tooled around at hotel conventions. He would get the lay of the land and figure out how best to get to rooms because there wasn't always an easy, wheelchair accessible path to them. I remember following behind him at the Chicago Hilton, down into the basement, through the kitchen, past various hotel staff, to end up where we were supposed to be.

I never once heard him complain about his disability. It was only in recent years that somebody else mentioned to me that polio was the cause. But that's the point of Ken Viste's whole life. He refused to let his disability take center stage. He had too many important things to do. This doctor was as determined as they come.

In 1988, the Milwaukee Journal *ran a feature on him shortly before he became president of the Wisconsin Medical Society, at age 44. The story reported that, from his wheelchair, Viste used a periscope to observe surgery during medical school. It was just one example of how he overcame hurdles.*

To give you a sense of who this man was, I've pulled excerpts from a memorable speech he gave. Keep in mind, Viste had to be persuaded to tell the story you're about to read because he didn't think anybody would find it of interest. "Why would anybody care?" he asked me.

{*Speech to colleagues, Madison 1999*}

Remember, as a child, what it was like to have big dreams? Didn't you dream of being some great super hero or movie star that you were going to be when you finally became an adult? I had really big dreams. But these wonderful dreams of being the next legendary Green Bay Packer super hero ended in one night. I remember it as if it were yesterday. September 17, 1955. What began as a headache and muscle stiffness, which I thought was from freshman football practice, became a nightmare, as I woke up. When I tried to get out of bed, I fell flat on my face. Something terrible was happening to me but I didn't know what. I never walked again.

The unthinkable became a reality when our family doctor came to my house and he told my parents and me, "Ken—you have polio." Polio. The finality of that word, especially in 1955, just sank into your soul and your bones. As a 13-year old boy, it sounded like I had been sentenced to life in prison. However, despite this horrific news, something else happened to me during my year of treatment and rehabilitation. I became absorbed with medicine and the many doctors who treated me. I was in awe of what they did, how they helped others and the respect in which they were held. They had the compassion and patience to tell me that I—Ken Viste—wasn't any less of a person than I was before polio struck. Eventually, I believed them.

Just watching and coming to know how dedicated and compassionate these physicians were, how consumed they were by their work, made a powerful impression on me. Because of the difference they made in the lives of so many other people, they changed my dream. I decided I would make my life count by learning how to help heal others, help ease their pain and give people back their hope—every day. Believe me, I understand with every fiber of my body how crucial it is to have hope, to have physicians who care—someone willing to take the time to listen to concerns.

As a poor farm boy living in northern Wisconsin, our only hope for me was access to care. We all need and deserve that. Today, 42 million uninsured individuals are hoping we will not forget them. They hope we are listening to their unmet needs to have access to quality care. We must renew our commitment to help those who are poor, isolated, living in rural parts of this country, unemployed, underemployed. Their access to health care is their access to hope.

During my polio treatment many of the doctors became my friends. I shared many confidences with them. I remember laughing with my doctor one time when I told him how I had escaped from the hospital for an afternoon. He sat and listened to me, as if he had all the time in the world. I told him I was so sick and tired of being cooped up and going to therapy all the time. I had craved some excitement. I had been in and out of hospitals for over a year by now, confined to a bed most of the time or stuck in my house. The kind of excitement I was seeking was beyond the walls of the therapy rooms. I came up with an idea. Since I was in the hospital that happened to be in the same town as the Governor—I'd go see him. Getting in to see the Governor became the goal.

For one thing, even when I made it to the Capitol, why would the Governor want to see me? He was a very important, busy man with a lot of demands on his time. I was a gangly, 14-year old kid with heavy leg braces in a wheelchair, wearing mischief all over my face. A challenge, not an obstacle. I was very determined.

Secondly, I didn't have a plan of exactly how I could possibly travel the three miles from the hospital to the State Capitol. Keep in mind, as a farm kid it never occurred to me that I could have called a cab. The shortest distance between the hospital and the State Capitol was a lot of hills, a lot of curbs, a lot of traffic.

So how did I get there? With these. {Raises his hands}

These hands took me up and down city streets. I grew more and more excited, as I arrived at the Capitol and found myself knocking on the door of the executive office. A secretary well trained in getting rid of people like me, asked the perfunctory questions. "May I help you?"

"Why yes," I said. "I don't vote yet, but I'm here to see our Governor." I looked her right in the eye.

She didn't say a word. She looked me up and down with the precision of a CT scanner. Then she asked her next question.

"Do you have an appointment?"

I hesitated. I sat up a little taller in my chair and looked her right back in the eye. Then, I locked the brakes on my wheelchair in place—a clear signal to her that I wasn't going anywhere, and said, "Well, I'm sure he would want to see me if he knew I was here. My name is Ken Viste."

Minutes later, Wisconsin's Governor Kohler came out of his office and shook my hand. Then, he invited me into his office and we spent the next 45 minutes talking. I asked him a lot of questions. He asked me a lot of questions. But most important, he took the time to listen—to me. Yes, I did get my picture taken with him. My mother still has the picture on a shelf back on the farm to prove it.

The story, however, illustrates how impossible some goals first seem when we first get started on the journey. But something happens to you in the process of taking on a goal. You develop momentum, belief, courage, and the raw power that helps you keep moving toward the finish line. The strength and determination I had even as a 14-year old kid is something that still pushes me today. As I look out in this room, I know that each and every one of you have this strength and determination, too.

Leaders need drive and determination to make things happen. But they also need to know how to listen to others. Governor Kohler was a great listener. We must encourage participation, do a better job of listening to one another and find the best solutions through consensus. If we do this, we will achieve great things.

We need to remember that difficult challenges won't be solved over night. After all, even overnight success takes time.

For another six years, Dr. Ken Viste would be involved in numerous medical projects, organizations and issues. In 1994, he was selected to serve on the prestigious Practicing Physician's Advisory Council, which advises the U.S. Health and Human Services Secretary regarding Medicare issues. Over his career, Dr. Viste headed his national neurology society, served as an AMA Delegate and was an advisor to three Wisconsin Governors, before cancer quickly ceased his adventures.

The day after his funeral, in Oshkosh, my wife, our one-year old and I left our hotel to relax at a local park. We were enjoying a gorgeous, clear day, while our daughter played on the swings. Soon, we struck up a conversation with a friendly guy setting up for a large picnic. When he heard we were from Madison, he asked what brought us to town.

"We attended a funeral for a good friend last night," I explained.

"Ken Viste's?"

Incredulous, I just said, "Yeah."

"Great guy–saved my mom's life."

The doctor whom I knew to be a leader on the state, national and international levels, was also a giant at home. Imagine, we pick a park at random and the first stranger we meet the morning after his funeral is somebody whose mother he saved! Local residents also admired Ken Viste because he was a generous benefactor for disability groups, as well as for other causes, including political candidates of both parties.

Tommy Thompson, the longest serving Governor in Wisconsin history and the former Secretary of the U. S. Department of Health and Human Services, was among the notables who called to express their concern and appreciation during Viste's final days. I can't help but wonder whether Kenneth Martin Viste, Jr., MD, was reminded of that time almost 50 years ago, when he was the one calling on a Wisconsin Governor.

POSTSCRIPT

Many of the voices in these chapters played in my head as my father lay dying in the intensive care ward at St. Luke's Hospital in Milwaukee, the same hospital where he was born 88 years before. I was better equipped to deal with the decision-making and angst when he fell fatally ill as the result of progressive heart disease. Our medical options were all poor, but at least I realized that the worst thing would have been to require dad to be laden with tubes, gasping uncomfortably for the last hours of his life when there was no reasonable chance for recovery. Instead, he rested easily with his entire adoring family surrounding him. About six hours after we removed the tubes, he quietly slipped away to the afterlife.

Of course, knowing dad's thoughts about end-of-life care was extremely helpful. I recall a dinner I had with my parents a few years before he passed away where we discussed the prospect of lingering indefinitely on tubes in a nursing home. "A fate worse than death," I said. Everybody agreed. Jokingly, I held up glass and said, "To death." Dad laughed and clinked glasses with me. My mother, on the other hand, looked at us as if we were mad.

"I'm not drinking to that," she said.

However difficult contemplating death is, the lessons taught by Doctors Heggestad, Dougherty, Whitcomb and Schwartzstein—helped me recognize that dying really is part of the life cycle. Accepting death, rather than forcing life, no matter its quality, makes little sense to me. I've probably felt that way for a long time, but these interviews confirmed such sentiments.

But I appreciated the value of these conversations long before my dad fell ill. In fact, I was filled with exhilaration as I drove back to Madison in June, 2005, from the small, rural community of Dodgeville, where I had just finished an electrifying discussion with a surgeon. It had been almost one year since I had conducted my first interview for *White Coat Wisdom*, but only then did I fully realize what potential this oral history might have on people, as well as on me. I was always sure of the worthiness of this project, but it became so apparent after my lengthy conversation with physician musician Adam Dachman, DO, that I could hardly contain myself. I was in the presence of an exceptional person—somebody who sees and experiences things many of us miss or dismiss. *I've got a tiger by the tail here,* I thought, as I drove home glancing at my digital audio recorder lying on the seat.

Unlike Dachman, I interviewed most of the doctors at their homes so they'd be as relaxed as possible when discussing what medicine means to them. It was interesting to see that almost everyone lived in surprisingly modest homes. Maybe that's why money rarely came up as a reason for pursuing the profession or why they enjoyed it so much. That's not to say that they don't appreciate the lifestyle they lead. It just didn't appear to be the driving motivation for their career choice. Instead, their success as doctors and as content people appears inextricably linked to the fact that they are doing something they enjoy, that requires them to continually learn and hone their skills, and perhaps most critically, connect intimately with a great variety of human beings on a regular basis.

Interview after interview, I was mining great material. In fact, at times I was shocked at how much they were willing to reveal. So many times during the course of these conversations I had to bite my tongue because I instinctively felt an obligation to share something from my life since they were being so open with theirs. But of course, this wasn't about me and I didn't want to derail the conversation just as they were getting revved up.

Each person was different, but equally substantial in what he or she was communicating. Talking to each for two to three hours was without question the most satisfying part of the whole process. The similarities between these physicians, no matter their race, gender or age, were striking. Each had a drive to succeed and a true passion for medicine. Their profession was their life.

I've always been fortunate to have good, often fascinating jobs {literally millions of people heard my stories on National Public Radio}, but none of mine compared to theirs. I remain a bit jealous of doctors when it comes to career fulfillment. "Love" is the word most of them used to describe how they feel about practicing medicine.

However, I do not envy them for the sacrifices they've had to make—or at least thought they had to make—with respect to their loved ones, especially when their kids were growing up. As the father of two toddlers, it is indeed a special time, one which I wouldn't want to miss for any job. But that's the whole point of *White Coat Wisdom.* They're not talking about a job. Medicine is something much more than employment to them.

The differences I noticed among these physicians were mainly those associated with their individual personalities and particular experience in their specialty. It made me realize how much physicians can learn from each other because depending on where they they've practiced, their perspective and knowledge can vary tremendously.

Engaging as these doctors are, one of the most difficult tasks in preparing this book was in the transcribing, which I found to be a chore, until I was seduced into each conversation again when I hit the play button. At first, I only planned to transcribe the first three chapters and then hire a professional after I secured a publisher. Unfortunately, interesting an agent or publisher was much more involved and time consuming than I had anticipated. Understandably, they want a specific road map of where you are going with a book, but that's hard to deliver when you're writing an oral history and haven't interviewed everybody yet! I had a good idea of what I wanted to discuss, but I never could have predicted what these physicians told me.

For a short time, I put the whole project on hold, awaiting the verdict from the publishing world. But a good friend, Tammy Ripp, and a literary agent, Scott Edelstein, convinced me to just write it and worry about publishers later. Others, however, in the writing community insisted the traditional route of waiting before investing time and labor in a book was the most prudent course. The former turned out to be excellent advice for me, as I was already too charged up to put everything on hold at the whim of people I didn't know and didn't necessarily trust. I carried on, nonetheless. As I continued working on the chapters, I realized that some of these very accomplished physicians told me about people in authority who told them as young people, that they weren't good enough, smart enough or determined enough to make it in medical school. It turned out these doctors used that negativity to their advantage and empowered themselves to prove their detractors wrong. Now, I was on a similar quest.

Soon, I was rising every day at 5:00 a.m., eagerly ready to either transcribe the interviews or edit them. The passion I felt for this project was much like what I feel before leaving for a vacation or playing a round of golf. I looked forward to these early mornings because it was the only time I could concentrate continuously for an hour and a half without interruption. I had become so on task, devoting most free moments to slowly, but surely moving the ball forward, my wife, Maureen, told me numerous times that I was "obsessed with that book." She wasn't too far off base with that assessment, though I prefer the word "passionate" to describe my interest in seeing this through.

Whenever it seemed that completing the task was too overwhelming, given my full-time job and family responsibilities, I kept thinking back to the lives of those whom I was profiling. Each of them persevered in depth and duration far beyond anything I was confronting with my literary challenges. *If they can plow through 36-hour shifts in residency, I can certainly finish this manuscript,* I would tell myself.

In doing so, I was learning new things all the time *from* these doctors and *about* these doctors, even though I've known almost all of them for many years. How could I work regularly with an orthopedic surgeon for seven years and not know that he was in a car accident that ended his career in the OR? The answer lies in the fact that none of us knows people as well as we think. Until you sit down for an extended period with a pen in hand or a recording device and ask people questions about their lives, you won't stand a chance of getting below the surface. Some doctors revealed to me that their own children will learn things about them in the book because their kids never asked these kinds of questions. If their own children don't know the major stories of their lives, patients certainly know less.

The overarching lesson for me after having heard more than 55 hours of conversations with these extraordinarily accomplished people, multiple times through the editing process, is that true success and fulfillment comes when doing something you love in service to others. Yes, medicine is hard work that requires dedication and compassion. They provide an important service, but they're sharing themselves in the process. They're developing tight, caring relationships with entire families, and that's a return that doesn't accumulate in a bank account.

Other lessons were more concrete. My family and I now eat more blueberries and pop more fish oil pills than we did before, as we are savvier about the lack of omega 3 in our diets. We will most certainly be especially encouraging to our young daughters, being hypersensitive to not dismissing an interest they may develop as they grow, no matter how far fetched it may seem.

I also live more of my life now. We watch less television, though we never watched a lot to begin with. Self-described workaholic Dr. Dan Wik convinced me that too many of us watch our lives pass by in front of a big screen instead of getting in the fray and actually living it. And he's right.

As I contemplate this book going to press, I wonder what readers will take away from it? Will they find each doctor has something important to share, even though he or she isn't necessarily famous or may not have a personality that jibes with their own? Will they love some doctors and be turned off by others? For me, each chapter is very special, something akin to the love one has for his or her children—you don't love one more than another.

Yet another lesson involves the meaning of success. I learned from my friend Darold Treffert, MD, the savant expert psychiatrist, and author, that in the publishing world, success is all about how you define it. If success only means a best seller and a guest appearance on "*Oprah*," then I may well be disappointed, as few titles catch fire like that. Easy for him to say, though, because he's been on "*60 Minutes*," as well as numerous other national and international television programs discussing his books!

But what if success means a few young people are inspired by these accounts and pursue a career in medicine? How many thousands of patients might they treat in their lifetimes? How many lives could they save or improve? What if readers, no matter how many, learn things that improve their lives and those of their families? What if readers decide to help Dr. Julian De Lia save more identical twins or assist Dr. George Schneider in caring for the working poor? When you think about it like that, the implications for the ideas presented in *White Coat Wisdom* may be quite profound, indeed.

What Dr. Dachman helped me realize is that we're all connected in one way or other. What we do affects others and vice versa. It's in these relationships where we find meaning.

Had I not attended that Super Bowl party where I struck up a conversation with a new friend who ardently encouraged me, not acted on the opportunity to delve into the established relationships I have with so many impressive physicians and not received advice from others inside and out of the publishing world who helped me figure out how to do this, *White Coat Wisdom* might well have been nothing more than an unfulfilled, albeit interesting, idea.

So what are *you* waiting for?

Share *White Coat Wisdom*
With Friends, Colleagues and Students

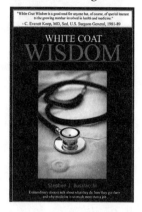

To order a copy/copies of *White Coat Wisdom,* see www.whitecoatwisdom. com, or via U.S. Mail:

Name _____

Address _____

City _____Phone# _____

State _____ Zip _____ e-mail address _____

_____copy/copies of *White Coat Wisdom* x $34.95 =   _____

Wisconsin residents add 5% sales tax =   _____

Shipping $3.50 (U.S. locations)   _____

Additional Books add $1.00 each   _____

Enclose check made out to Apollo's Voice, LLC or CC for a **total** of: _____

MC _____   Visa _____   Card #_____ exp. _____

Signature _____

Apollo's Voice, LLC
P.O. Box 628044,
Middleton, WI

Apollo's Voice

Another Book by Stephen J. Busalacchi

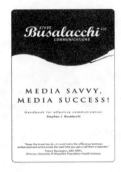

"Keep this book handy—it could make the difference between
embarrassment and success the next time you get a call from a reporter."
Patrick Remington, MD, MPH
Director, University of Wisconsin Population Health Institute

To order a copy/copies of *Media Savvy, Media Success!* see
www.Apollosvoice.com or via U.S. Mail:

Name _____

Address _____

City _____Phone# _____

State _____ Zip _____ e-mail address _____

_____copy/copies of *Media Savvy, Media Success!* x $9.95 =   ___ ___

Wisconsin residents add 5% sales tax =   _____

Shipping $1.50 (U.S. locations)   _____

Additional Books add $.50 each   _____

Enclose check made out to Apollo's Voice, LLC or CC for a total of: _____

MC ____   Visa ____   Card #_____ exp. _____

Signature _____

Apollo's Voice, LLC
P.O. Box 628044,
Middleton, WI

Apollo's Voice

INDEX

high heels, 191
Hoffman, Dustin, 495–496. See also savant
    syndrome
homosexuality, 375–379
hospice care, 554–558, 560, 563–565
house calls, 406–407, 549
human body, 227

I

identity as surgeon, 82, 85
"I'm sorry" laws, 389. See also law
Indiana University, 240
Indiana University School of Medicine,
    240–243
"infertility" specialist, 275
injury, dealing with, 81–95
inner city, 358–359
insurance industry, 450–455. See also
    health care system; law
internal medicine, 125, 349, 392
Internet, 152–153, 297

J

Jaeger, Robert, 275–282
Jalalabad, Afghanistan, 310–312
Jensen, Norman, 383–395
Joe Camel, 168
Johns Hopkins University, 362–363
Judaism, 420. See also spirituality

K

Kalayoglu, Munci, 467–479
Kanner, Leo, 494
Karofsky, Peter, 408
"Keys of Hope," 210
King, Russ, 143
Kohler, Walter J., 572
Koop, C. Everett, 172–173, 176
Korpi, Esa, 287
Kriss, Fred, 430

L

La Crosse, 293
laparoscopy, 267. See also surgery
laser surgery, 100–105, 110. See also
    surgery
lasik, 483. See also surgery
law
    apology law, 389
    degree, 430–431
    insurance industry, 450–455
    malpractice suits, 89–90, 279–280, 384–

386, 433–434, 437–439
    medical liability insurance, 281
    school, 432–433
    Supreme Court, 454
    United States Department of Justice
        lawsuit, 168–169, 177
lawyers. See law
Lemke, Leslie, 495–496, 502
Lemke, May, 495, 507
lens implants, 483–484. See also surgery
levity, use of, 267
liability crisis, 450–455. See also law
life expectancy, 117
Life Magazine, 468
lifestyle, effects of, 298–300
lifestyle, medicine as, 50–51, 78
liver transplant, 468–479. See also surgery
Locum tenens, 411
Loyola University Chicago Stritch School of
    Medicine, 124
Luckman, Jack, 241
lumpectomy, 259. See also surgery

M

Madison, Wisconsin, 145
Magiera, Christopher, 449–463
malpractice suits, 89–90, 279–280,
    384–386, 433–434, 437–438.
    See also law
Manley, Jack, 548
Marcus Welby, 412. See also television
Marines, 542–543. See also armed forces
marketing, 245
Marquette University School of Medicine,
    349
MASH, 364. See also television
maternal fetal medicine, 103
Mayo Clinic, 225–228, 283, 403
McCarthy, Jack, 487
McDonald, James, 486
media, 140–141, 253, 255. See also
    television
medical advancements, 265
Medical College of Virginia, 456–457
Medical College of Wisconsin (MCW), 10,
    349, 540
Medical Examining Board, 31–32
medical liability insurance, 281. See also law
medical missions, 220. See also
    philanthropy
medical record systems, 234–235, 293,
    307–308, 416
medical refugees, 450